# OPHTHALMIC GENETICS

First Edition Published in 1951 as
"Genetics in Ophthalmology"

# OPHTHALMIC GENETICS

SECOND EDITION

ARNOLD SORSBY
C.B.E., M.D., F.R.C.S.

EMERITUS RESEARCH PROFESSOR IN OPHTHALMOLOGY, ROYAL COLLEGE OF SURGEONS AND ROYAL EYE HOSPITAL: EMERITUS SURGEON, ROYAL EYE HOSPITAL, LONDON

LONDON
BUTTERWORTHS

ENGLAND: BUTTERWORTH & CO. (PUBLISHERS) LTD.
LONDON: 88 Kingsway, W.C.2

AUSTRALIA: BUTTERWORTH & CO. (AUSTRALIA) LTD.
SYDNEY: 20 Loftus Street
MELBOURNE: 343 Little Collins Street
BRISBANE: 240 Queen Street

CANADA: BUTTERWORTH & CO. (CANADA) LTD.
TORONTO: 14 Curity Avenue, 374

NEW ZEALAND: BUTTERWORTH & CO. (NEW ZEALAND) LTD.
WELLINGTON: 49/51 Ballance Street
AUCKLAND: 35 High Street

SOUTH AFRICA: BUTTERWORTH & CO. (SOUTH AFRICA) LTD.
DURBAN: 33/35 Beach Grove





Suggested U.D.C. Number: 617.7–056
Suggested Additional Number: 575:617.7

Standard Book Number: 407 34450 0



*Printed in Great Britain by R. J. Acford Ltd., Chichester, Sussex.*

# CONTENTS

# PREFACE TO THE SECOND EDITION

THE NAME *Genetics in Ophthalmology*, under which title the first edition of this book appeared, implied a proselytising effort. The emergence of genetics as an outstanding discipline during the past two decades, and the increasing significance of clinical genetics in medical practice, now make missionary zeal superfluous. In this new edition it was also thought superfluous to devote a whole introductory section to an account of elementary genetics. The present edition is therefore a more direct and factual exposition than was possible 20 years ago. This in itself warrants a new name for the book.

The new title of *Ophthalmic Genetics* is readily justified by the fact that the subject now takes its place along with ophthalmic pathology, ophthalmic surgery and other established disciplines as an essential aspect of the specialty. For the present, its major contribution is still in accurate diagnosis and in the planning of rational treatment. But increasingly it is effective in prophylaxis, whilst the therapeutic measures already possible are no longer merely the shadows cast before by coming events.

ARNOLD SORSBY

## EXTRACT FROM PREFACE TO THE FIRST EDITION

AT THE beginning of the last century, smallpox was the dominant cause of blindness and towards the end of the century it had been replaced by ophthalmia neonatorum. Some two-thirds of those who sought relief at the earliest institution for the blind —the one established at Liverpool in 1791—are said to have been blinded by smallpox, whilst an inquiry conducted in 1884 by the Ophthalmological Society revealed that some 30–41 per cent of all inmates at different institutions and schools for the blind had been blinded by ophthalmia neonatorum. In the nineteenth century, infections would therefore appear to have overshadowed all other causes of blindness.

The causes of blindness as seen today cannot readily be interpreted in terms of extraneous causative agents. Neither cataract, nor glaucoma, nor myopia, nor the senile degenerative changes, nor the hereditary anomalies are explicable in terms of bacteriology. The therapeutic revolution we have witnessed in our generation has brought into relief a more complex and varied pathology than was envisaged by the pioneers of bacteriology or by our predecessors at the beginning of the century. Throughout the history of medicine there has been a shifting of emphasis, now on the extraneous factor, now on the constitutional factor, and whilst the results of bacteriology—with its stress on the extraneous factor—have been immense, it has become apparent that the constitutional factor, as opposed to the extraneous factor of disease, has now come to be the starting point for further advance.

Constitution is as yet an ill-defined concept. The reactions of an individual to his environment are likely to be a complex process, immensely difficult to unravel. An individual's reactions may be determined by the past experiences of his body, but also by his inherent anatomical and physiological structure. That, in turn, may have been conditioned by extraneous factors such as an abnormal maternal environment during development but also by an inherent genetic structure, and this, again, may well have been moulded by extraneous circumstances.

Medical genetics is an aspect of the study of constitution. The concept of the genetic constitution of an individual presents a sharp antithesis to the concept of environmental factors. But disease is generally the result of the disharmonious interaction of constitution and environment, so that study of the genetic constitution of man is as significant as the study of the environmental pathogen. At the two extremes, either factor by itself may produce disease, as shown respectively by the lesions produced by mechanical injury and that produced by an inherited gene for retinitis pigmentosa. Frequently, however, other environmental or constitutional factors have to come into play for a disease process to become established. Not every individual exposed to tuberculous infection develops tuberculosis; not every carrier of the gene for, say, the Laurence-Biedl syndrome, develops the full syndrome. Medical genetics is therefore not merely a study of the modes but also of the nature of inheritance.

Contrary to the widespread belief, medical genetics is not concerned with collecting curious pedigrees of the unconsidered trifles of pathology. At the very least, it is an attempt to elucidate some aspects of the constitutional basis of disease.

## EXTRACT FROM PREFACE TO THE FIRST EDITION

In some affections the genetic factor is obvious. In others, it can be revealed only by exhaustive investigations aided by an understanding of genetic theory. The genetic anomalies have assumed greater significance with the recognition of modes of inheritance other than the simple autosomal recessives and dominants of the past. Isolated cases of genetic disease are no longer clinical puzzles and unusual modes of inheritance are more readily recognized. A further significant development has been the recognition of the abiotrophic character of many of the genetic anomalies, so that many affections coming on late in life and previously regarded as of environmental origin are now recognized as genetic in type. It is not unlikely that some of the so-called senile degenerations are late abiotrophic manifestations, and evidence is accumulating that senile cataract and primary glaucoma are essentially genetic affections. Indeed, the congenital anomalies and classical forms of abiotrophic defects constitute only a small part of the inherited abnormalities or inherited potentialities towards abnormality of the eye. The scope of ophthalmological genetics is, in fact, very much wider than was suspected by the pioneers of the study, and this enlarged scope has an immediate bearing on the causes of blindness and ocular disease generally, as seen today. And if the scope of ophthalmological genetics has become larger, so has the prospect of the eventual control of the genetically determined affections. The fatalism with which genetic affections are generally regarded is as unfounded in reason as it is unjustified by achievement already reached.

ARNOLD SORSBY

# CHAPTER 1

## INTRODUCTION

A sharp antithesis between environmental and hereditary affections is fallacious and misleading. Even the effects of such a well defined environmental factor as trauma may be influenced by the genetic constitution of the patient. A blow which would give little pathological disturbance in one individual may lead to fracture of the femur in a patient with fragilitas ossium of genetic origin. None the less, it would be merely an exercise in logic to stress the genetic factor in conditions in which environmental factors are the main causative agents. Moreover, such exercises would be clinically misleading, particularly if the environmental factors are readily amenable to correction, and the hereditary factors are not.

Such considerations do, however, emphasize the fact that only in extreme cases can hereditary and environmental factors be clearly disentangled in the effect they produce. At the one extreme there are clinical conditions, such as, say, Tay-Sachs disease, which are always genetic in origin; at the other extreme there are such lesions as a stab wound which are always environmental. In many clinical conditions both environmental and genetic factors may be equally significant, and—what is as important—the appearances of an affection definitely of genetic or definitely of environmental origin may be indistinguishable. Optic atrophy, whether derived genetically or caused by injury to the optic nerve, will look very much alike and will give the same blindness. Lamellar cataract may be genetic in origin or caused by nutritional disturbances in the mother: a macular lesion cannot always be readily distinguished as of genetic or environmental origin.

The hazy demarcation clinically between genetic and environmental affections is partly caused by the fact that genetic anomalies do not constitute rigid entities uninfluenced by other physiological mechanisms. For practical purposes the significant thing is that some genetic anomalies arise from disturbance in intra-uterine life, producing congenital anomalies, whilst others, the abiotrophic group (or heredo-degenerations), occur in apparently fully formed tissues which do not live out their normal span. The abiotrophic group presents at the moment the more hopeful line of approach, as the congenital anomalies are unlikely to be reversed to normalcy. The control of congenital anomalies requires a far fuller understanding of embryological physiology than is possessed today, while the control of abiotrophic anomalies raises complex problems of post-natal development.

### CLINICAL VARIETIES OF GENETIC DISEASE

Broadly speaking the following varieties of genetic affections may be recognized: congenital anomalies; abiotrophic anomalies; phakomatoses; neoplasms; metabolic disorders; and syndromes. In some, at least, of these groups there are examples which merge on to the disturbances of environmental origin, or are indistinguishable in appearances, whilst, as discussed more fully below, few of the syndromes are exclusively either congenital, abiotrophic or phakomatous in origin, and the distinction between congenital and abiotrophic can be very tenuous indeed.

### Congenital anomalies

There are clearly established environmental causes of congenital anomalies. The conception of intra-uterine infection favoured by the older clinicians is valid, but not in the extreme form which was previously held. Congenital syphilis is the classical example of intra-uterine infection. It is one of the exceptions to the general rule that maternal infections are kept back by the placental barrier from reaching the embryo. Depending upon the stage of development at which intra-uterine infection with syphilis occurs, and the severity of the infection, the range of effects extends from miscarriage, stillbirth, or a child born with all the stigmata of congenital syphilis, to a child apparently normal at birth and developing the manifestations of congenital syphilis later in life. Syphilitic anomalies that may be present in a child born at term include opacification of the cornea from intra-uterine interstitial keratitis, gross malformation of the eye, and possibly chorio-retinal lesions. Buphthalmos has occasionally been observed. The more recent recognition of the significance of transmitted maternal infection by the virus of rubella and of the protozoon of toxoplasmosis has emphasized the significance of pre-natal infection as a cause of maldevelopmental defects.

Apart from infection, toxic factors may induce maldevelopmental defects, as shown tragically by the recent experience with thalidomide and less convincingly by the older experiences with quinine. Prematurity—or the factors inducing it—may be a cause of serious congenital defect: retrolental fibroplasia is mainly the ocular counterpart of a wide variety of congenital defects seen in the premature infant kept alive by the fine methods developed in recent years.

Experimentally, a great variety of ocular abnormalities have been produced ranging from cyclopia and anophthalmos to minor defects. Such anomalies have been particularly studied in the developing fish, where relatively slight changes in the temperature, oxygen, and salt concentration of the fluid in which the embryo grows give widespread effects. The younger the embryo is, the more marked are these effects. It would seem that once the tissue is fully formed the effects of environmental factors are slight; it is the developing tissue which is particularly prone to be affected. With fuller knowledge the clinical appearance of the lesion might be used as a time scale indicative of the height of activity of the disturbing factor. Environmental factors disturbing a normal process may therefore be infective as in syphilis, rubella and toxoplasmosis, "developmental" as in prematurity, or chemical as probably in some of the mass of congenital anomalies for which no infective agent or genetic causation can be established.

Many, perhaps most, congenital anomalies are determined genetically. The clinical similarity of many of the congenital anomalies of genetic origin with those of environmental origin—such as buphthalmos and lamellar cataract, to mention only two—raises the question whether ultimately a common mechanism underlies both types. Only a fuller knowledge of the physiology of the embryo and of gene action will make it possible to answer such speculations. For the present all that can be done is to distinguish in extreme cases those anomalies that are clearly of one or other type. Many of the congenital anomalies do not definitely fall into one or other group. A genetic anomaly may be suspected if two or more children in a sibship show fundamentally similar lesions; or if the family history supports the diagnosis, but frequently the family history is negative or incomplete.

On clinical appearances a lesion in an isolated case is more likely to be genetic rather than environmental in origin if there is a striking symmetry in the two eyes and inflammatory reactions are lacking. Symmetry, however, is not conclusive; in a frank pedigree of anophthalmos one eye may show microphthalmia and the other anything ranging from normalcy to anophthalmos.

**Abiotrophies**

Abiotrophic lesions have not been studied to any extent in animal genetics. Abiotrophy is, however, an undoubted clinical phenomenon: a classical example is retinitis pigmentosa. Here the children are born apparently normal and retain normal vision until the onset of the genetically determined disturbance of the fundus. Abiotrophies affecting children and young adults have been recognized for many years, but it is only lately that there has been any clear appreciation of the fact that genetically determined anomalies may not become manifest until well in middle life, or even possibly in old age. In general medicine Huntington's chorea stands out as an important example of an abiotrophic process frequently coming on in middle life. The blood dyscrasias are less clearly recognized as genetic anomalies of late onset. In ophthalmology there is some evidence that macular dystrophy may develop in middle life and later, and definite evidence of "generalized fundus dystrophy" which begins as a macular lesion at about the age of 40 years and leads to subtotal blindness by the age of 70 years. The conception of abiotrophy implies not only hereditary transmission of a disease process, which is sometimes latent for many years, but also carries the implication that the hereditary disturbance becomes manifest in a tissue that had developed normally and had functioned normally for some years. Evidence that the tissue was in fact normal is unlikely to be available from human observations. An excised eye showing retinitis pigmentosa gives no information as to the state of the retina before the affection developed.

An increasing number of abiotrophic processes are being isolated. Outstanding amongst these are the corneal dystrophies, the macular dystrophies, Leber's optic atrophy, and the group of affections known as retinitis pigmentosa. It is also likely that many cases of optic atrophy, and some, if not the bulk, of glaucoma and senile cataract and ill-differentiated fundus lesions, including the fundus lesions of high myopia, are genetically determined abiotrophies.

Clinically four features are generally ascribed to the abiotrophies.

*Familial stamp*

Within the same family there is said to be a striking similarity in onset, clinical course, and appearances of the particular affection, such as say retinitis pigmentosa or macular dystrophy. This is true to a large extent, but is no absolute rule. Affected members of a family share not only the same pathogenic gene, but to a large extent a similar total genetic constitution, and to a certain extent also a similar environment. These are all factors that tend to produce uniformity and similarity in clinical manifestations within a particular group, and help to explain variations as between different family groups. Individual variations within a group, however, do occur not infrequently, as different members do not, of course, have an identical total genetic constitution or environment. In assessing dissimilarity as between different members of a group, it must be borne in mind that the abiotrophies are generally progressive and strictly comparable stages are not frequently seen within a sibship.

*Symmetry*

Symmetry as to site, general appearance and effects is frequently present in abiotrophic lesions. The bilateral onset of retinitis pigmentosa or macular dystrophy, and the parallel course in the two eyes are indeed characteristic aspects of these two and of other typical abiotrophies. Departures from this strict symmetry are, however, not uncommon, particularly as to onset and the early stages in some other abiotrophies. Sometimes, as in the dominant generalized fundus dystrophy setting in at about the age of 40 years, there may be an interval of several years between the onset of the affection in the two eyes, and even at a later stage the two eyes are not necessarily identical in appearance.

*A characteristic reaction*

The pigment reaction in retinitis pigmentosa, the mottling in one form of macular dystrophy and the hard granular aspect of dominant corneal dystrophy are generally unmistakable. They are, however, unmistakable of the particular affection and not of abiotrophic lesions generally. To regard as abiotrophic only those appearances which satisfy the somewhat well defined lesions in the better recognized abiotrophies is to ignore the fact that such undoubted abiotrophies as Leber's disease, or generalized fundus dystrophy show features that are ophthalmoscopically indistinguishable from inflammatory or oedematous reactions. It is true that frankly inflammatory reactions, such as vascularization of the cornea and vitreous opacities, are not commonly seen in the abiotrophies, but any suggestion that the abiotrophies have specific and characteristic reactions is an oversimplification and a diagnostic pitfall.

*Anticipation*

Glaucoma in particular is frequently given as an example of anticipation—or the belief that in dominant abiotrophies the affection appears at successively earlier ages in the younger generations. There is little support for this view in well-established and easily recognized abiotrophies, and it is likely that the concept of anticipation has emerged in the study of such affections as are not readily diagnosed (such as chronic glaucoma) and that early cases are discovered incidentally as a result of a systematic study of affected families. It is true that occasionally an individual may be affected at an earlier age than his affected ancestors, but the opposite has also been observed.

**Phakomatoses**

The classical examples of the phakomatoses (van der Hoeve) are neurofibromatosis, tuberose sclerosis, and the haemangiomatosis group. Here the lesion, as in the hereditary congenital anomalies and in the abiotrophies, is genetically determined. In contrast to the congenital anomalies there is no congenital defect, and in contrast to the abiotrophies the individual is not altogether normal at birth. Minor blemishes such as *café au lait* spots and moles are present on the skin, and these or parallel hidden lesions burst into activity with growth or later in life. It is thus that neurofibromatosis develops as a widespread affection, or the signs of tuberose sclerosis become obvious. Sometimes phakomatoses, or rather a particular phakoma, may become malignant—a good example of the old theory of Cohnheim, which postulated development of cancer from congenital cell-nests. As yet only the more extreme forms of the phakomatoses have been recognized, and they are generally dominant. They are of interest not only as a link between the congenital anomalies and abiotrophies, but also as a link with the hereditary tumours.

**Neoplasms**

An outstanding example of hereditary tumours is presented by retinoblastoma. There is nothing to suggest that retinoblastomata are malignant phakomas for there are no associated general conditions as in phakomatoses. Direct transmission of glioma over two generations has been observed repeatedly, and there are several authenticated examples of transmission over three generations.

The line of demarcation between simple and malignant melanomas of the iris and choroid is not always clear. There are several pedigrees on the occurrence of choroidal sarcoma; there is as yet little information on the genetic background of melanomas generally.

**Metabolic disorders**

Apart from diabetes and the lipoid disturbances—the classical metabolic disorders—the inborn errors of the metabolism to which Garrod drew attention at the beginning of the century have attracted considerable studies during the recent decades. Biochemical genetics is now a firmly established discipline, concerned with molecular biochemistry as well as with the biochemistry of tissue fluids and storage in tissues. The subject is dealt with in Chapter 12. Here it is only necessary to stress that exploratory developments are steadily increasing. Thus, it is possible that some forms of optic atrophy may result from glucose-6-phosphate dehydrogenase deficiency. In functional disturbances like night-blindness, the visual purple cycle is now explicable in terms of anomalous vitamin A metabolism, whilst colour vision and its aberrations are now interpreted in terms of tangible visual pigments. The study of "biochemical lesions" is opening up in our generation paths as significant in pathology as the study of histological lesions did in the last century.

**Syndromes**

The term syndrome has no precise meaning clinically or genetically. It was a landmark in general medicine when the hypertrophied heart and the contracted kidney could be visualized as different aspects of the same underlying vascular disturbance. In the absence of the necessary knowledge by which the changes in the two organs could be correlated, Bright's disease might well have been regarded as a syndrome in modern terminology. In the present-day use, the term syndrome does not always carry a genetic implication, though there is an increasing tendency for the term to be limited in this sense. The syndrome of macular coloboma and apical dystrophy of hands and feet is clearly congenital in nature. The syndrome of angioid streaks, pseudo-xanthoma elasticum and vascular hypertension consists of components that become manifest in postnatal life. In the Laurence–Moon–Biedl syndrome some of the components, such as polydactyly, are clearly congenital, whilst others, such as the retinal lesion and obesity, might perhaps be regarded as abiotrophic. Some syndromes are, therefore, a combination of congenital anomalies, others are essentially abiotrophic, whilst yet others are a mixture of both. The phakomatoses illustrate this further still, in so far as malignant changes may occur late in life on the basis of minimal congenital anomalies. These considerations emphasize the tenuous nature of any attempt to sort out different varieties of genetic disease on a chronological basis. Such attempts break down as the attempts to classify syndromes as of ectodermal or mesodermal origin have broken down. Until a clearer understanding of the mechanism of the gene is obtained, the clinical groupings employed currently serve a useful purpose in classification and description.

## OBSERVATIONS ON ANIMALS WITH HEREDITARY EYE DISEASES

Although there is much yet to be done in establishing the modes of inheritance in the recognized genetic disturbances, and in establishing criteria for the clinical recognition of as yet ill-defined affections with a genetic basis, further progress lies essentially in the development of experimental studies in embryology and genetics. The study of patients with genetic disease has difficulties considerably greater than the study of patients with disturbances of environmental origin, for the full investigation of a patient with a genetic anomaly involves an extensive study of many relatives. This is not always possible, nor does medicine allow the experimental situations obtainable in animal investigations. For this reason it is essential that the counterparts of human genetic disease, when met in animals, should be submitted to the controlled techniques of the laboratory. Both congenital hereditary defects and abiotrophic anomalies occur in animals no less frequently than in man, and planned breeding can give an unlimited supply of experimental material. Ophthalmology in particular is suitable for such developments. Hereditary anophthalmos is known in mice (Fig. 1), buphthalmos in rabbits (Fig. 2), aniridia in cats, a lesion similar to retinitis pigmentosa in the Irish setter and in many other animals. Embryological, histological and biochemical studies on such animal disorders have helped to elucidate the nature of the congenital defects, and of the abiotrophic anomalies.

### Congenital hereditary defects

In general terms two types of disturbance may occur. In one there may be arrested development, giving at birth a feature that is normal at an earlier stage of development; thus, coloboma of the choroid does in fact represent a normal appearance in embryonic life. The other type represents something outside the normal range of development; thus the opaque lens of congenital cataract, transmitted from generation to generation, does not find its counterpart in normal development. Malformations of this type come close to the pathological deviations seen with disturbances of environmental origin damaging the embryo: these are embryopathies in the narrower sense of the term (restricted to imply super-added disease).

Recessive anophthalmos in the mouse is a good example of a congenital defect consequent on arrested development. This proceeds normally half-way through pregnancy, when no further differentiation occurs and regressive changes set in (Fig. 3). Anophthalmos is not inherited as such but results from an inherited inability of the vesicle to grow to maturity.

**Abiotrophic defects**

An older generation regarded abiotrophic disorders in rather mystical terms—failure of vitality in a fully developed tissue. Paget, and later Gowers who popularized this concept, stressed the similarity to premature senescence. Such views raise difficult questions on the nature of senescence and of life itself. Fortunately the position is rather simpler, as shown by actual observation in strains of animals affected with retinal dystrophy, discussed in Chapter 9. The essential findings were that at birth the mouse retina is undifferentiated into its various layers; these become established by the eleventh day after birth. In

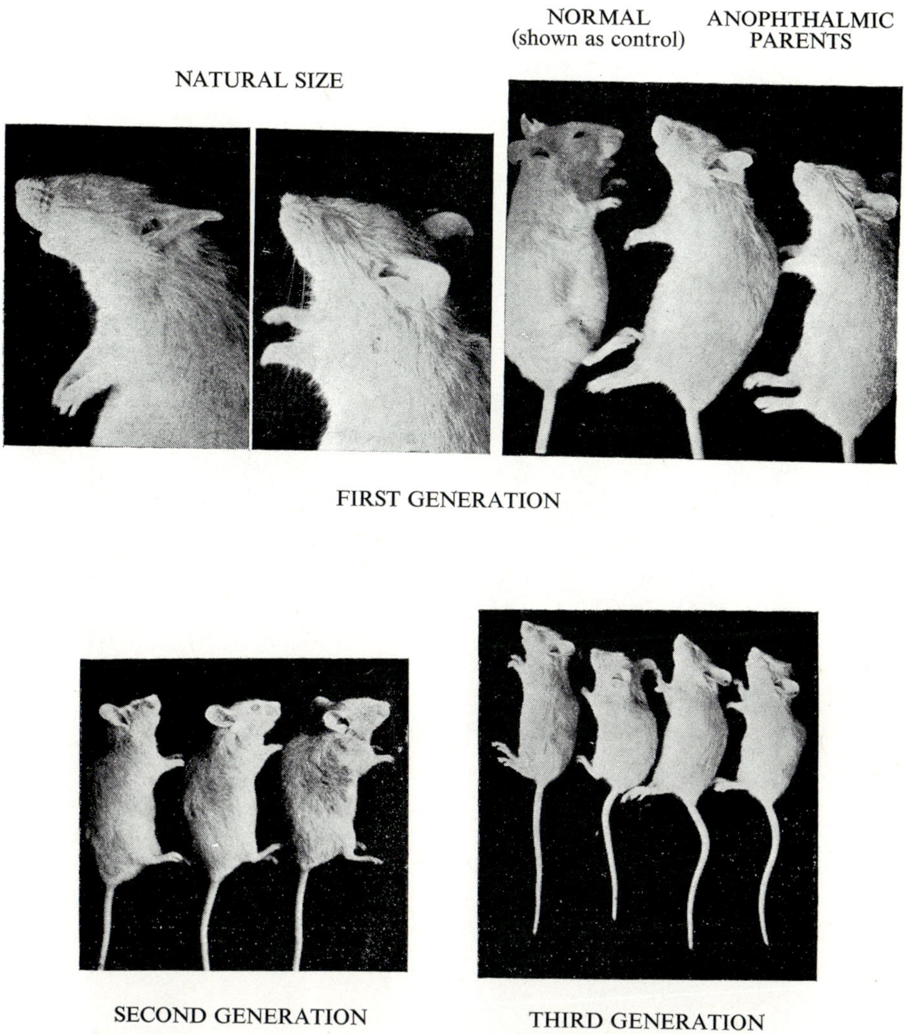


FIG. 1.—Anophthalmic mice. Anophthalmos in mice is inherited in a recessive manner. This photograph shows three successive generations in an inbred colony. (*Animals derived from stock kindly supplied by Dr. Herman B. Chase, Brown University, Providence, U.S.A.*)

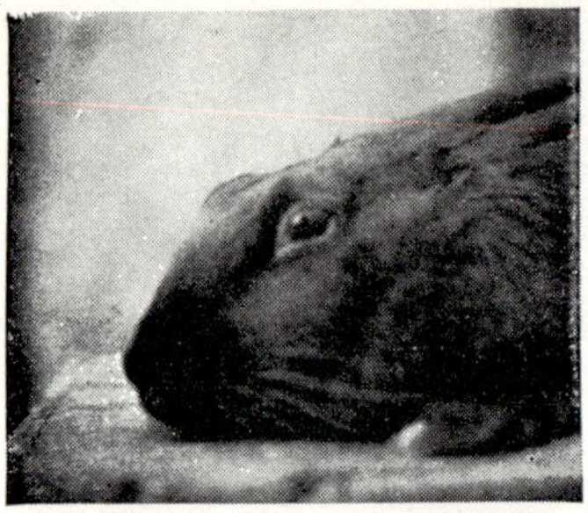

FIG. 2.—Buphthalmos in rabbits. This is also a recessive affection. The photograph shows a normal rabbit for contrast (left) and three successive generations in which the abnormality varied greatly in severity. In all animals the buphthalmos was obvious at birth and became intensified in growth. (*Animals derived from stock kindly supplied by Dr. R. Brückner of Basle.*)

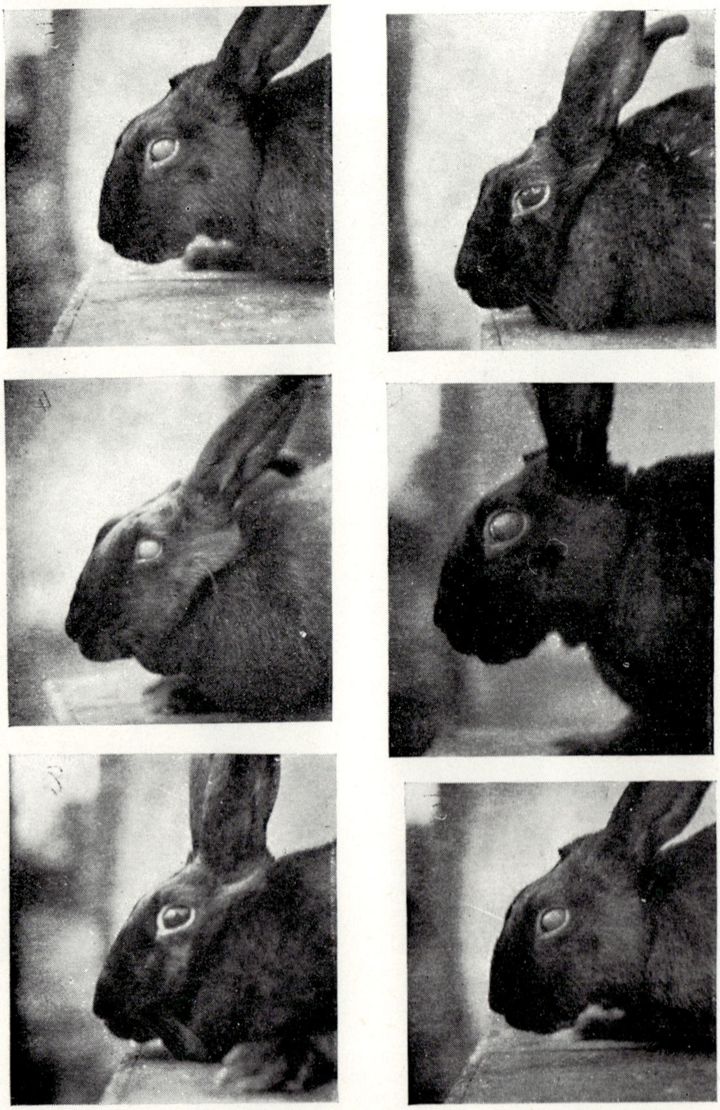

retinal dystrophy (a recessive affection simulating human retinitis pigmentosa) development proceeds normally till the eleventh day and all layers of the retina are differentiated. But whilst in the normal mouse further post-natal development occurs in the rods, no such finer differentiation occurs in the dystrophic strain; on the contrary, regressive changes set in. Prior to the occurrence of these regressive changes the retina is, however, normal only to a superficial view; in fact it

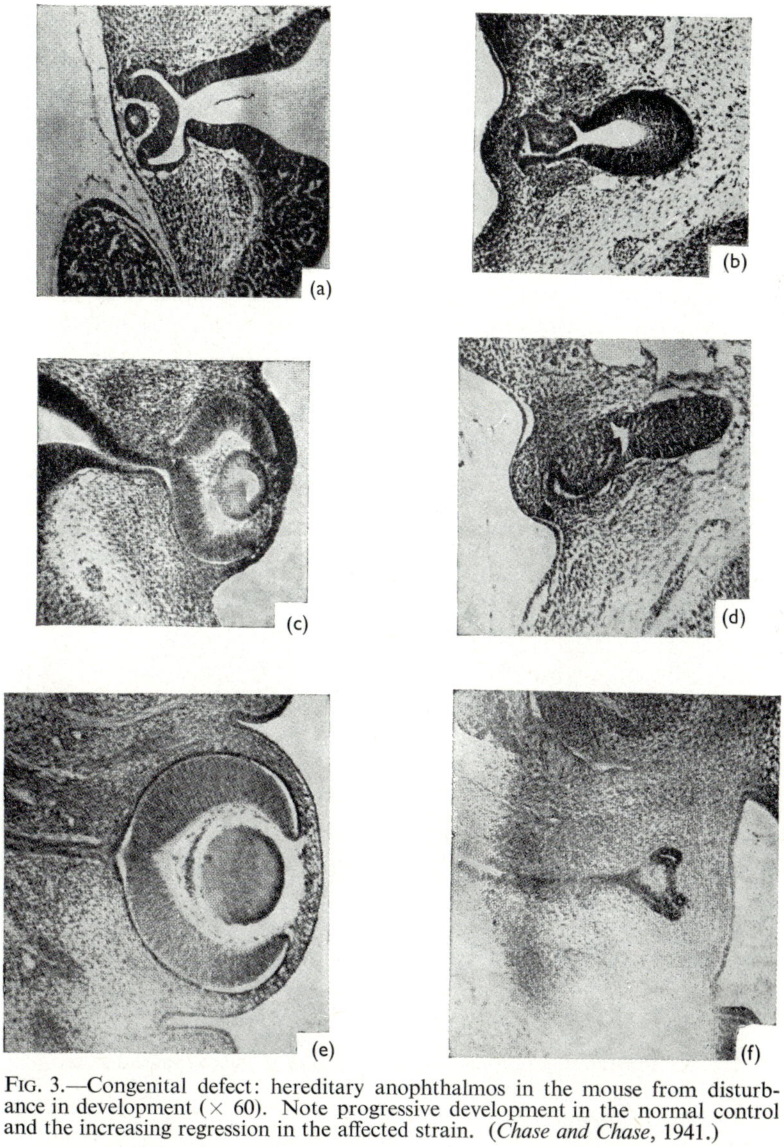


FIG. 3.—Congenital defect: hereditary anophthalmos in the mouse from disturbance in development (× 60). Note progressive development in the normal control and the increasing regression in the affected strain. (*Chase and Chase*, 1941.)

| Control: | at: | Anophthalmic strain: |
|---|---|---|
| (*a*) Left eye | 10 days 23 hours | (*d*) Left eye |
| (*b*) Right eye | 11 days 20 hours | (*e*) Left eye |
| (*c*) Right eye | 13 days 2 hours | (*f*) Right eye |

shows the mildest of congenital defects—arrest of development in the terminal stages of post-natal development. Similar observations on strains of rats and Irish setters also affected with retinal dystrophy, suggest therefore that this defect represents a developmental anomaly in which the regressive changes occur in post-natal life instead of in intra-uterine life as with anophthalmos (*see* p. 166).

**Relationship between a congenital and an abiotrophic defect**

It is clear that there is no fundamental difference between a congenital defect and an abiotrophic malformation. In the congenital defect the hereditary anomaly has run its course in intra-uterine life, whilst in the abiotrophic disturbance normal post-natal development is lacking or faulty and is replaced instead by a hereditarily determined degeneration. This unification of hereditary congenital defects and abiotrophic disorders is borne out by the fact that not all congenital abnormalities are indeed stationary and non-progressive (as will be seen in the description given below of congenital macular cysts and similar disorders), whilst some abiotrophic defects are only mildly progressive. The congenital defect is essentially a macroscopic defect, and the abiotrophic disorder a microscopic defect; the first is often stationary, the second is always progressive to some degree; and both are present at birth.

That a sharp contrast between congenital hereditary disturbances and abiotrophic disorders is artificial is borne out by such disorders as the phakomatoses, retinoblastoma, and the occasional hereditary sarcoma of the choroid. In these disorders, some of which become manifest in childhood and others in adult life, an obvious congenital anomaly of a minor character is often present at birth, almost always in the phakomata and probably also in retinoblastoma (Fig. 4 illustrates the essential aspects).

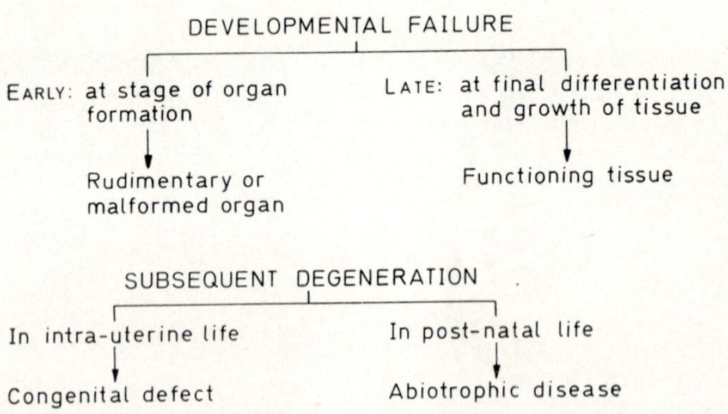


FIG. 4.—Relationship between congenital defects and abiotrophic disease.

**Biochemical studies on such defects**

As yet only tentative explorations have been undertaken mainly in retinal dystrophy (pp. 166–175) and to some extent in cataract.

## SOME NEWER CLINICAL TRENDS

### Polymorphic appearances of the abiotrophies

Although the distinction between congenital and abiotrophic defects is slight on pathological grounds, it is all important clinically. The congenital defect, which generally has little or no significant post-natal development, shows a fairly characteristic appearance which hardly varies from patient to patient. In contrast, the abiotrophic defect is frequently polymorphous, and the different stages of development frequently show marked differences, not readily recognized as different stages in one and the same disorder. The abiotrophic disorder has not one face, but many. Recognition of the polymorphic character of these defects has greatly facilitated diagnosis of fundus lesions, for in the past many intermediate aspects of the fundus dystrophies were confused with inflammatory and other environmental disorders.

### Biochemical anomalies

The increasing number of genetic defects that are becoming related to biochemical disorders is well illustrated in ophthalmology by the relatively recent recognition of such affections as the cataract of galactosaemia, the lens dislocation of homocystinuria, the retinal lesions in haemoglobin S anaemia and such disturbances as the Lowe syndrome with its characteristic amino-aciduria. The replacement of the older manual methods of analysis in chemistry by automation procedures has opened an immense and rapidly expanding field of observation.

### The detection of the carrier state

Of late, the search for minimal manifestations of pathogenic genes—that is, the recognition of the carrier state—has extended to biochemical and serological as well as to morphological traits. This search has been helped by the appreciation of the fact that genes are pleiotropic in effect; that is, they influence more than one trait, and these not necessarily morphological. The recognition of the carrier state is an obvious first line of defence in the control of genetic disorders. It is a matter of some interest that some of the tell-tale minor clinical anomalies now recognized as evidence of the carrier state were known to earlier generations of clinicians, and because of their innocuousness were regarded by them as "physiological variations".

The term carrier state—with its suggestion of similarity to the carrier of infectious disease—is not altogether satisfactory; furthermore, it has no precise meaning. Partial manifestations in heterozygotes in recessive autosomal disorders are more strictly aspects of intermediate rather than recessive inheritance. Likewise, partial manifestations in women carriers of recessive sex-linked affections are aspects of intermediate rather than recessive sex-linkage. The partial manifestations seen with dominant genes are aspects of expressivity, and are often not considered in discussions on the carrier state. The carrier state is sometimes even advantageous: the sickle cell trait carries with it greater resistance to infection by malignant tertian malaria. In strict logic the term could be applied to the possessor of any pathogenic gene, whether manifest or silent. Here the term is used in its clinical context: the search for minimal anomalies (morphological, serological or biochemical) which indicate that the individual carries a pathogenic gene.

In autosomal dominant affections, incomplete expression is often seen in the colobomatous defects, in aniridia, macular cysts, keratoconus and glaucoma. In consequence relative minor anomalies in a particular patient may carry grave genetic implications for his family as a whole. These tell-tale anomalies are generally morphological in character, as is the mild loss of pigment said to be present in carriers of recessive generalized albinism; a non-ocular morphological feature —a peculiar vacuolation of lymphocytes—has been recorded for the carrier's recessive juvenile amaurotic idiocy, and mild changes in the leucocytes in the Higashi–Chediak leucocyte anomaly. An increasing number of biochemical anomalies are being recorded in the carriers of other recessive disorders such as a low galactose–transferase activity in galactosaemia and possibly also diminution of β-lipoprotein in the Bassen–Kornzweig syndrome.

The fullest information yet available is that for a series of sex-linked affections; the carrier women can readily be recognized by the characteristic and innocuous fundus appearances in choroideraemia, in the sex-linked form of retinitis pigmentosa, in ocular albinism and possibly also in retinal aplasia. The carrier state can also be recognized by the mild skin and corneal anomalies in the sex-linked palmo-plantar keratosis described by Siemens.

With the increasing range of recognizible stigmata of the carrier state, genetic counselling should become more precise than is as yet possible in many affections.

**Chromosome anomalies**

Whilst a number of chromosome anomalies have been reported in isolated cases of sporadic congenital ocular anomalies, little has as yet emerged that can be systematized. No one particular congenital ocular anomaly can be ascribed exclusively to a chromosomal aberration (François, 1966, 1968; Keith, 1966, 1968; Warburg and Andersen, 1968).

Of the six well established trisomy syndromes ocular anomalies are not common in the three sex-chromosomal syndromes: XXX "super" or triplo females, XXY Klinefelter syndrome and in XYX syndrome. The incidence of colour blindness has been found to be lower in Klinefelter males than in normal males, presumably because both X chromosomes would have to carry the pathogenic gene before it can be expressed. In the autosomal trisomy syndromes, ocular anomalies are probably common in the 13–15D trisomy syndrome, microphthalmos with coloboma, cataract and a retinal maldevelopment being present in most cases, though in some the eyes are normal. In trisomy 17–18E syndrome, severe ocular anomalies are rare, and mild lesions may not be uncommon.

In trisomy 21G (the Down syndrome, mongolism)—the commonest of trisomic syndromes—ocular anomalies are common, though relatively mild. They are well known and are discussed more fully elsewhere (p. 235).

Ocular defects are apparently rare in monosomy syndromes. In Turner's syndrome (XO females), colour blindness is as common as in normal males, for in these females a pathogenic gene on the single X chromosome is expressed as it is in normal males.

**Polygenic inheritance**

It is likely that we are entering a new phase in the study of modes of inheritance. Until now medical genetics has been largely concerned with monofactorial transmission. In discontinuous variation—as seen in most physiological traits—the additive actions of many genes come into play. The study of polygenic inheritance as applied to disease starts not with Mendelian ratios but with the concentration of particular disorders in given families. Rigid statistical criteria are clearly needed if there is to be no confusion with environmental influences. Family studies in ophthalmological disorders are as yet few, mostly limited to the anomalies of refraction, glaucoma and squint.

## FOR FURTHER READING

Hsia, D. Y. (1968). *Human Developmental Genetics.* Chicago; Year Book Publishers.

Roberts, J. A. F. (1967). *An Introduction to Medical Genetics*, 4th ed. Oxford University Press.

Thompson, J. S. and Thompson, M. W. (1966). *Genetics in Medicine.* Philadelphia; Saunders.

SECTION I

# THE GLOBE AS A WHOLE

Arrested development as a cause of congenital anomalies is most clearly seen in the series of defects that arise from faulty closure of the embryonic choroidal fissure; normally closure occurs at the 16 mm. stage, i.e. at 6 weeks. The anomalies consequent on arrested development of the primary optic vesicle originate at a yet earlier phase of embryonic life, whilst such an anomaly as aniridia is an example of arrested development at a later stage. But many congenital defects (such as the atypical colobomata) are not readily explained on this simple basis. Anomalous rather than arrested development comes into question.

These morphological difficulties are compounded by the complexities as to aetiology, so that at present all classifications of congenital anomalies are rather arbitrary and tend to overlap in their embryological, pathological and clinical aspects. Even the line of demarcation between congenital and congenitally determined anomalies is distinctly tenuous. Of the four groups of disorders discussed in this section only that in the first chapter, which deals with arrested development, has a clear embryological basis; the remaining chapters—those on buphthalmos and glaucoma, the errors of refraction, and on the motor anomalies—are essentially clinical concepts.

# CHAPTER 2

## AFFECTIONS MAINLY DUE TO ARRESTED DEVELOPMENT

### The typical colobomata complex

That incomplete closure of the embryonic choroidal fissure was responsible not only for typical colobomata of the iris and choroid but possibly also for coloboma of the optic nerve and some forms of microphthalmos was well recognized by the end of the nineteenth century. In the first decades of the present century observations on inbred strains of rabbits with colobomatous defects brought experimental confirmation of these findings, and further revealed that inferior conus, nasal conus and circumpapillary ectasia belong to this group.

These studies tallied well with family histories reported by clinicians during those years. Pedigrees then recorded showed the occurrence within one and the same family of such affections as typical colobomata of the iris and choroid and microphthalmos (Fig. 5 *a*). Later observations have brought coloboma of the optic nerve, extreme microphthalmos with cyst formation (orbito-palpebral cyst) and rudimentary formation of the globe (spurious or secondary anophthalmos) within a range that extends from minimal notches at the site of a typical iris coloboma to clinical anophthalmos (Fig. 5 *b*, *c* and *d*).

Several considerations emerge from pedigrees of this type and many less extensive observations over one or two generations. In the first place the whole group of affections must be regarded as dominant. Second, assuming the affections to be monofactorial the pathogenic gene has a wide range of expression extending from anomalies with little or no effect on vision to spurious bilateral anophthalmos. Third, the occasional records (particularly in the older literature) of irregular dominance might be genuine or might represent instances of overlooked minimal colobomata. There is at present little information on penetrance and expression. Fourth, reports of the affection in some sibships raise the possibility of a recessive form; but the infrequency of parental consanguinity in these records and the undoubted occurrence of readily overlooked minimal defects in the ascendants, make this unlikely. Finally, it is likely that within given families only coloboma of the iris, or iris and choroid, will be observed (Figs. 6 and 7), whilst in others the more serious variants may be seen frequently. What is not clear is whether constancy or variation in these manifestations of the gene is the more frequent.

Typical colobomatous anomalies may be associated with defects that arise from less well understood disturbances that occur simultaneously in the developing eye. Thus any of these defects may be seen in such non-colobomatous anomalies as aniridia, buphthalmos, congenital cataract and opaque nerve fibres. They may also occur in generalized congenital anomalies, as is shown by their occasional presence in many syndromes. In other words, typical colobomatous anomalies may be strictly localized lesions, but not uncommonly they are indicative of more widespread lesions in the globe or the body as a whole.

### The microphthalmos complex

The ocular affections in which microphthalmos is a cardinal component are a

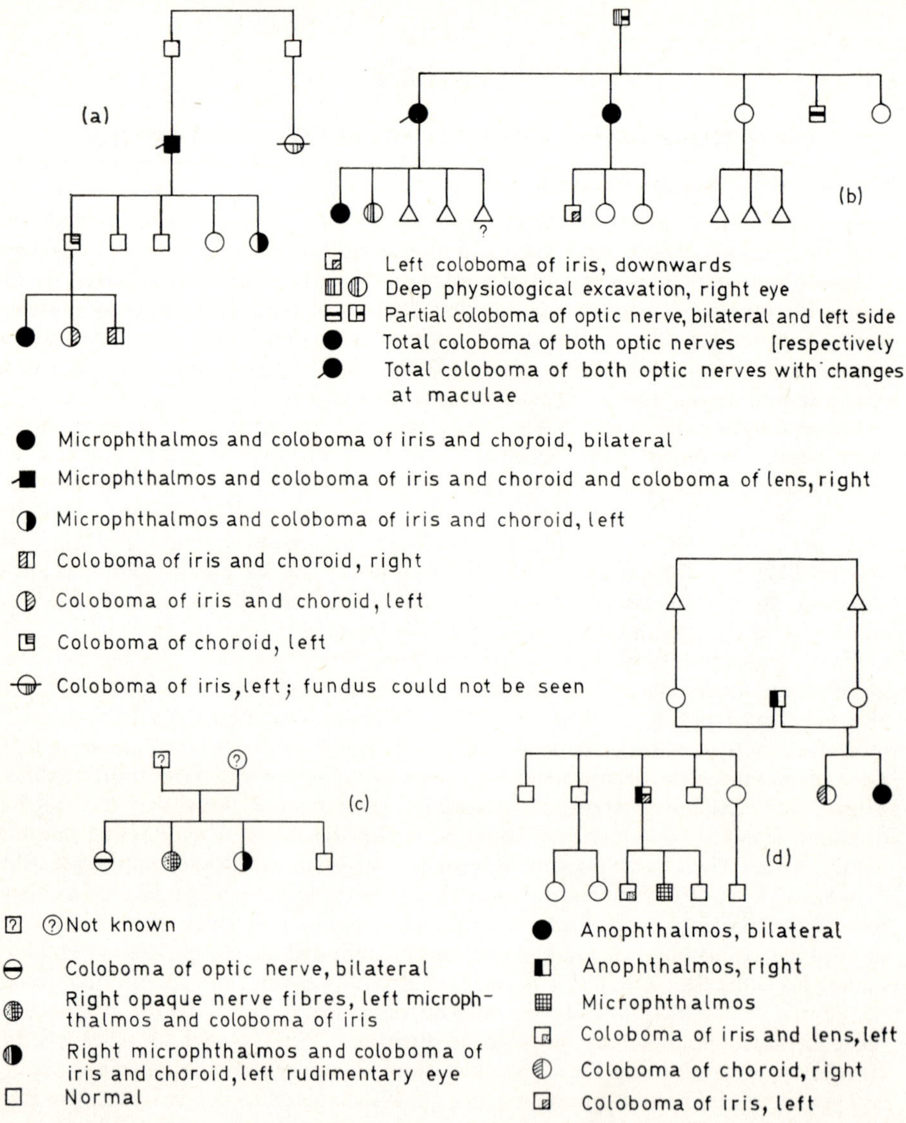


FIG. 5.—Four pedigrees illustrating intrafamilial range of typical colobomatous defects.
(*a*) A family showing anomalies extending from coloboma of the iris and of the lens to microphthalmos. (*After Selz*, 1900.)
(*b*) A family, one member of which shows coloboma of the iris and the other members various degrees of coloboma of the optic nerve. (*After Weyert*, 1890.)
(*c*) A sibship showing bilateral coloboma of the iris with microphthalmos in two members, and coloboma of the optic nerve in a third member. (*After Pfanmüller*, 1894.)
(*d*) A family showing a range of defects from unilateral coloboma of the iris to bilateral anophthalmos. (*After Fleischer*, 1938.)

highly complex group. Whilst some cases of microphthalmos are determined by faulty closure of the embryonic fissure, most are not so readily defined embryologically. Nor is microphthalmos itself always readily recognized. It is assessed on clinical grounds rather than on precise measurement. An axial length of about 20 mm. is probably the lower limit of a normal eye, whilst 10 mm. is the lowest value for the transverse diameter of the cornea (*see* Figs. 32*d* and 59). Some well-defined types stand out.

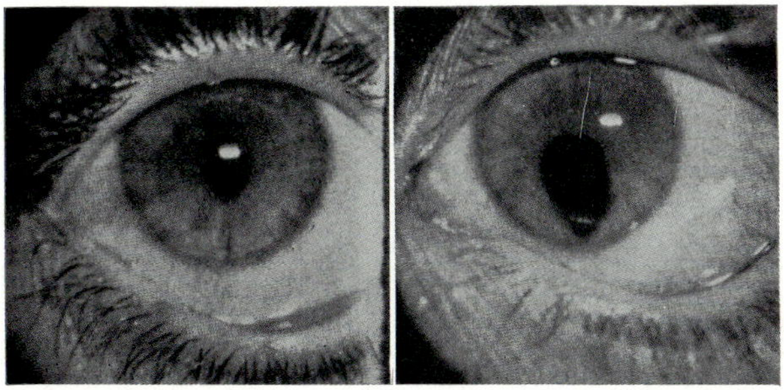

FIG. 6.—Rudimentary coloboma of iris in a woman and fully developed typical coloboma in her son. (*After Fleischer*, 1938.)

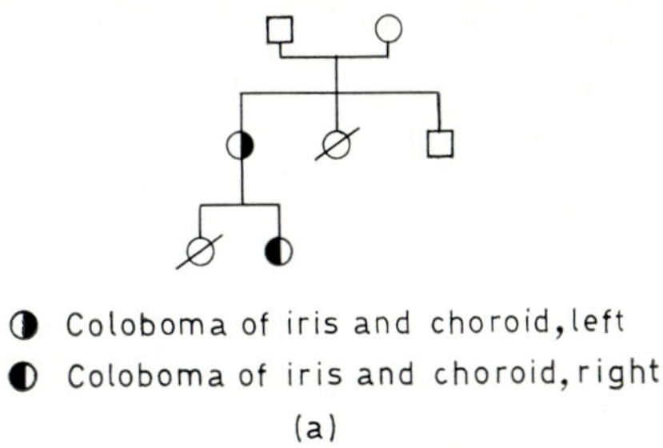


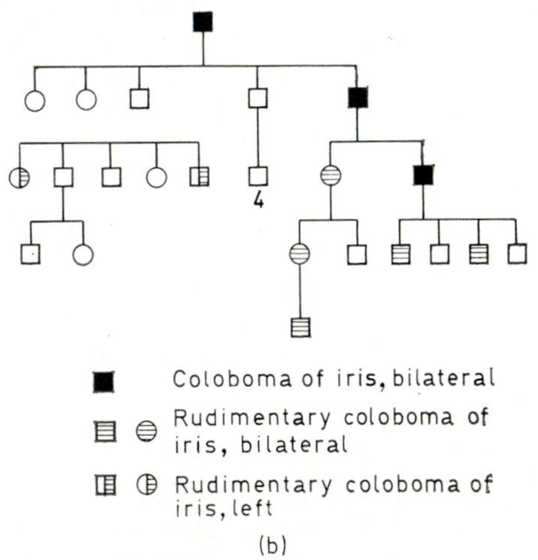


FIG. 7.—Pedigrees illustrative of similarity of colobomatous defects within the same family.

(*a*) Unilateral coloboma of iris and choroid in mother and daughter. Contralateral. (*Personal observation.*)

(*b*) Dominant inheritance of bilateral coloboma of iris, apparently with little variation. (*After Møllenbach*, 1947.)

*Anophthalmos and microphthalmos consequent on anomalous development of the primary optic vesicle*

Suppression of the primary optic vesicle inevitably leads to anophthalmos. More frequently there is anomalous development which leads to severe microphthalmos in which a varying degree of ocular development is present: such eyes may undergo regressive changes in embryonic life ending in clinical anophthalmos—a mere stump with rudimentary ocular tissue. Such regressive changes have been observed experimentally in an inbred strain of anophthalmic mice illustrated in Fig. 1; in some mice the regressive changes were slight so that microphthalmos rather than anophthalmos was present. Both clinically and in the experimental mouse, cyst formation may also occur from distension of an invaginated primary optic vesicle, so that orbital cyst, anophthalmos and microphthalmos need to be regarded as a continuous range of disorders. Pathological records have shown that the optic nerves, chiasma and tracts are often absent in anophthalmos.

This type of anophthalmos is recessive. This is suggested by an early pedigree (Fig. 8) and by a series of familial occurrences in which the parents were consanguineous, and by sibships without consanguinity but equally without such anomalies in the antecedents.

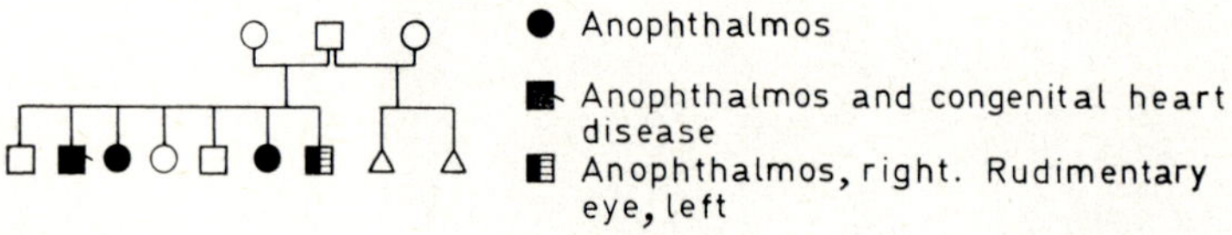


FIG. 8.—Anophthalmos. An early pedigree. (*After Briggs* (1813). In *Sorsby*, 1934.)

*Cryptophthalmos*

Gross microphthalmos is generally present. The affection is not uncommonly unilateral; and the lid anomaly is not a cardinal aspect for it may be limited to one side whilst the microphthalmos is bilateral. Associated systemic anomalies are frequent and are often lethal before or after birth.

Affected sibships with consanguinity in the parents suggest that commonly the affection is recessive, but transmission over two generations has been observed (Coover, 1910; Magrader, 1921).

*Sex-linked pseudoglioma*

This individualized form of microphthalmos, known by many different designations (such as sex-linked microphthalmia, sex-linked congenital detachment, sex-linked congenital non-attachment of the retina, Norrie's disease and Heine–Norrie disease) was recognized as a distinct entity by W. M. G. Wilson in 1949 and is discussed elsewhere (p. 130).

*Colobomatous microphthalmos*

In contrast to the preceeding forms, this type of microphthalmos is generally dominant and less severe. Individual cases may occasionally simulate anophthalmos clinically, but usually the colobomatous nature of the microphthalmos will be obvious from the presence of typical colobomata. In cases where detailed examination is precluded owing to degenerative changes—such as in a shrunken disorganized eye which carries an opaque cornea—only collateral evidence from the examination of relatives will establish the nature of the affection.

*Microphthalmos in association with circumscribed non-colobomatous affections*

*Microphthalmos with congenital cataract.*—Different varieties of congenital cataract are frequently associated with microphthalmos. Harman in 1910 recorded pedigrees of lamellar, coralliform, discoid, anterior and posterior polar cataract in association with microphthalmos. Clinically, congenital cataract is frequently seen in small eyes, and successful operative procedures often give disappointing results. It is almost a matter of personal taste whether such cases are regarded as congenital cataract with small eyes or microphthalmos complicated by cataract. In the considerable literature on the subject, almost all the pedigrees show clear dominant inheritance. The evidence for recessive inheritance and for sex-linked inheritance is slight. Detailed studies combining genetic investigations with present-day measurement and slit-lamp examinations are lacking. It is not known whether congenital cataract with microphthalmos constitutes a clinical entity different from congenital cataract without the associated disturbance of the globe.

*Microphthalmos with retinitis pigmentosa.*—The older literature records a number of families showing the association of retinitis pigmentosa with glaucoma (*see* Fig. 135*a*). More recent reports have stressed microphthalmos as a further association (Hermann, 1958).

*Microphthalmos with ectopic pupils.*—An extensive pedigree of this dominant form of microphthalmos is that given in Fig. 9. In this family the microphthalmos

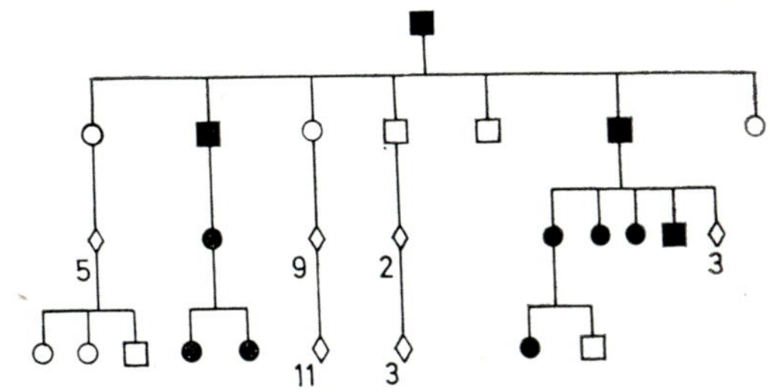


FIG. 9.—Microphthalmos with other ocular lesions. Pedigree showing dominant inheritance of microphthalmos with myopia and ectopic pupils. (*After Usher*, 1921.)

was slight, whilst high myopia, mental defects and other systemic anomalies were frequent.

*Microphthalmos with high hypermetropia and partial amblyopia.*—The large number of sporadic cases on record, and the available pedigrees, of which Fig. 10 is illustrative, suggest that microphthalmos with high hypermetropia is a distinct

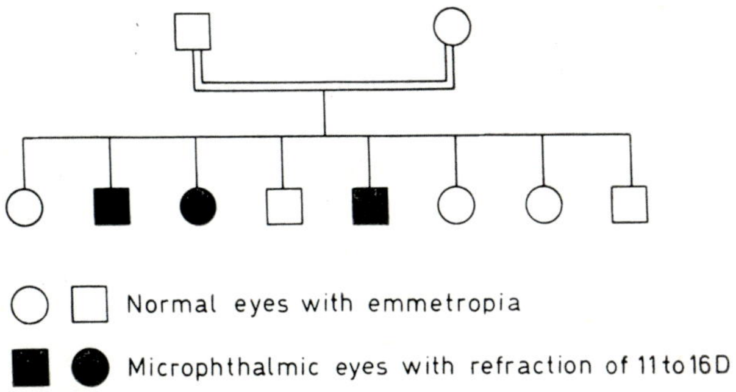


**FIG. 10.**—Uncomplicated microphthalmos. (*After Waardenburg*, 1913.)

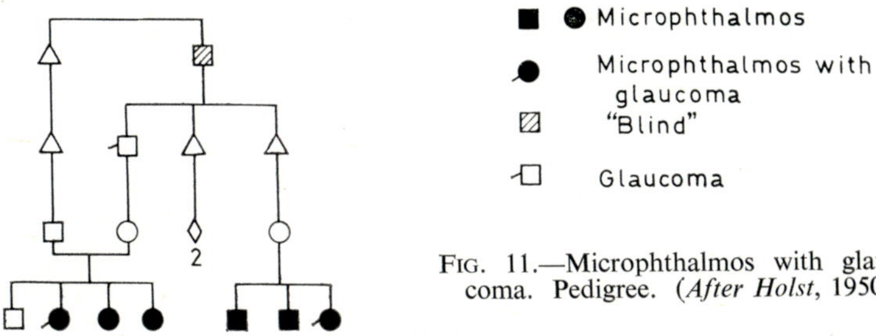


FIG. 11.—Microphthalmos with glaucoma. Pedigree. (*After Holst*, 1950.)

TABLE I

SOME TYPES OF MICROPHTHALMOS

| | *Pathological basis* | *Mode of inheritance* | *Clinical features* | *Remarks* |
|---|---|---|---|---|
| Anophthalmos–microphthalmos complex | Defective development of primary optic vesicle | Recessive | Very severe defects ranging from rudimentary eye to anophthalmos | |
| Pseudoglioma–microphthalmos | Non-attachment of layers of invaginated primary vesicle | Sex-linked recessive | Generally very severe | Probably a variant of sex-linked cystic detachment |
| Colobomatous microphthalmos | Failure of closure of foetal choroidal cleft | Dominant | Can be so severe that any typical colobomatous defects present may be obscured either by degenerative changes or by the microphthalmos being so extreme as to simulate anophthalmos | Associated cysts may be larger than the microphthalmos |
| Microphthalmos with non-colobomatous affections | Probably failure of normal growth of the eye following anomalous development of the lens, iris and retina | | | |
| (*i*) Microphthalmos with congenital cataract | | Dominant | Apparently different forms of congenital cataract may be present in different families | Operative results generally poor |
| (*ii*) Microphthalmos with retinitis pigmentosa and glaucoma | | Dominant | The full syndrome not always present | |
| (*iii*) Microphthalmos with ectopic pupils | | Dominant | Requires fuller elucidation | ? High myopia a constant feature |
| (*iv*) Microphthalmos with high hypermetropia | | ? Recessive | Poor vision from defective foveal development | |
| (*v*) Microphthalmos with glaucoma | | ? Recessive | Requires fuller elucidation | The significance of small eye in primary glaucoma is a comparable problem |
| (*vi*) Microphthalmos with various non-colobomatous disorders (aniridia, congenital opacities of the cornea, etc.) | | ? | ? | Only an occasional association; ? individualized genetic affections |

clinical entity and is inherited in a recessive manner. Presumed or visible foveal anomalies are held to be responsible for the frequently observed subnormal vision.

*Microphthalmos complicated by glaucoma.*—This association is well known clinically, but its genetic status is uncertain. Recessive inheritance is suggested by the pedigree in Fig. 11.

*Microphthalmos with other non-colobomatous ocular lesions.*—Microphthalmos is occasionally seen in aniridia, and in the different forms of congenital opacification of the cornea. It is likely that the microphthalmos in such cases is merely an extreme variant of the congenital defect rather than an individualized genetic entity. Table I summarizes the salient features of the more significant types of hereditary microphthalmos. Some of these have associated general disturbances, mostly of a non-specific type.

**The complex of anterior segment anomalies**

Both the anterior chamber cleavage anomaly and aniridia are affections that involve the anterior segment rather than the globe as a whole.

*The anterior chamber cleavage anomaly (Rieger; Falls; Reese)*

Under the designation of *dysgenesis mesodermalis iridis et cornea*, Rieger in 1934–5 grouped together a number of anomalies that had previously been reported as separate entities, such as posterior embryotoxon described by Axenfeld in 1920, some corneal opacities that had been designated as Peters' anomaly, and also various hypoplastic lesions of the iris. The complete picture was rarely seen in any one patient, but constituted a genetic entity. It is frequently referred to as Rieger's anomaly. Falls in 1949 reported independently on a "gene producing various defects of the anterior segment of the eye" in a family observed over three generations (Fig. 12); the anomalies seen ranged over corectopia, pseudopolycoria, slit pupil, iridotasis, dyscoria and ectopic pupil. The cornea in some members of the pedigree showed opacities and embryotoxon; the lens was ectopic, and occasionally anterior polar cataract was present. Buphthalmos was also observed. Members of this family differed considerably in the degree of involvement they showed. Figure 13 shows the range of anomalies that are often grouped as aspects of posterior embryotoxon.

Reese and Ellsworth have recently stressed that all these defects can be interpreted as the result of "faulty cleavage" of the syncythium of mesodermal cells which grow in from the margin of the optic cup in three more or less distinct waves and which are destined to form respectively Descemet's endothelium, the corneal stroma and the iris stroma. In the course of this differentiation (at about 7–10 weeks) the anterior chamber develops and becomes a completely closed space.

The corneal lesions, the angle lesions (including such affections as hyaline membrane), and the iris anomalies (including anomalies like anterior synechiae), are thus readily explained as aspects of arrested development with secondary effects (Figs. 14–16). It is likely that the glaucoma recorded in a family with sex-linked hypoplasia of the iris (*see* Fig. 111*b*) illustrated yet another aspect of the cleavage anomaly. A wide range of associated ocular and skeletal defects had been stressed by Collier (1962).

*Aniridia*

Aniridia is a major blinding affection generally associated with other extensive ocular anomalies, the most significant being aplasia of the macula. The lack of macular development has been brought forward to support the view that aniridia

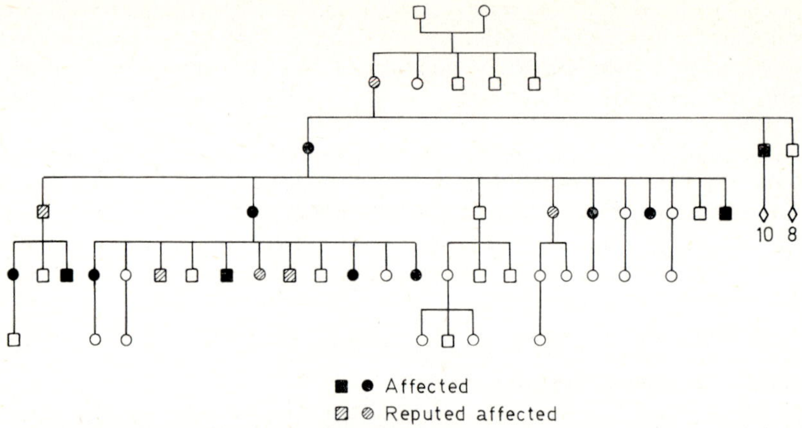


FIG. 12.—Widespread anomalies in the anterior segment of the eye. Pedigree of a family in which a wide range of anterior segment anomalies was inherited in a dominant manner. (*After Falls*, 1949.)

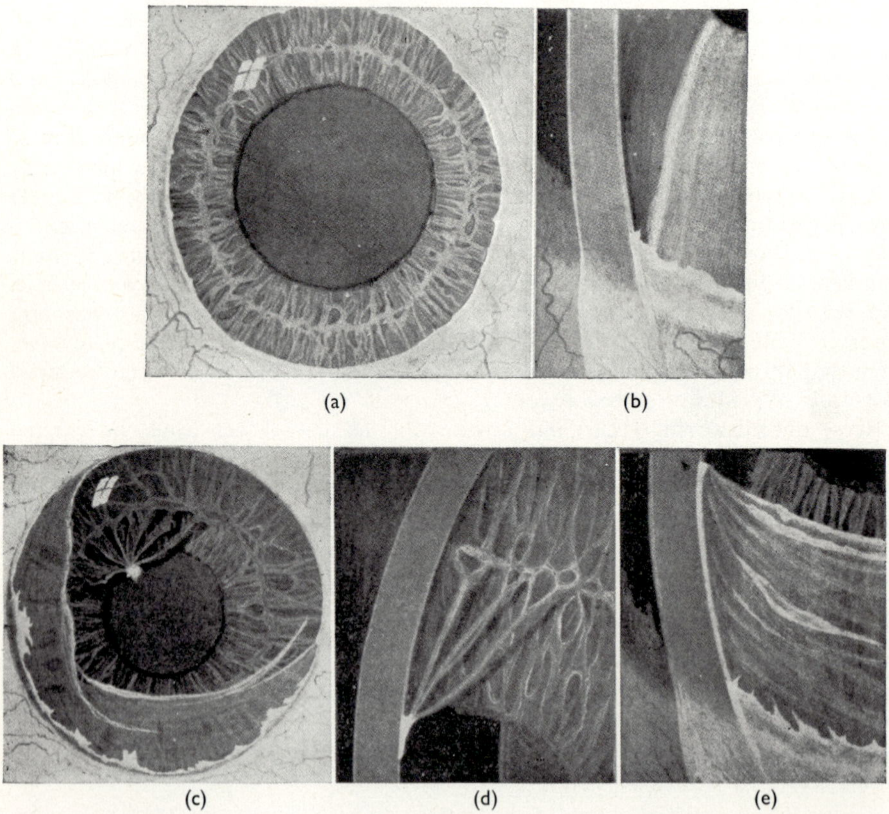


FIG. 13.—Range of appearances in posterior embryotoxon (posterior marginal dysplasia of the cornea): (*a*) and (*b*) face view and slit-lamp view respectively in a mild case; (*c*), (*d*) and (*e*) face view and slit-lamp views in a marked case in which the corneal capacity is well developed, and numerous filaments stretch from the collarette of the iris; microphthalmos was present (*From Streiff*, 1949.)

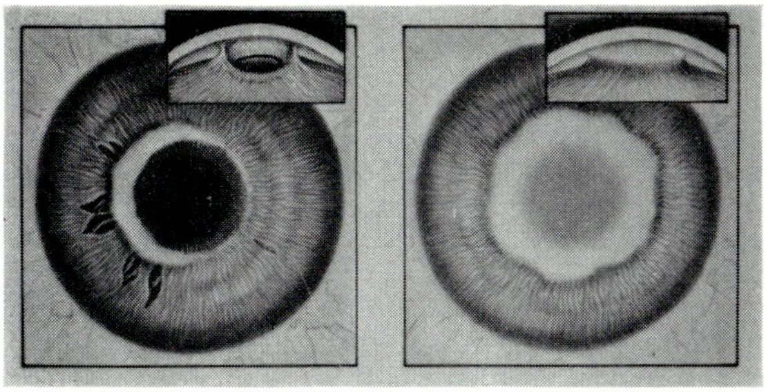

(a)

FIG. 14.—The anterior chamber cleavage complex. Examples of corneal opacities and synechiae. (*From Reese and Ellsworth*, 1966.) (*a*) Appearances in a baby three weeks old. The right eye shows an arcuate corneal opacity and a collarette of synechiae (inset gives the gonioscopic view). The left eye is more severely affected. The tension was high.

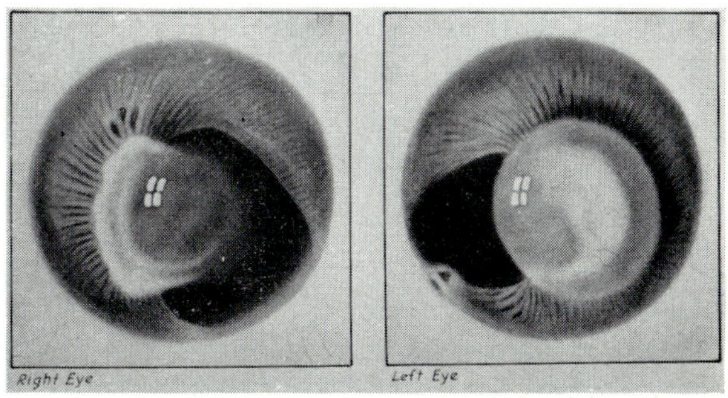


(b)

(*b*) More severe appearances in a baby nine months old. Central anterior synechiae and large corneal opacities necessitated optical iridectomy. Here, too, the tension was high.

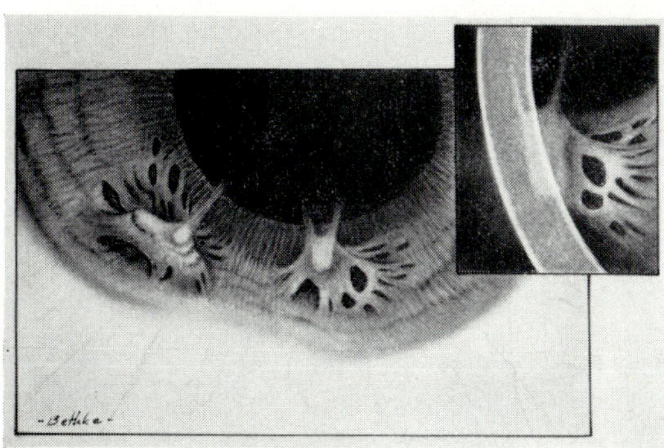

(c)

(*c*) Less severe appearances in a 12-year-old child. Paracentral anterior synechiae and localized corneal opacities.

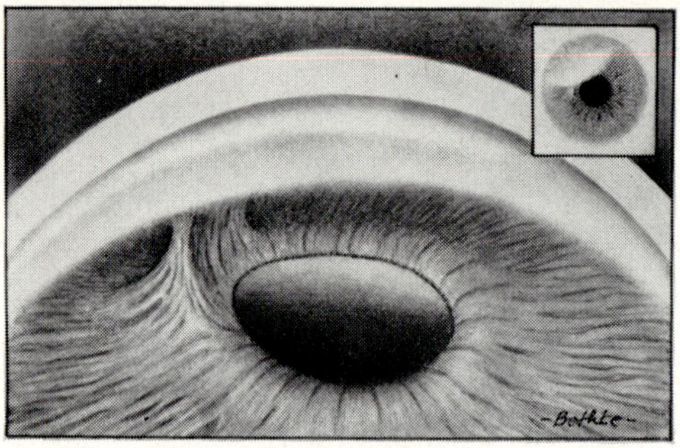

(a)

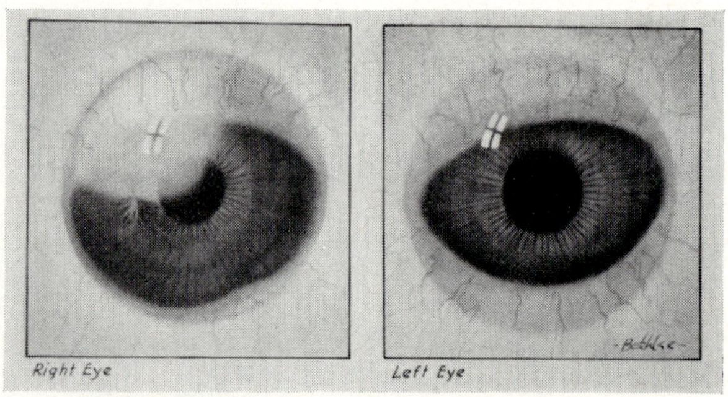


(a)

FIG. 15.—The anterior chamber cleavage complex. Further illustrations on the range of appearances. (*From Reese and Ellsworth*, 1966.) (*a*) The sclerosing keratitis type seen in a baby. Gonioscopic view and corneal changes.

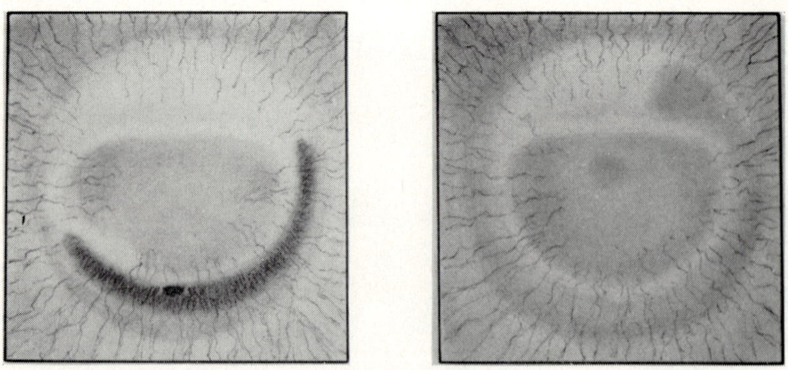

(b)

(*b*) Severe sclerosing keratitis seen in another baby. The tension was high.

(*c*) Appearances in a baby eight weeks old. There is an iris coloboma in addition to anterior synechiae and corneal opacity. The tension was high.

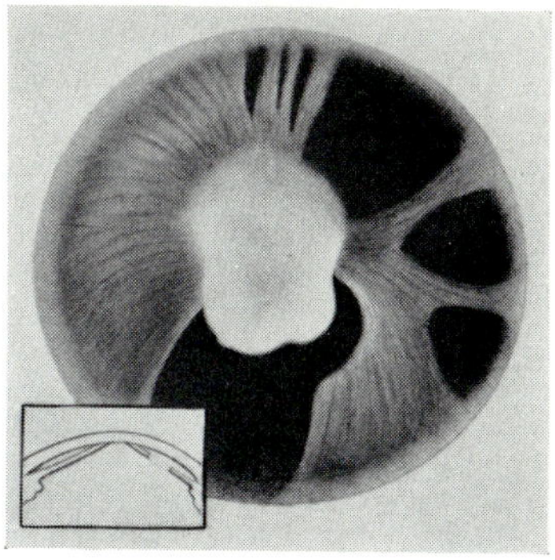

(c)

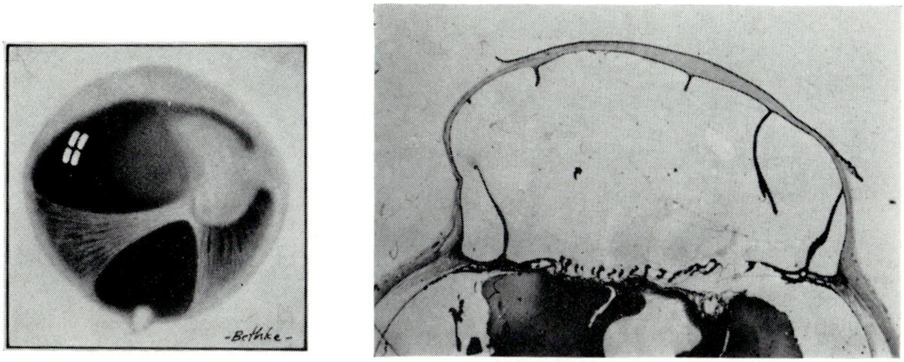

(d)

(*d*) Widespread anomalies in an eye which initially showed microphthalmos, and later buphthalmos from uncontrolled glaucoma, necessitating enucleation.

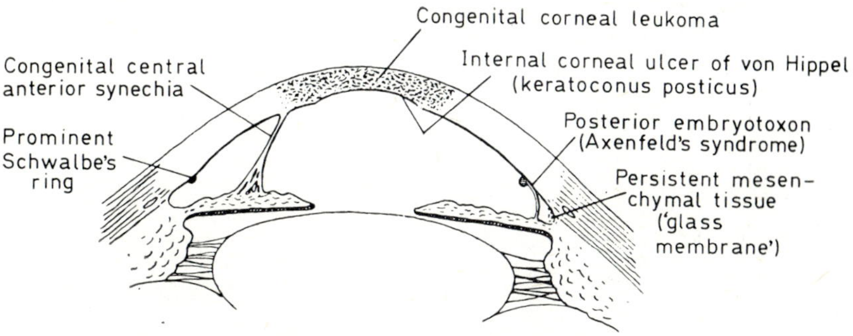


FIG. 16.—Composite drawing shows location of various cleavage defects. (*From Reese and Ellsworth*, 1966).

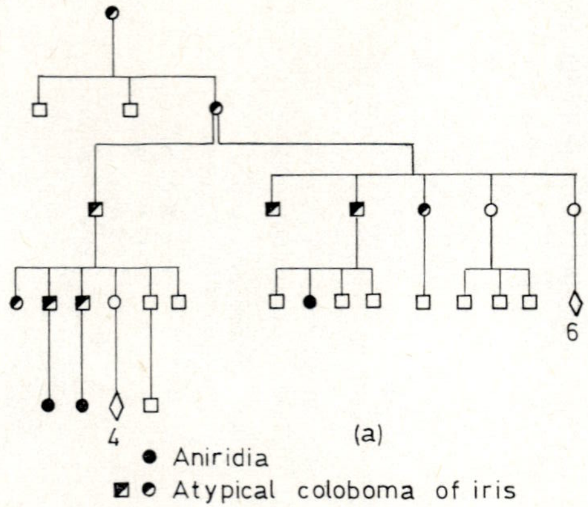


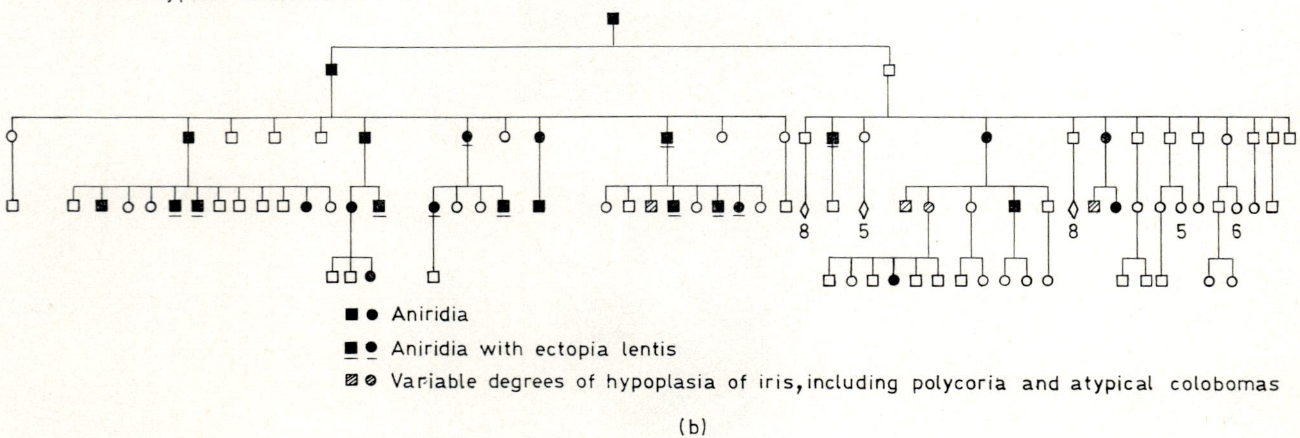


FIG. 17.—Aniridia. Two pedigrees illustrative of dominant inheritance and of the range of anomalies in families with aniridia. (*a*) Pedigree showing the occurrence of atypical coloboma of the iris in some members of the family and aniridia in others. (*After Snell*, 1908.)
(*b*) Pedigree showing different members of a family with aniridia, aniridia with ectopia lentis, and variable degrees of hypoplasia of iris including polycoria and atypical colobomas. (*After Beattie*, 1947.)

is determined by failure in ectodermal development at the 70–80 mm. stage (eleventh to twelfth week of embryonic life), when both the ectodermal layers of the iris and the fovea become differentiated. The frequent association of extensive lens opacities and of hypoplasia of the ciliary processes would fit this assumption. The occasionally associated buphthalmos and the frequent occurrence of secondary glaucoma are probably secondary features consequent on maldevelopment of the angle.

The concept of aniridia must be extended to include some atypical iris colobomas as well as fully formed aniridia. Even this latter type shows considerable variations, as a variable amount of tissue is present at the root. That atypical iris colobomas may be part of the picture of aniridia has been brought out by a number of pedigrees. Fig. 17 *a* is illustrative, showing three fully developed cases of aniridia in a family in which nine others showed extensive atypical colobomas. In other pedigrees, aplasia of the anterior mesodermal layer of the iris and small peripheral defects in the posterior layer, or polycoria, appear as a variant of complete aniridia (Fig. 17 *b*).

Aniridia is inherited in a dominant manner with penetrance of 85–90 per cent. Such pedigrees as are recorded to show irregular dominance may well have contained cases of rudimentary atypical colobomas. There is no evidence of mosaicism (Reed and Falls, 1955).

It is possible that there is also a recessive form of aniridia. Studies in Japan and elsewhere suggest that these recessive cases, in contrast to the dominant cases, have a fully developed macula.

## FOR FURTHER READING

**Colobomatous Defects**

Bell, Julia (1933). In *The Treasury of Human Inheritance*. Ed. by K. Pearson. Vol. II. Pt. V. London; Cambridge University Press.

Fleischer, B. (1938). In *Handbuch der Erbkrankheiten*. Ed. by A. Gutt. Vol. 5, pp. 1–34. Leipzig; G. Thieme.

Mollenbach, C. F. (1947). *Medfødte defekter i øjects Indre Hinder*. (Vol. 15, Opera ex Domo Biologiae Heredit. Human. Univ. Hafniensis.) Copenhagen; Munksgaard.

**The Microphthalmos Complex**

Bell, Julia (1933). In *The Treasury of Human Inheritance*. Ed. by K. Pearson. Vol. II. Pt. V. London; Cambridge University Press.

Sjögren, T., and Larsson, T. (1949). "Microphthalmos and Anophthalmos with or without Coincident Oligophrenia." *Acta psychiat., Kbh.*, Suppl. 56.

Usher, C. H. (1921). *Br. J. Ophthal.*, **5**, 289.

**Anterior Segment Anomalies**

*The Anterior Chamber Cleavage Syndrome*

Falls, H. F. (1949). *Am. J. Ophthal.*, **32**, 41.

Reese, A. B., and Ellsworth, R. M. (1966). *Archs Ophthal.*, **75**, 307.

Rieger, H. (1934). *Arch. f. Ophthal.*, **131**, 523.

— (1935). *Arch. f. Ophthal.*, **133**, 602.

Waardenburg, P. J. (1961). *Genetics and Ophthalmology*, p. 570. St. Louis; Mosby.

*Aniridia*

Beattie, P. H. (1947). *Br. J. Ophthal.*, **31**, 649.

Bell, Julia (1933). In *The Treasury of Human Inheritance*. Ed. by K. Pearson. Vol. II, Pt. V. London; Cambridge University Press.

# CHAPTER 3

## BUPHTHALMOS AND GLAUCOMA

### BUPHTHALMOS

Most cases of buphthalmos are sporadic. In an investigation on the family history of cases seen at Tübingen between 1875 and 1935 Brons found 19 affected sibs in seven families in the total of 172 cases. Westerlund's data for Denmark were similar: 11 familial cases in a total of 102. Less extensive series have given an average incidence of the same value.

A substantial difficulty in assessing the significance of heredity arises from the fact that, as in glaucoma, there are probably different pathological entities grouped under one clinical designation. This is suggested by the following considerations: (1) The developmental anomaly in the angle of the anterior chamber which gives rise to buphthalmos, may lead to a distended globe already present at birth or to distension that becomes manifest in infancy; there is thus a gradual transition to juvenile glaucoma in which there is no distension. (2) There is the classical distinction between primary and secondary buphthalmos. (3) The distinction between buphthalmos and megalocornea is not always readily made. (4) There is the recent recognition that buphthalmos may be an aspect of widespread ocular or even systemic disorders (such as the cleavage anomaly and Lowe's hyperaminoaciduria syndrome respectively).

The significance of heredity in buphthalmos must therefore await a finer differential diagnosis of the different types than we have at present. Twin material—though slight in extent—records concordance in monozygotic twins; in three pairs of monozygotic twins the affection was unilateral (Kiehle and Pugmire, 1934; Potts, 1950; Massimeo, 1956). The evidence for the existence of a recessive variety (Fig. 18) is considerable: apart from the many records of familial cases of the classical primary type of buphthalmos, there is an incidence of parental consanguinity of the order of 10 per cent in the more substantial series on record.

In a recessive disorder transmission is not to be expected (except in the unusual situation shown in the pedigree recorded in Fig. 19). What little information there is on this aspect supports this expectation (Fig. 20) but a few selected observations—such as those recorded in Fig. 21—suggest that the affection has been transmitted (without necessarily being fully expressed); it is possible, however, that some of the cases of direct transmission were examples of "pseudo-dominance". There is no record of transmission over three generations. Whether buphthalmos may occasionally be an early manifestation in families with dominantly inherited glaucoma cannot be decided on the available evidence; such occurrences have been reported (Heath, 1960; Jerndal, 1968) but may have been merely incidental.

### GLAUCOMA

Although the designation of glaucoma has a considerable history, the concept of glaucoma as a clinical entity in which ocular hypertension was the cardinal sign

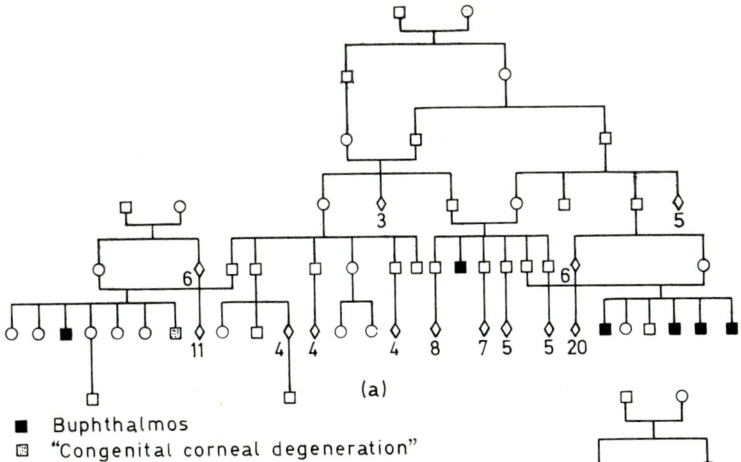


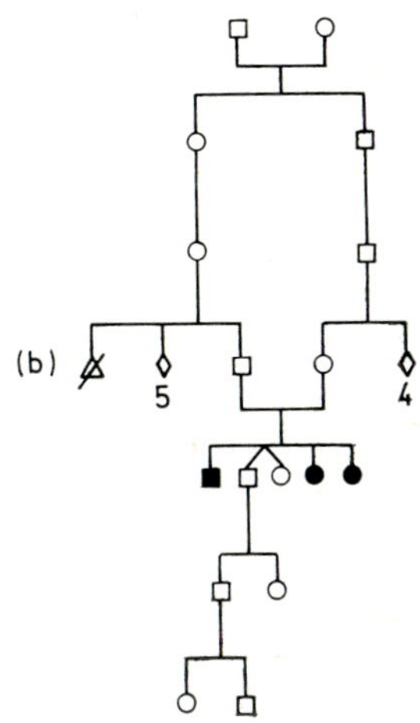


FIG. 18.—Buphthalmos. Pedigrees illustrative of recessive inheritance. (*After Westerlund*, 1947.)

(*a*) Buphthalmos in three collateral branches of a family heavily intermarried.

(*b*) Buphthalmos in the offspring of parents who were second cousins.

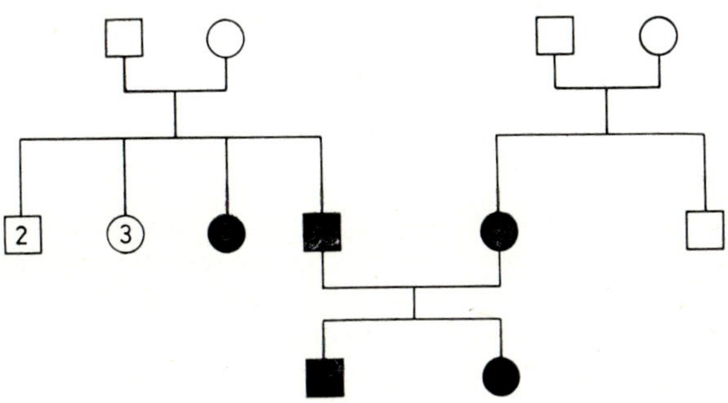

FIG. 19.—Buphthalmos. Recessive inheritance. (*After Algan*, 1957.)

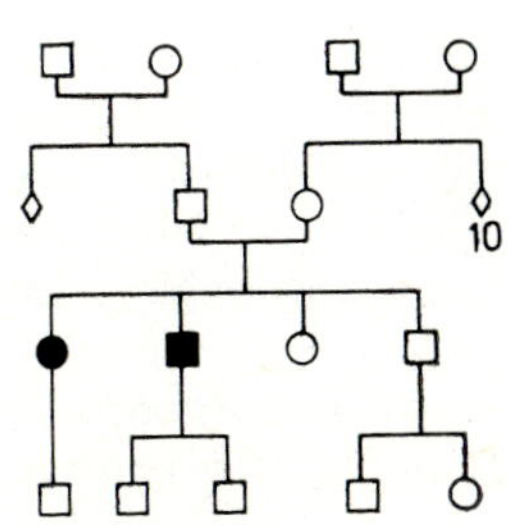

FIG. 20.—Pedigree showing normal offspring of an affected woman and also of her affected brother. (*After A. D. Griffith and L. H. Savin. Hitherto unpublished. Royal Eye Hospital No.* 0/6210.)

is of fairly recent origin. Mackenzie established this for acute glaucoma in 1830 in the first edition of his classical textbook, whilst the recognition of chronic glaucoma came some 30 years later following on the appreciation of cupping of the disc as observed by the then recent innovation of ophthalmoscopy.

The recognition of the hereditary character of glaucoma dates back to those formative years. Two incidental features in these early observations have influenced many later records. In the first place, the recognition of the transmission of glaucoma implied the occurrence of glaucoma fairly early in life (when the parents of an affected individual were still available for examination). Second, this material often showed the onset of the affection at an earlier age in the second generation

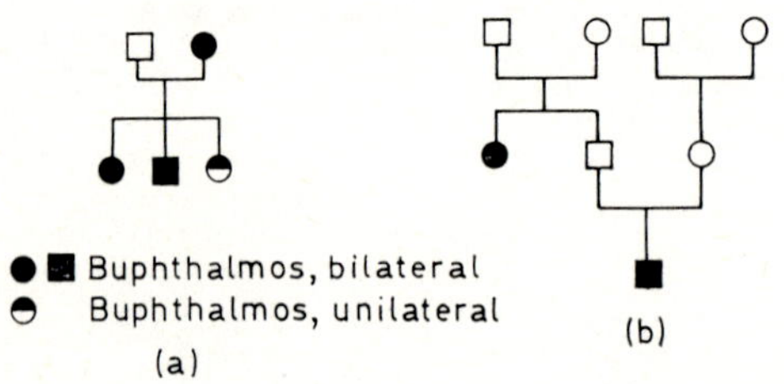


FIG. 21.—Buphthalmos. Pedigrees illustrative of a possibly dominant mode of inheritance of buphthalmos.
(*a*) Buphthalmos over two generations. (*After Argyll Robertson*, 1891.)
(*b*) Buphthalmos in an aunt and nephew. (*After Sourdille*, 1925.)

than in the first (for it was only with such cases that two or more generations would be seen). These incidental features have led to the concept of juvenile glaucoma as a distinct entity and to that of anticipation in succeeding generations. As shown below neither concept is valid.

In the study of inheritance in glaucoma three phases stand out. In the first, which goes back to the early days of the recognition of the affection and extends until the 1930s, a large number of family histories were recorded; this selected material showed that glaucoma could be hereditary. In the second phase a considerable frequency of a positive family history of glaucoma was established in unselected cases. In the third phase—one that is proceeding actively today—screening procedures for early or latent glaucoma are being applied to the families of affected individuals. These phases and several other aspects call for detailed consideration.

**Pedigrees of glaucoma**

Figures 22 and 23 are typical of many more which record the occurrence of congestive glaucoma and chronic simple glaucoma over several generations. Inheritance is clearly dominant. Irregular dominance is suggested by Fig. 24, but the possibility of an overlooked latent glaucoma cannot be excluded.

The recognition of open angle and narrow angle types of glaucoma has brought its quota of pedigrees showing dominant inheritance in both these types. Figs. 25 and 26 are illustrative, whilst Fig. 27 shows a pedigree of chronic closed angle glaucoma with acute or subacute crises.

It is likely that the two varieties of glaucoma as assessed by gonioscopy are genetically distinct, although the appearance of an open angle may be disturbed to simulate a narrow angle in an individual patient.

In recent years an increasing number of pedigrees suggestive of recessive inheritance have been recorded (Fig. 28), but adequate evidence for a high incidence of consanguinity of the parents is not yet available for any substantial series of cases.

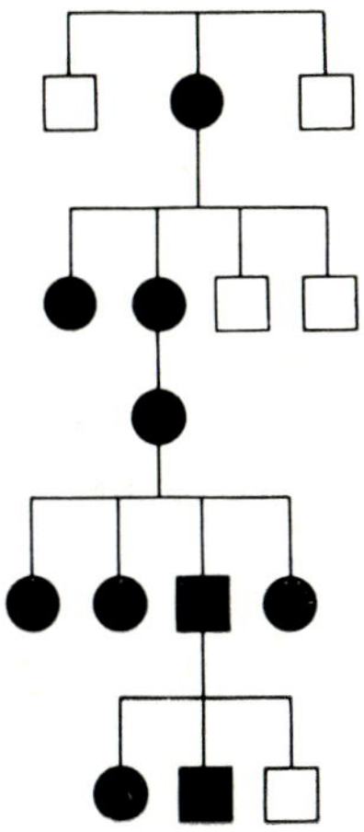

FIG. 22.—Congestive glaucoma. Dominant inheritance. (*After Sédan and Sédan-Bauby*, 1949.)

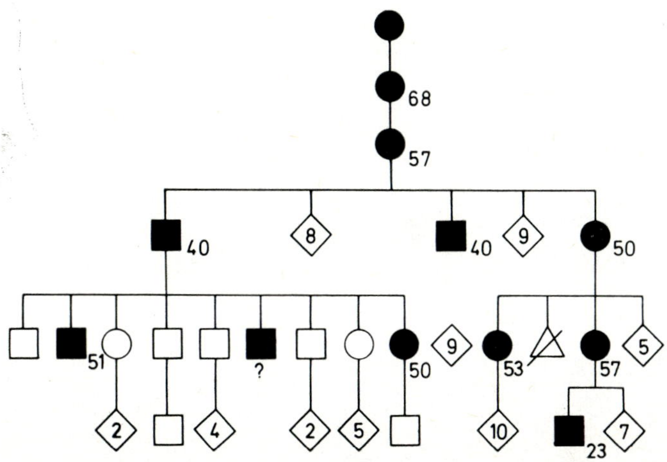


FIG. 23.—Chronic simple glaucoma. Dominant inheritance. (*After François*, 1961.)

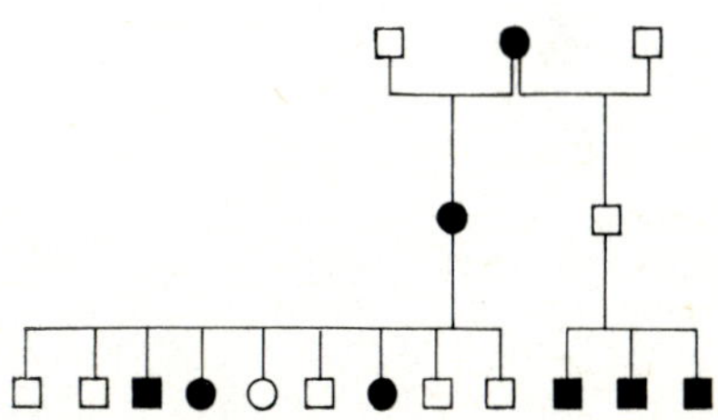

FIG. 24.—Glaucoma. A pedigree suggestive of irregular dominance. (*After Biro*, 1939.)

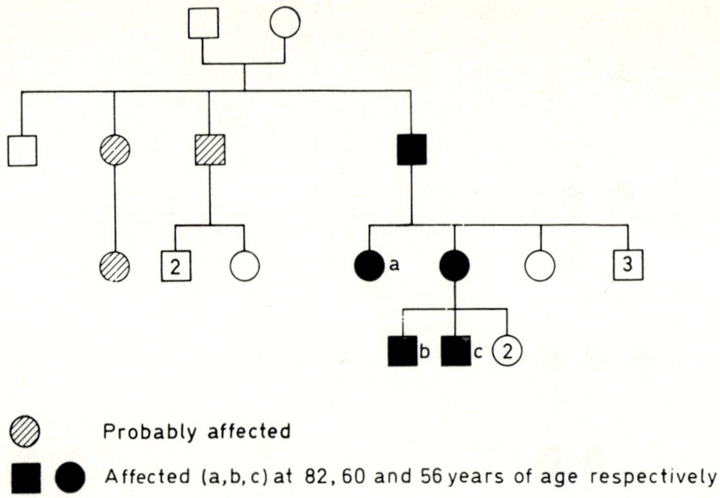


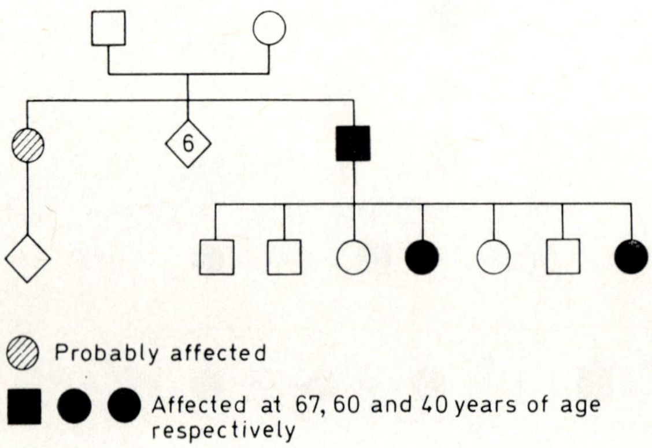


FIG. 25 (*above*).—Open angle glaucoma. (*After Weekers, Gouguard-Rion and Gouguard,* 1955.)

FIG. 26 (*left*).—Narrow angle glaucoma. (*After Weekers, Gouguard-Rion and Gouguard,* 1955.)

FIG. 27 (*below*).—Chronic closed angle glaucoma with acute or subacute crises. (*After François,* 1961.)

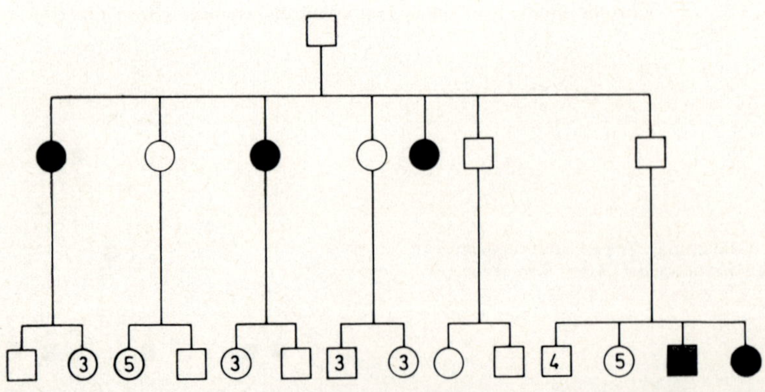

FIG. 28.—Glaucoma. Pedigrees suggestive of recessive inheritance.

(*a*) "Juvenile glaucoma". (*After Holst*, 1950.)

(*b*) "Presenile intermittent glaucoma": recessive. (*After Waardenburg*, 1949.)

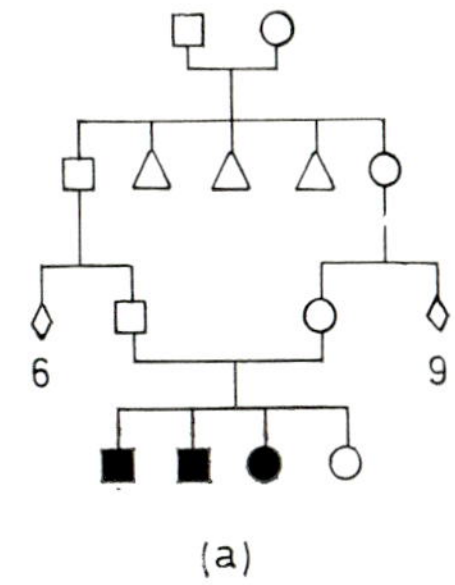


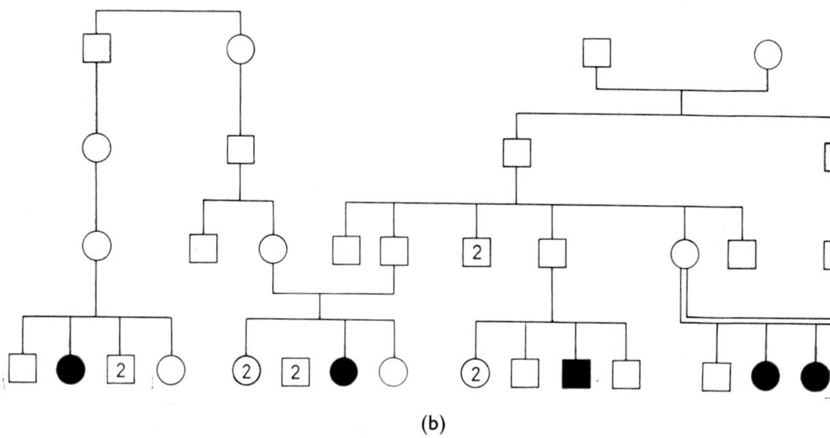


**Family history in unselected cases**

The conflicting views as to the significance of heredity in isolated cases of glaucoma could not be assessed until the family histories in unselected series of cases were available. The earliest of such studies, that of Biro in 1939, found that 5·6 per cent of patients (43 out of 761) gave a family history. A later and more intensive study by the same author gave an incidence of 12·8 per cent in 125 cases. This agreed closely with the 13 per cent in 82 cases studied by Westerlund in 1947. Since then a number of other observers have recorded somewhat similar findings. Most substantial series show a family history in 15–20 per cent of cases, but Waardenburg has recorded 46 per cent in 104 consecutive cases.

**Latent glaucoma in the families of affected individuals**

Since Brav and Kirber in 1951 found an incidence of 1·53 per cent of previously undetected hypertension in a mass tonometric investigation of some 10,000 persons aged 40–65 years, similar findings have been reported by other observers. Other unmasking procedures, such as tonography, provacative applications of tropical corticosteroids and central field screening, have since been used singly or in combination, and it would seem that no single test is adequate to establish potential glaucoma whilst the diagnosis of early glaucoma still presents difficulties. With these uncertainties the application of these procedures in family studies has given rather variable results. An incidence of "latent" glaucoma of up to 20 per cent, and even more in the relatives of glaucoma patients, has been recorded by some observers (Miller and Paterson, 1962). Becker and Hahn (1964) have found an increase in applanation pressure of more than 6 mm. Hg in 73 per cent of the offspring of glaucoma patients; this they interpreted as showing that glaucoma is a recessive affection, and that a response is characteristic of the heterozygous as well as the homeozygous state.

On the available evidence, it is clear that glaucoma—both the open angle and the narrow angle type—is genetically determined in a high proportion of cases, even if precipitated by environmental factors. Whether all glaucoma is always thus determined, and if so whether it is monofactorial or polygenic, are still open questions; and little is as yet known as to the degrees of penetrance and expression of the pathogenic factors.

**Sex-linkage in glaucoma**

It is likely that recessive sex-linked inheritance applies to two unusual forms of glaucoma.

*Pigmentary glaucoma (Sugar)*

Since Sugar first described this affection in 1940, some 150 cases have been reported. In Sugar's series of 19 cases, only two were females, although the collected literature gives an incidence of 23·4 per cent in 128 cases. Fig. 29 shows a pedigree recorded by Stankovič (1961); it is interpreted by him as showing

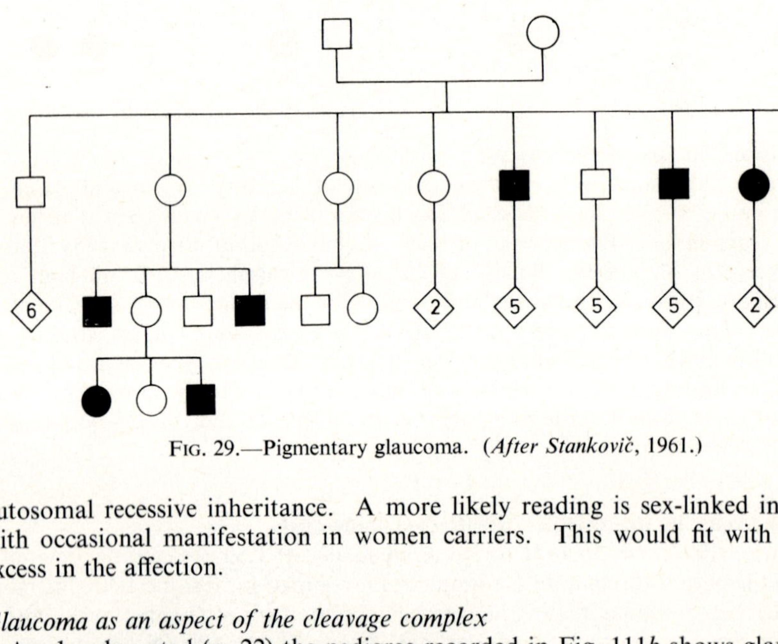


FIG. 29.—Pigmentary glaucoma. (*After Stankovič*, 1961.)

autosomal recessive inheritance. A more likely reading is sex-linked inheritance with occasional manifestation in women carriers. This would fit with the male excess in the affection.

*Glaucoma as an aspect of the cleavage complex*

As already noted (p. 22) the pedigree recorded in Fig. 111*b* shows glaucoma as an aspect of sex-linked "hypoplasia of the iris".

**Juvenile glaucoma**

The conception of juvenile glaucoma as a distinct clinical entity, elaborated by Löhlein, is based on a statistical fallacy consequent on the use of selected material.

Drawing mainly on cases recorded in the literature, Löhlein held that juvenile glaucoma was a clinical entity because in the group as a whole—extending from the artificial limits of the ages of 5–35 years—something like 40 per cent occurred between the ages of 16 and 20; in addition, some 50 per cent were myopic, and there was a familial occurrence in some 20 per cent. He also held that this type of affection occurs most often in men. These are hardly valid criteria. The concentration of cases within the age group of 16–20 years in material collected from the literature obviously carries an element of selection; in patients over 20 years of age, the condition is less likely to be recorded. The sex difference noted in Löhlein's series was not statistically significant. Any excess in the incidence of myopia is easily explained by the fact that the eye was still expansile at the ages under consideration. A familial occurrence in 20 per cent of cases is not strikingly different from the percentage obtained for other forms of glaucoma. What is true in Löhlein's conception is the fact—already observed by the older ophthalmologists—that glaucoma is not exclusively a disease of the aged, although its frequency increases with age. Reports abound on these early cases because of the exceptional interest they have aroused. Furthermore, as in many other affections, the "familial stamp" applies: within given families glaucoma tends to have the same onset and to run the same course.

**Anticipation**

The most striking instances of anticipation are those recorded in the older literature. Later workers dealing with unselected material have found a few impressive instances, but also instances of the affection becoming manifest at a later date in descendants. Generally the pattern as to age is not at all consistent (*see* Fig. 23).

## FOR FURTHER READING

Bell, Julia (1933). In *The Treasury of Human Inheritance.* Ed. by K. Pearson. Vol. II, Pt. V. London; Cambridge University Press.

Brons, H. (1937). *Uber die Vererbung des Hydrophthalmus Congenitus.* Thesis; Tübingen.

Hunt, N. B. (Ed.) (1966). *Glaucoma* (Proceedings of a Symposium, 1965). Edinburgh; Livingstone.

Posner, A., and Schlossman, A. (1949). *Archs Ophthal.*, **41**, 125.

Stokes, W. H. (1940). *Archs Ophthal.*, **24**, 885.

Waardenburg, P. J. (1961). In *Genetics in Ophthalmology*, p. 578. Ed. by P. J. Waardenburg, A. Franceschetti, and D. Klein. Oxford; Blackwell.

Westerlund, E. (1947). *On the Primary Glaucoma Diseases.* (Vol. 12, Opera ex Domo Biologiae Heredit. Human. Univ. Hafniensis.) Copenhagen; Munksgaard.

# CHAPTER 4

## REFRACTION

The biomathematical approach to the problems of refraction initiated by Steiger in the early years of the century and developed since by a number of workers, has established that the emmetropic eye results from the co-ordination of the components of refraction (essentially the powers of the cornea and of the lens and the axial length of the eye) and ametropia generally form inadequate correlation (Figs. 30 and 31).

The components of refraction are not optical constants but have values that follow a statistically Normal (i.e. binomial) distribution (Fig. 32 *a–d*).

Were these components to show free variation, the distribution of the different refractions in the general population would also follow a Normal distribution. As can be seen from Fig. 32 *e* the curves of the distribution of refraction show a marked excess around emmetropia—the result of adequate correlation. But such curves also show an excess of high myopes; these, as also the cases of high hypermetropia, are determined by the fact that in some 4 per cent of the population the axial length of the globe falls outside the range seen in emmetropia (22·0 to 26·0 mm. in one series—Sorsby and colleagues, 1957).

Eyes with high refractive errors are abnormal if only because they possess axial lengths that cannot be compensated by the range of values in the cornea and lens. In other words, in contrast to emmetropia (in which the optical components are fully correlated) and low and medium degrees of hypermetropia and myopia (in which the same components are less adequately correlated), high myopia and hypermetropia result from an abnormal component—an anomalous axial length. These considerations make it possible to regard refractions roughly between +4·0 D and −6·0 D as a continuous variation (similar to the distribution of normal stature) and the higher refractive errors as discontinuous variations (similar to the place dwarfs and giants occupy in the distribution of height in the general population).

The data obtained from the different methods of investigation recorded below are sufficiently definite to have established the paramount significance of heredity in refraction, but the different modes of inheritance and their frequencies, as also the possible significance of contributory environmental factors, are still to be determined.

### Pedigree material and its limitations

There are a large number of pedigrees illustrative of the fact that some refractive states may be hereditary. Most pedigrees show dominant transmission of myopia or of hypermetropia; the degrees of the refractive error when recorded may be fairly similar within a given family, but often enough show a substantial range. Many pedigrees are suggestive of recessive inheritance and some of the offspring tend to show values intermediate between those seen in the parents. In some pedigrees, anisometropia is shown as transmitted over two or more generations, whilst others record it in sibships. There is no convincing record or sex-linked inheritance in uncomplicated refractive errors.

FIG. 30 (*right*).—The significance of correlation in emmetropia and ametropia: (*a*), (*b*) and (*c*) emmetropic eyes possessing unequal lengths; axial (*d*), (*e*) and (*f*) eyes with identical axial lengths but markedly different refractions. (*After Sorsby, Benjamin, Davey, Sheridan and Tanner*, 1957.)

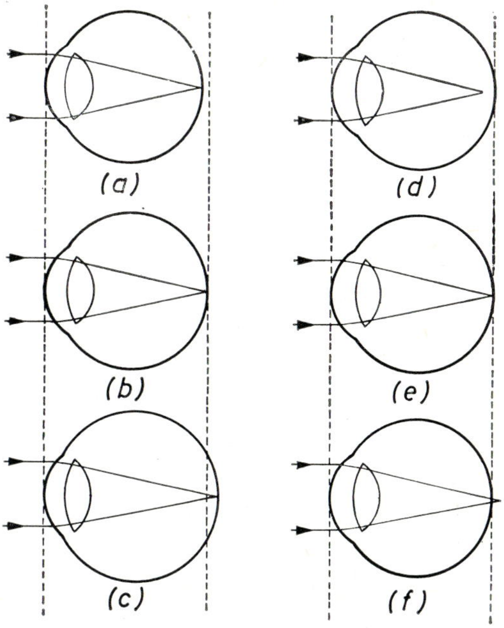


FIG. 31 (*below*).—Diagrammatic construction of the relationship between axial length and corneal power in (*a*) emmetropia and (*b*) ametropias up to 4·0D. (*After Sorsby, Benjamin, Davey, Sheridan and Tanner*, 1957.)

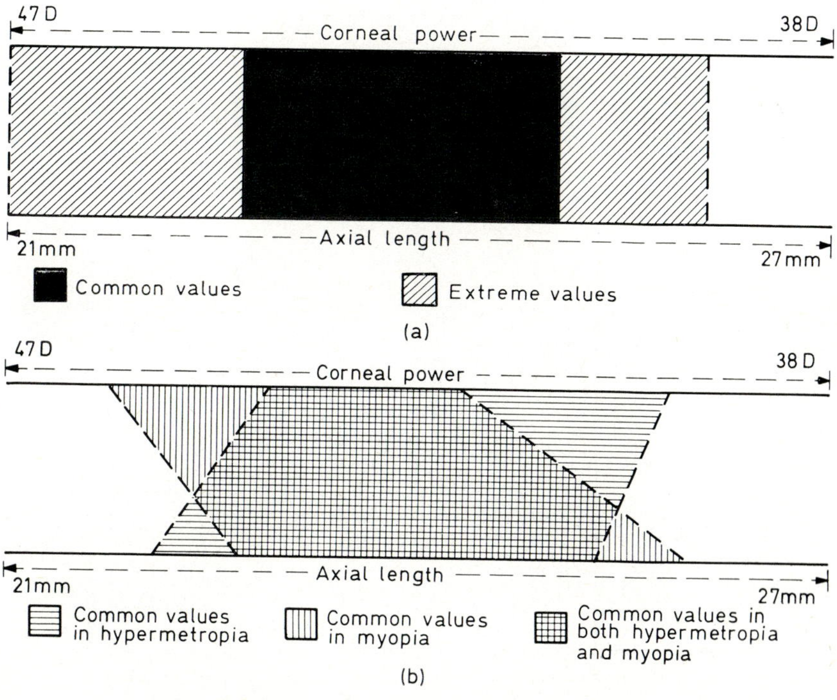

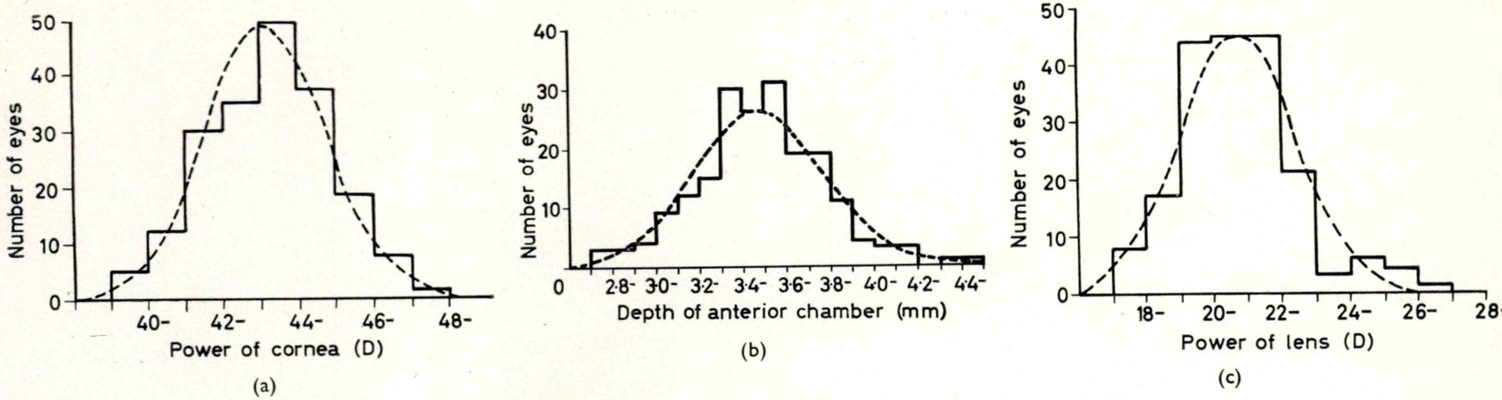

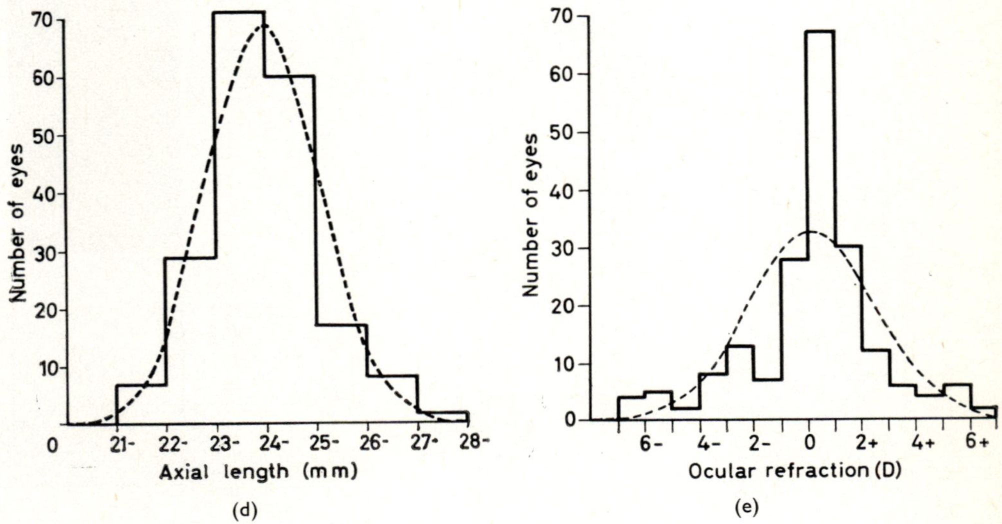


FIG. 32.—Curves of distribution of refraction and its components in 194 eyes: (*a*) ocular refraction (D); (*b*) power of cornea (D); (*c*) depth of anterior chamber (mm); (*d*) power of lens (D); and (*e*) axial length (mm). (*After Sorsby, Benjamin. Davey, Sheridan and Tanner*, 1957.)

## Studies on twins

*Isolated cases*

In the individual pairs of uniovular twins there are many reports on concordance as to unusual spherical errors or of astigmatism of a high degree or at unusual axes. Occasionally the concordance is of the mirror type or it extends only to the type of refraction (such as high myopia) without actual agreement as to the degree of error, and exceptionally such concordance is lacking altogether. These unusual findings only emphasize the high degree of concordance that is commonly seen. Thus in one uniovular pair, one of the twins showed −20·0 D and −1·50 D, whilst the other showed −1·50 D and −1·60 D, the mirror symmetry in this case extending to the presence of posterior staphylomatous changes in the two highly myopic eyes (Münch, 1922).

*Unselected series*

Since Jablonski's pioneer investigation in 1922 on unselected twin material—28 pairs of uniovular twins and 23 pairs of binovular twins—a number of such studies have been reported, which together give data on well over 200 uniovular pairs with adequate controls from binovular pairs of twins. Since most of the refractions in this material show modal values, considerable concordance is to be expected in the material as a whole, but marked concordance for uniovular twins was an outstanding finding. On the evidence of these data all refractive states—including myopia—are genetically determined.

*The components of refraction in an unselected series*

Utilizing the procedures they have elaborated for measuring the individual components of refraction, Sorsby and his associates studied 78 pairs of uniovular twins, 40 pairs of like-sexed binovular twins and 48 pairs of unselected control pairs. In the uniovular twins (with a distribution of refraction fairly similar to that in the general population) concordance by the fine criteria used was high: 70·6 per cent for refraction and 66·7 per cent and 70·5 per cent for the depth of the anterior chamber and the thickness of the lens respectively, 85·9 per cent and 53·8 per cent for the powers of the anterior and the posterior surfaces of the lens and 83·3 per cent for the axial length. Fairly similar values were obtained when the modal and non-modal refraction groups were considered separately, and hypermetropia and myopia showed essentially the same pattern as emmetropia. In no less than 16·7 per cent of the uniovular pairs there was concordance of all six components studied when all refraction groups were taken together, and much the same result was obtained when the different groups were considered separately (Fig. 33). By contrast, in the 40 pairs of binovular twins and the 48 unrelated control pairs there was only slight concordance for refraction and its components. When the control pairs did have identical refractions, similarity in the values of the components was lacking. Table II gives a statistical summary of this work.

## Family studies

*Selected families*

Apart from a study by Wold (1949) on myopic families there is a short series of 21 families selected because of an unusual refraction in either the parents or the offspring, and studied not only for refraction as a whole but also for the individual components.

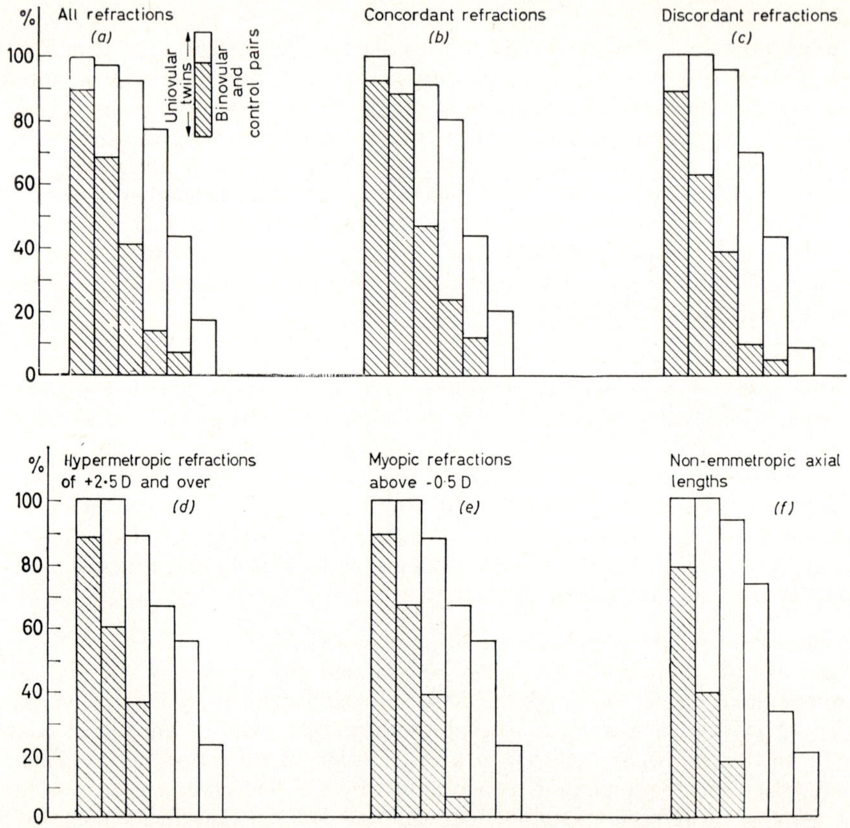


FIG. 33.—Similarity of the structure of the eye in uniovular twins. Components studied: corneal power, depth of anterior chamber and thickness of lens, radius of curvature of anterior and posterior surfaces of the lens, and axial length. In any two persons, it is likely that at least one of the six components of refraction will be similar (for example, in one pair the axial length will be concordant, in another the anterior surface of the lens), but when two or more components are considered—as in the second, third and subsequent columns of each of the diagrams—the incidence of concordance declines steeply. The control material (40 binovular pairs and 48 control pairs taken together) shows this clearly, but in the uniovular twins (78 pairs) the decline is very much less, for uniovular twins tend to have not only similar refractions, but similar individual components. This pattern applies to the whole range of refractions: (*a*) the controls show concordance in only a small percentage of cases when four or five components are considered; not a single pair shows concordance for all six components. In contrast, in uniovular twins, concordance is high for four components (almost 80 per cent), over 40 per cent for five components and nearly 20 per cent for all six components; (*b*) very much the same pattern persists. In the control material, though the pairs show identical refractions, they do not show any such similarity in components; (*c*) the only substantial difference is some decline in the incidence of concordance for all components in the uniovular series; (*d*) uniovular twins show a high degree of concordance; in the control material the incidence of concordance is low; (*e*) essentially the same findings as are seen with hypermetropia are observed; (*f*) the contrast between the high concordance for uniovular twins and the poor concordance for the control material is striking. (*After Sorsby, Sheridan and Leary*, 1962.)

TABLE II

COMPONENTS OF REFRACTION IN TWINS

**(a) Coefficients of Correlation in the Different Refraction Groups**

| *Refraction group (D)* | *No. within refraction group* | *Coefficient of correlation* | | | |
|---|---|---|---|---|---|
| | | *Power of cornea* | *Depth of anterior chamber* | *Power of lens* | *Axial length* |
| **Uniovular Pairs** | | | | | |
| *All* | 156 | 0·934 | 0·827 | 0·831 | 0·919 |
| + 4·01 and over | 13 | 0·858 | 0·917 | 0·911 | 0·755 |
| + 2·26 to + 4·00 | 6 | 0·931 | 0·890 | 0·976 | 0·619 |
| + 0·51 to + 2·25 | 61 | 0·921 | 0·749 | 0·761 | 0·902 |
| 0·00 to + 0·50 | 40 | 0·899 | 0·926 | 0·879 | 0·875 |
| − 0·01 to − 0·50 | 12 | 0·879 | 0·856 | 0·944 | 0·839 |
| − 0·51 to − 2·25 | 16 | 0·922 | 0·836 | 0·930 | 0·570** |
| − 2·26 to − 4·00 | 3[1] | | | | |
| − 4·01 and over | 5[1] | | | | |
| **Binovular Pairs** | | | | | |
| *All* | 80 | 0·591 | 0·452 | 0·507 | 0·482 |
| + 4·01 and over | 4[1] | | | | |
| + 2·26 to + 4·00 | 11 | 0·761 | 0·306 | 0·385 | 0·615 |
| + 0·51 to + 2·25 | 37 | 0·494 | 0·474 | 0·568 | 0·317 |
| 0·00 to + 0·50 | 17 | 0·659 | 0·471 | 0·398 | 0·344 |
| − 0·01 to − 0·50 | 4[1] | | | | |
| − 0·51 to − 2·25<br>− 2·26 to − 4·00 | 4 }<br>3 } | 0·755 | −0·290 | 0·647 | 0·203 |
| − 4·01 and over | 0 | | | | |
| **Control Pairs** | | | | | |
| *All* | 96 | 0·075 | 0·358** | 0·303** | 0·037 |
| + 4·01 and over | 8 | −0·051 | 0·550 | −0·401 | −0·420 |
| + 2·26 to + 4·00 | 11 | −0·311 | 0·212 | −0·034 | −0·501 |
| + 0·51 to + 2·25 | 32 | 0·050 | 0·431* | −0·182 | −0·148 |
| 0·00 to + 0·50 | 30 | 0·356 | 0·401* | 0·575** | 0·473** |
| − 0·01 to − 0·50 | 4[1] | | | | |
| − 0·51 to − 2·25 | 6 | 0·147 | −0·396 | 0·190 | 0·451 |
| − 2·26 to − 4·00 | 5[1] | | | | |
| − 4·01 and over | 0 | | | | |

**(b) Coefficients of Correlation for the Components of the Major Refraction Groups in the Three Series of Pairs**

| *Refraction group* | *No. within refraction group* | *Coefficient of correlation* | | | |
|---|---|---|---|---|---|
| | | *Power of cornea* | *Depth of anterior chamber* | *Power of lens* | *Axial length* |
| *All Refractions* | | | | | |
| Uniovular pairs | 156 | 0·934 | 0·827 | 0·831 | 0·919 |
| Binovular pairs | 80 | 0·591 | 0·452 | 0·507 | 0·482 |
| Control pairs | 96 | 0·075 | 0·358** | 0·303** | 0·037 |

*Notes:* Tests of significance were performed using Fisher's $z$ transformation. In the case of binovular twins difference from 0·5 is tested and in the case of controls the difference from zero. In the case of uniovular twins each sub-group is tested to determine whether the correlation coefficient is lower than in the group as a whole.

One asterisk denotes significance at 5% level of probability, two at 1% level.

[1] Coefficients not calculated for groups of less than six.

**Table II b (continued)**

| *Refraction group* | *No. within refraction group* | *Coefficient of correlation* | | | |
|---|---|---|---|---|---|
| | | *Power of cornea* | *Depth of anterior chamber* | *Power of lens* | *Axial length* |
| *Emmetropes* (0·0 to 0·50 D) | | | | | |
| Uniovular pairs | 40 | 0·899 | 0·926 | 0·879 | 0·875 |
| Binovular pairs | 17 | 0·659 | 0·471 | 0·398 | 0·344 |
| Control pairs | 30 | 0·356 | 0·401* | 0·575** | 0·473** |
| *Low Hypermetropes* (0·51 to 2·25 D) | | | | | |
| Uniovular pairs | 61 | 0·921 | 0·749 | 0·761 | 0·902 |
| Binovular pairs | 37 | 0·494 | 0·474 | 0·568 | 0·317 |
| Control pairs | 32 | 0·050 | 0·431* | −0·182 | −0·148 |
| *High Hypermetropes* (2·26 D and over) | | | | | |
| Uniovular pairs | 19 | 0·882 | 0·892 | 0·925 | 0·735* |
| Binovular pairs | 15 | 0·759 | 0·317 | 0·351 | 0·607 |
| Control pairs | 19 | −0·126 | 0·346 | −0·263 | −0·511* |
| *All Myopes* over −0·51 D | | | | | |
| Uniovular pairs | 24 | 0·926 | 0·947 | 0·843 | 0·735** |
| Binovular pairs | 7 | 0·755 | −0·290 | 0·647 | 0·203 |
| Control pairs | 11 | −0·235 | −0·265 | 0·305 | −0·127 |

*Notes:* Tests of significance were performed using Fisher's *z* transformation. In the case of binovular twins difference from 0·5 is tested and in the case of controls the difference from zero. In the case of uniovular twins each sub-group is tested to determine whether the correlation coefficient is lower than in the group as a whole.
One asterisk denotes significance at 5% level of probability, two at 1% level.
[1] Coefficients not calculated for groups of less than six.

### (c) Coefficients of Correlation in Some Specific Groups

| *Groups* | | *No. of pairs* (one or both of which fall within group) | *No. of subjects* | *Coefficient of correlation* | | | |
|---|---|---|---|---|---|---|---|
| | | | | *Cornea* | *Depth of anterior chamber* | *Lens* | *Axial length* |
| Non-modal refractions[2] | U | 23 | 41 | 0·886 | 0·878 | 0·853 | 0·935 |
| | B | 19 | 24 | 0·675 | 0·237 | 0·473 | 0·239 |
| | C | 23 | 28 | −0·049 | 0·278 | −0·186 | −0·315 |
| Eyes with axial length outside the emmetropic range[3] | U | 12 | 20 | 0·886 | 0·928 | 0·862 | 0·970 |
| | B | 8 | 9 | 0·787 | 0·054 | 0·570 | 0·167 |
| | C | 14 | 15 | 0·616 | 0·442 | −0·236 | −0·146 |
| Discordant refractions[4] | U | 23 | 46 | 0·880 | 0·890 | 0·898 | 0·793** |
| | B | 28 | 56 | 0·533 | 0·463 | 0·404 | 0·405 |
| | C | 34 | 68 | −0·042 | 0·169 | 0·091 | −0·225 |

[2] Spherical errors of ± 2·25 D or more, or cylindrical errors of more than ± 1·25 D.
[3] Taken here as 22·5 to 25·9 mm.
[4] Refractions differing by ± 0·5 D in the pair of twins (or controls).

(*After Sorsby and Fraser*, 1964.) U = Uniovular; B = Binovular: C = Control.

Table IIIa shows that there was a high degree of correlation between the parents and children for refraction and all components except axial length. These results leave open the significance of heredity in unusual axial lengths.

*Unselected families*

Twenty-eight unselected families with a total of 106 subjects were studied for ocular refraction and its components. In contrast to the expected lack of correlation between the parents there was a substantial degree of correlation for parent/offspring and for mid-parent/offspring coefficients. Table IIIb sets out the findings statistically.

Although the coefficients fall short of the values of 0·50 and 0·71 expected under the hypothesis of additive effects on a number of genes without dominance, they are none the less substantial. Further elucidation from larger studies is needed.

TABLE III

FAMILY STUDIES ON THE COMPONENTS OF REFRACTION

**(a) Coefficients of Correlation for Refraction and its Components in 21 Families with Unusual Refraction in either the Parents or the Offspring**

| | *Father/mother 21 pairs* | *Parent/child 56* | *Mid-parent/ offspring 28* | *Sib/sib 7* |
|---|---|---|---|---|
| Refraction | 0·339 | 0·285 | 0·342 | −0·104 |
| Axial length | 0·321 | 0·062 | 0·076 | −0·122 |
| Corneal power | −0·039 | 0·271 | 0·401 | −0·289 |
| Lens power | −0·099 | 0·416 | 0·580 | 0·349 |
| Anterior chamber | 0·111 | 0·323 | 0·412 | 0·615 |

**(b) Coefficients of Correlation for Refraction and its Components in 28 Unselected Families**

| | *Father/mother 28 pairs* | *Parent/child 100* | *Mid-parent/ offspring 50* | *Sib/sib 24/22* |
|---|---|---|---|---|
| Refraction | −0·119 | 0·227 | 0·348 | 0·358 |
| Axial length | 0·108 | 0·314 | 0·434 | 0·492 |
| Corneal power | 0·138 | 0·378 | 0·542 | 0·093 |
| Lens power | −0·288 | 0·155 | 0·278 | 0·553 |
| Anterior chamber depth | −0·098 | 0·265 | 0·388 | 0·019 |

(*After Sorsby, Leary and Fraser*, 1966.)

## Some clinical considerations

Clinically both myopia and hypermetropia are seen in mild, moderate or marked degrees. These are indefinite and arbitrary divisions in a continuous range, but the classification has some justification in so far as the higher degrees of refractive error tend to carry characteristic complications. Most clinicians would regard myopia up to 4 D as of the low variety in which fundus complications are unlikely; between 4 and 6 D as medium myopia in which fundus lesions may occur; whilst myopia over 6 D would qualify for high myopia in which the tendency to chorio-retinal atrophy, macular haemorrhages or retinal detachment increases with increase in refraction. In hypermetropia, errors of refraction under 3 D are usually of little significance apart from the optical aspect, whilst errors between 3 and 6 D may not correct fully, and errors over 6 D tend to be seen in eyes that verge on mild microphthalmos.

The associated defects seen with the refractive errors also present considerable difficulties. The following schematic classification is of some value in that it emphasizes the sketchy state of our knowledge on the heredity of the common clinical types of refractive error.

*Hypermetropia*

*Uncomplicated hypermetropia.*—There are many pedigrees illustrative of recessive or of dominant inheritance of hypermetropia in its different degrees—low, medium or high (Fig. 34). The refractive errors seen in any particular family do

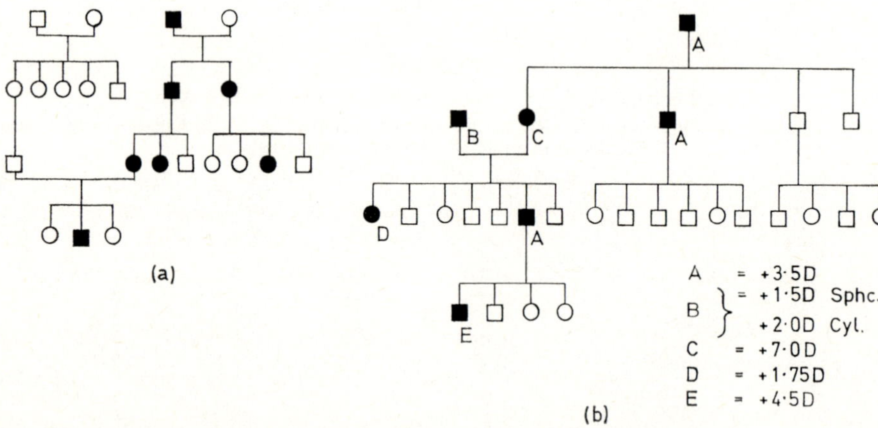


FIG. 34.—Hypermetropia. Pedigrees illustrative of dominant inheritance.
(*a*) Inheritance of low degrees of hypermetropia. (*After Jablonski*, 1924.)
(*b*) Variable degrees of hypermetropia within the same family. (*After Waardenburg*, 1932.)

not necessarily fall within the same clinical group, and the relative frequency of the different modes of inheritance is not known.

*Hypermetropia with squint.*—Fig. 35 records a dominant pedigree, but polygenic rather than simple dominant inheritance is the likely mode of transmission. This is discussed on p. 58. It is also likely that in such families the hypermetropia is merely a precipitating factor.

*Hypermetropia with glaucoma.*—The association of moderate and high hypermetropia with glaucoma is well established. The genetic aspects are obscure; they are likely to be similar to those suggested for squint.

*Hypermetropia with partial amblyopia.*—Most of the pedigrees of high hypermetropia with partial amblyopia appear to be recessive, but as these cases border on to microphthalmos with its dominant inheritance the exact status is not clear.

*Myopia*

*Uncomplicated myopia.*—As with hypermetropia there are many pedigrees showing either dominant or recessive inheritance, and different pedigrees show either very much the same degree of myopia or a considerable range of myopic errors (Fig. 36). Wold has emphasized the frequency of recessive inheritance.

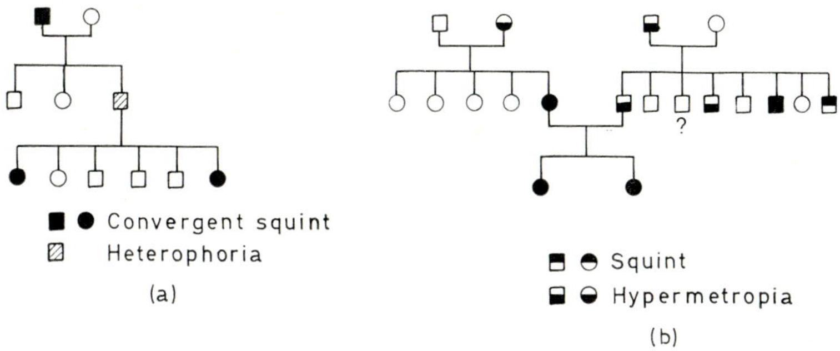


FIG. 35.—Convergent squint.
(*a*) Dominant inheritance in a family showing heterophoria as an incomplete form of squint. (*After Waardenburg*, 1948.)
(*b*) A pedigree showing the dominant inheritance of squint and hypermetropia independently. (*After Waardenburg*, 1932.)

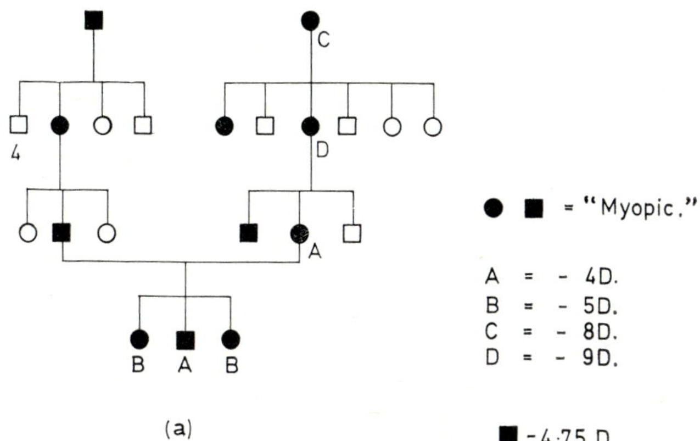


FIG. 36.—Myopia. Pedigree suggestive of dominant inheritance.
(*a*) Pedigree showing some range in the degree of myopia. (*After Jablonski*, 1922.)
(*b*) Pedigree showing a fair consistency in the degree of myopia. (*After Wolfflin*, 1949.)

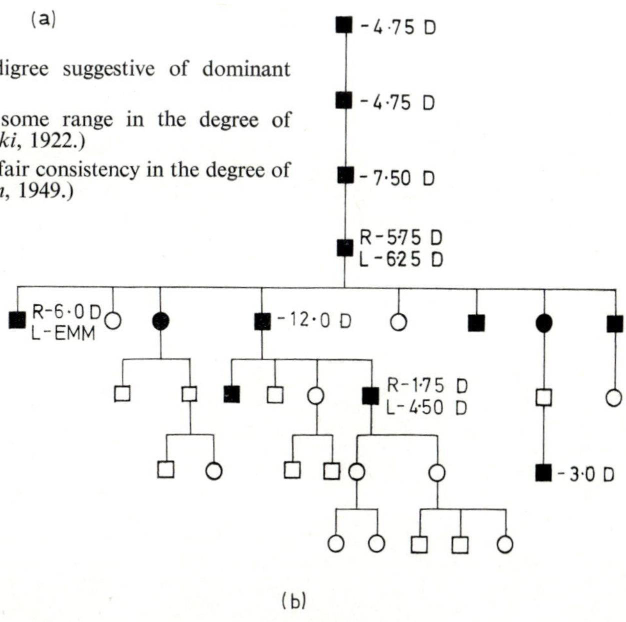

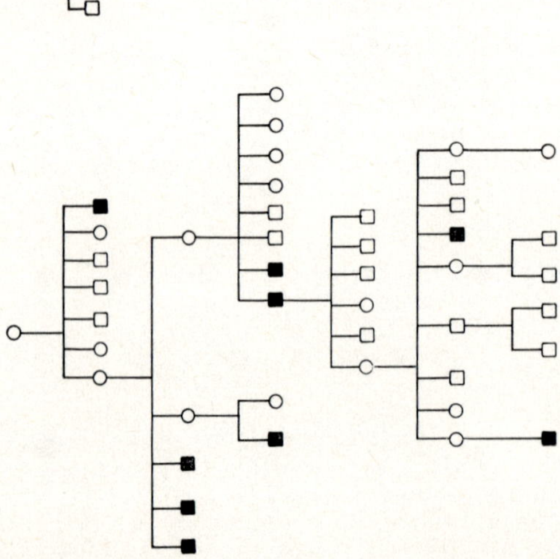

(a)

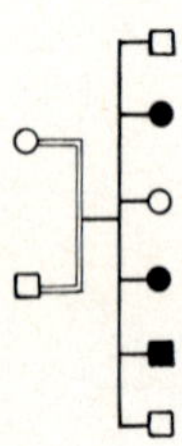

(c)

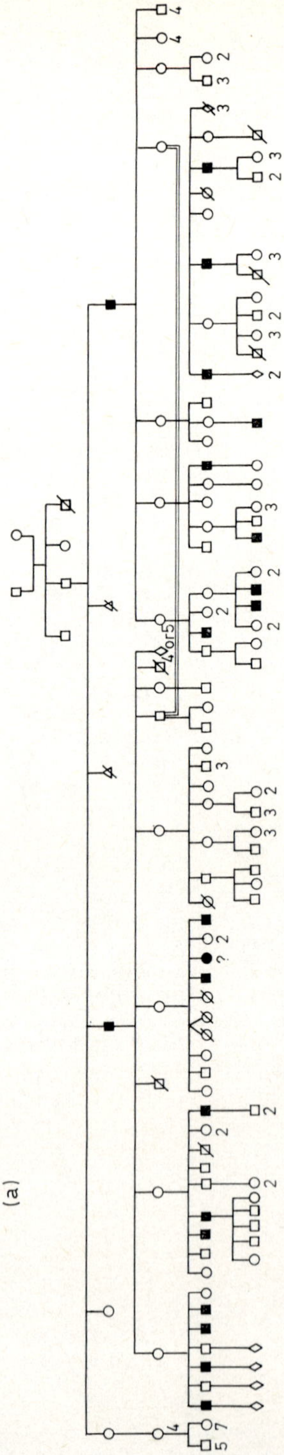

(b)

FIG. 37.—Night-blindness with myopia.

(*a*) Recessive sex-linkage. (*After Kleiner*, 1923.)
(*b*) Recessive sex-linkage. (*After Nettleship*, 1912.)
(*c*) Autosomal recessive inheritance. Extract from an extensive pedigree. (*After Gassler*, 1925.)

*Myopia with night-blindness.*—There are two clearly established genetic types with ill-defined, if any, clinical differences:

(1) Sex-linked recessive inheritance. Fig. 37 *a* shows the well-known Pflüger–Amman–Kleiner pedigree. A characteristic in this pedigree—as in some pedigrees recorded by Nettleship (Fig. 37 *b*)—was the degree of myopia which ranged between 6 and 11 D. Astigmatism, and also some degree of visual defect, was not uncommon. (It is not unlikely that the pedigree of apparently uncomplicated sex-linked recessive inheritance of myopia recorded by Worth (1906) falls into this group.)

(2) Autosomal recessive inheritance. In the large family recorded in Fig. 37 *c* the myopia varied between 9 and 16 D and corrected vision between 6/60 and 6/18.

*Congenital and childhood forms of myopia.*—Congenital myopia appears to be not uncommon in markedly premature infants and possibly represents the persistence of a normal foetal condition. Whether there is also a genetically determined congenital or infantile myopia is not known. It is certain, however, that some forms of myopia seen in young children are due to environmental causes: the interstitial keratitis of congenital syphilis often leads to myopia and it is likely that measles keratitis seen in the past also did so. The common type of myopia seen in children is the uncomplicated low myopia which develops towards puberty (the so-called school myopia).

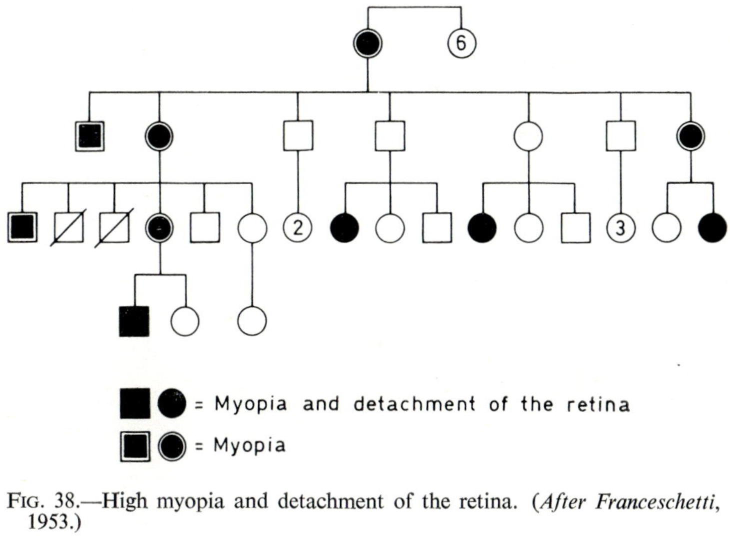


FIG. 38.—High myopia and detachment of the retina. (*After Franceschetti*, 1953.)

*Myopia with late complications.*—The complications of myopia generally come on many years after any increase in myopia has ceased. Mechanical explanations such as "stretching of the choroid" can hardly apply. To what extent the different types of complications represent genetic entities is not known. The most definite group is medium myopia with retinal detachment: a number of pedigrees suggest that bilateral retinal detachment at various periods in life has a familiar distribution—probably dominantly inherited as recorded in Fig. 38.

There are no adequate studies on a possible genetic background for the chorio-retinal atrophy and for the macular haemorrhages seen in middle life in some cases of medium and high myopia, nor on the lens opacities and actual cataract not uncommonly seen in middle-aged high myopes.

*Myopia with congenital anomalies.*—Myopia often of a high degree is not uncommon in eyes with congenital anomalies. Sometimes the congenital defect is well-defined—such as microphthalmos (*see* Fig. 9), microphakia (*see* Fig. 97), microcornea and external ophthalmoplegia (*see* Fig. 47). In some families no structural anomaly can be seen, but severe nystagmus is present (Fig. 39). In others, the structural defect, though severe, is not readily classified and may perhaps fall into the cleavage anomaly. A peculiar association—not always seen—is the high myopia in the affected eye in unilateral extensive opaque nerve fibres.

In this highly complex group of disorders dominant, recessive and sex-linked modes of inheritance have been met, but in many instances no genetic background can be established.

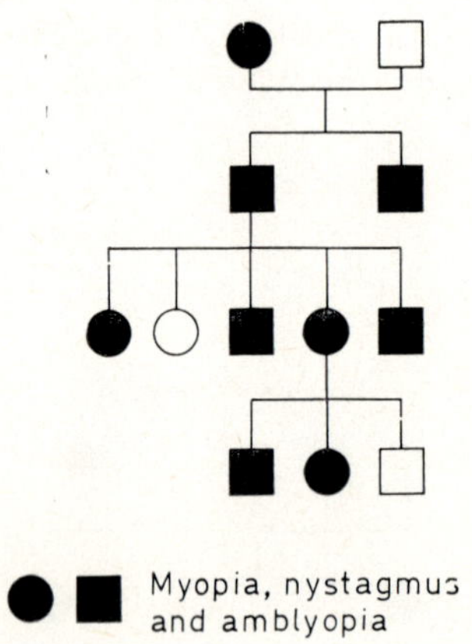


FIG. 39 (*left*).—Association of myopia, nystagmus, and amblyopia. (*After Vogt*, 1924.)

FIG. 40 (*below*).—Anisometropia. Pedigrees. (*a*) Pedigree suggestive of dominant inheritance. (*After Blatt*, 1924.) (*b*) Pedigree suggestive of recessive inheritance. (*Personal observation.*)

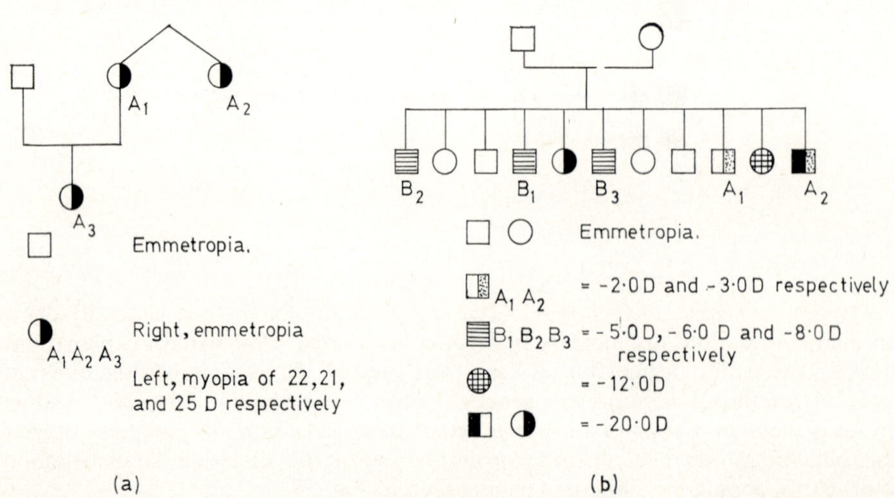

*Myopia in abiotrophic chorio-retinal disorders.*—It is likely that low degrees of myopia are unduly frequent in retinitis pigmentosa with its many different modes of inheritance. A rather more definite association is seen in choroideraemia—a sex-linked disorder. Gyrate atrophy, generally regarded as a recessive disorder, is said to be associated with high myopia.

*Myopia in systemic disorders.*—Systemic disorders such as mongolism, albinism and arachnodactyly are said to have a high incidence of myopia. Critical data are not available.

### *Anisometropia*

Usually the differences in the powers of the cornea and lens between the two eyes in anisometropia are slight, and though some of the milder cases of anisometropia are determined by such differences, most cases are the consequence of unequal axial lengths. Axial anisometropia is generally sporadic but there are pedigrees showing transmission over two generations (Fig. 40 *a*); recessive inheritance is suggested by the pedigree shown in Fig. 40 *b*.

### *Astigmatism*

This is discussed elsewhere as an aspect of abortive keratoconus (p. 73).

## FOR FURTHER READING

Sorsby, A., Benjamin, B., Davey, J. B., Sheridan, M. and Tanner, J. M. (1957). *Emmetropia and Its Aberrations.* Medical Research Council Special Reports Series, No. 293. London; H.M. Stationery Office.

— — and Sheridan, M. (1961). *Refraction and Its Components During the Growth of the Eye from the age of Three.* Medical Research Council Special Reports Series, No. 301. London; H.M. Stationery Office.

— Sheridan, M. and Leary, G.A. (1962). *Refraction and its Components in Twins.* Medical Research Council Special Reports Series, No. 303. London; H.M. Stationery Office.

— and Leary, G. A. (1969). *A Longitudinal Study of Refraction and its Components During Growth.* Medical Research Council Reports Series. London; H.M. Stationery Office. In the Press.

Steiger, A. (1913). *Die Enstehung der sphärischen Refraktionen des menschlichen Auges.* Berlin; Karger.

Stenström, S. (1946). "Untersuchungen ueber die Variation und Kovariation der optischen Elemente des menschlichen Auges." *Acta ophthal. Kbh.*, Suppl. XXVI (also English translation by D. Woolf (1948). *Am. J. Optom.*, **25,** 218, and reprinted as monograph 58).

Tron, E. J. (1948). "The Optical Elements of the Refractive Power of the Eye". In *Modern Trends in Ophthalmology*, Ed. by F. Ridley and A. Sorsby, Vol. 1, p. 245. London; Butterworths.

Weekers, R., Watillon, M. and Thomas-Decortis, G. (1961). *Arch. d'Ophtal. (Paris)* (N. S.), **21,** 217.

# CHAPTER 5

## MOTOR ANOMALIES

### PTOSIS

**The congenital varieties of ptosis**

*Simple ptosis*

Simple uncomplicated blepharoptosis is one of the more common congenital defects. It is usually unilateral and it may be so mild as to be barely noticeable or so severe that the pupil is covered by the drooping lid. In about 25 per cent of all cases the affection is bilateral; and in these, more commonly than in unilateral cases, varying degrees of defective action of the superior trectus may be present.

The lesion in both the levator and the superior rectus is essentially that of atrophy. In some cases this atrophy results from a nuclear or supranuclear congenital anomaly, but more commonly it is the consequence of a muscle dystrophy originating in the embryonic mass from which the two muscles are developed. Cases showing the full clinical picture of bilateral ptosis with deficient elevation of the globe are exceptional; in most instances there are varying degrees of partial manifestation.

The affection is dominant and, as can be seen from Fig. 41, both unilateral and bilateral cases occur within the same family and that manifestation can be even completely suppressed. Penetrance has been estimated at 60 per cent (Franceschetti, Klein and Guttman, 1950). Pedigrees recording the occurrences of exclusively unilateral cases may be merely examples of chance occurrences in an affection with low penetrance.

*Ptosis with epicanthus and other lid anomalies*

This is a well defined type. Inheritance is dominant. The pedigrees in Fig. 42 *a* and *b* are typical of many similar records. In some families, the epicanthus is slight, being of the *epicanthus inversus* type. In others the anomalies are more extensive: there are present a widened root of the nose, outward displacement of the inner epicanthi with elongation of the canaliculi and displacement of the puncta towards the cornea; in consequence of these changes there is diminution of the palpebral fissure—one of the varieties of blepharophimosis. Waardenburg regards these appearances as due to persistence of the normal embryonic state as at the beginning of the third month, and it is likely that many of these cases are part of the wider Klein–Waardenburg syndrome (*see* p. 206) with its dominant inheritance.

*Ptosis with external ophthalmoplegia*

Congenital external ophthalmoplegia, whether total or partial, is always accompanied by ptosis. As the ophthalmoplegia is the more significant defect this group is best considered with the palsies of the extra-ocular muscles. Some 10 per cent of all ptosis cases show these palsies; and these, in contrast to the ptosis, are frequently unilateral.

*Ptosis with jaw-winking (Marcus Gunn phenomenon)*

Jaw-winking, the most common of the congenital synkinetic anomalies, is typically unilateral and associated with ptosis. The ptosis is present at birth and

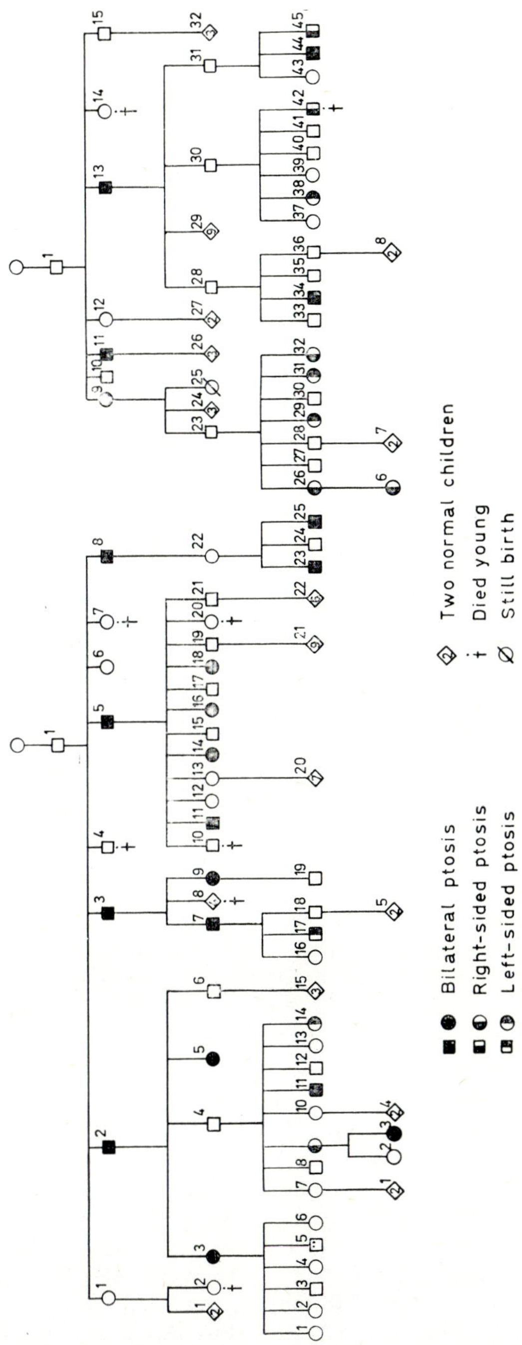


FIG. 41.—Simple ptosis. Pedigree showing variable expression and penetrance. (*After Guttman*, 1948–50.)

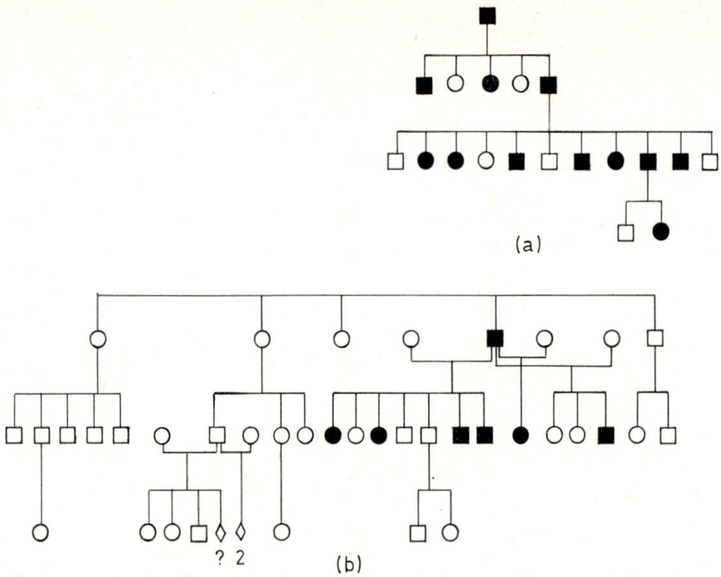


FIG. 42.—Ptosis with epicanthus. Pedigrees showing dominant inheritance.

(*a*) Pedigree showing direct transmission over four generations. (*After McIlroy*, 1930.)

(*b*) Pedigree showing transmission by an affected man to his children by three marriages. (*After Usher*, 1935.)

is clearly not paretic for the drooped lid shoots up each time the jaws are opened on sucking. It is believed that the ptosis is central in origin and the jaw-winking is determined by the existence of connecting fibres between the nucleus of the levator muscle and that of the motor branch of the trigeminal nerve.

Fig. 43 is typical of the dominant character of most of the hereditary cases reported. Irregular dominance has been recorded.

*Ptosis as part of widespread systemic defects*

Ptosis is an incidental and inconstant finding in many hereditary syndromes. In the context of the general disorder it is relatively insignificant.

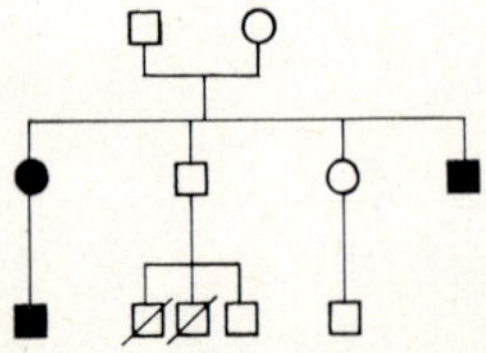

FIG. 43.—Marcus Gunn syndrome. Inheritance over two generations. (*After Falls, Kruse* and *Cotterman*, 1949.)

**The late developing varieties**

Ptosis arising late in post-natal life may be genetically determined and run a progressive course. The available pedigrees of this late developing—or abiotrophic—type of ptosis suggest a dominant inheritance (Fig. 44). The older observers tended to regard these disturbances as nuclear in origin, but it is more likely that

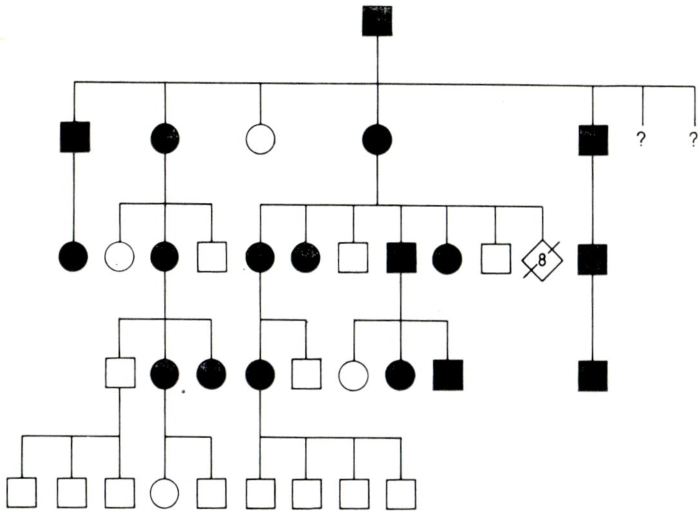


FIG. 44.—Delayed hereditary ptosis. In the fifth generation, the subjects are still too young to show signs of the disease. (*After Cameron*, 1950.)

hereditary ptosis and the allied oculo-pharyngeal dystrophy discussed elsewhere (*see* p. 248) are primary myopathies.

## OPHTHALMOPLEGIA

**The congenital varieties**

It is likely that most of the different varieties of ophthalmoplegia are myopathic rather than neurogenic in origin (Kiloh and Nevin, 1951). The pathology and genetics of this complex group are both obscure.

*Total ophthalmoplegia*

In none of the few families on record was the ophthalmoplegia quite total, although there was obvious involvement of the third, fourth and sixth cranial nerves. Fig. 45 is typical of the recessive inheritance seen in such families; this particular pedigree is of further interest in bringing out the possible relationship of this disorder to more widespread muscle anomalies.

*Internal ophthalmoplegia*

This is rare. The two families on record raise the possibility of sex-linked inheritance (Sédan and Roux, 1933; Handmann, 1943).

FIG. 45.—Total ophthalmoplegia with ptosis and miosis. (*After Waardenburg*, 1963.)

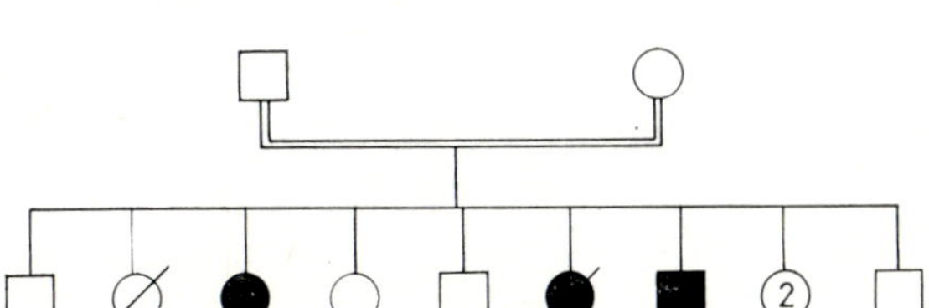

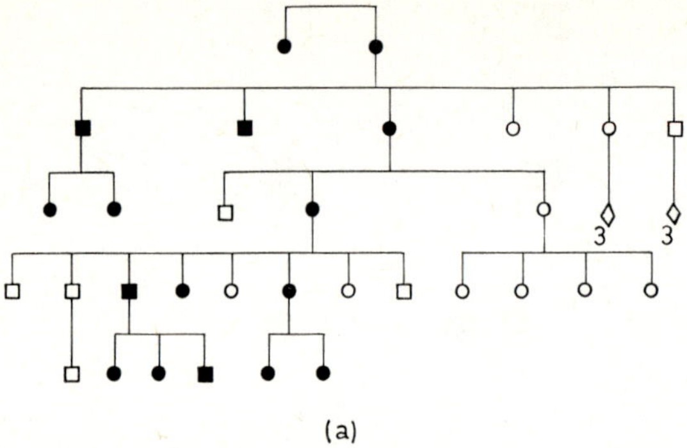


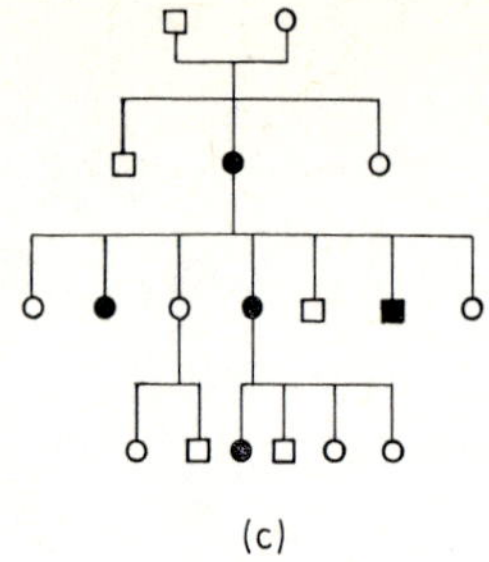


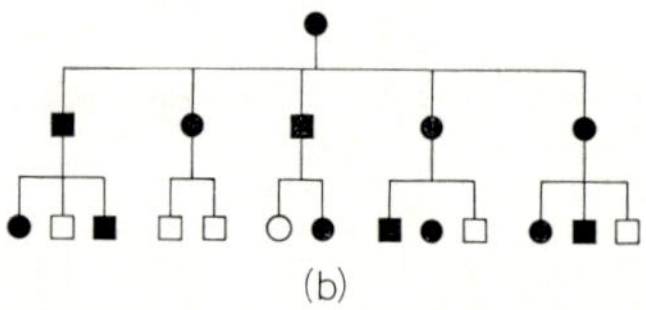


FIG. 46.—External ophthalmoplegia. (*a*) Pedigree showing dominant inheritance in a family in which the affection was present at birth. Ptosis was marked. (*After Bradburne*, 1912.) (*b*) Pedigree showing dominant ophthalmoplegia externa with considerable variability. (*After Jonkers*, 1950.) (*c*) Pedigree showing dominant inheritance in a family in which ptosis and nystagmus were marked additional features. (*After Crouzon and Béhague*, 1920.)

*External ophthalmoplegia*

This is generally incomplete for usually there is some action in one or more of the muscles, although the levator palpebrae is not often spared. Whilst a familial stamp is the rule, there may be considerable variation in expression within a given family not only as to the extent of the palsy but even to the possibility of a post-natal onset in some cases. Fig. 46 is typical of the dominant inheritance reported. Sex-linked inheritance is shown in the unique pedigree recorded in Fig. 47; here pupil anomalies and myopia, and also various neurological stigmata, were present in the affected males, whilst the carrier women showed absence of the knee and ankle jerks.

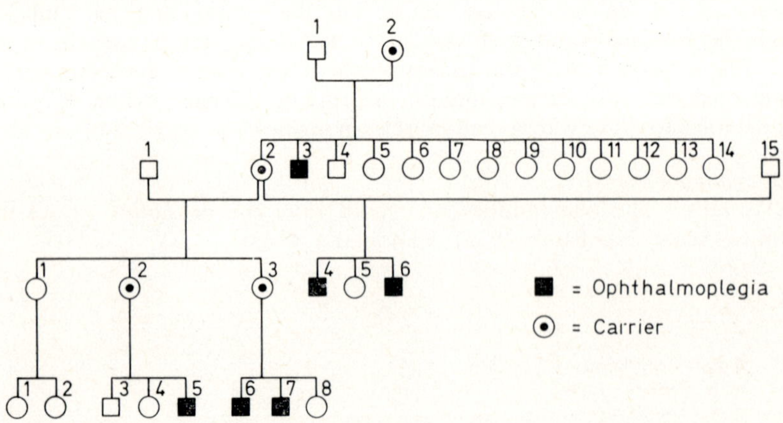


FIG. 47.—Sex-linked form of ophthalmoplegia externa with myopia, dyscoria or anisocoria, and lack of the lower tendon reflexes. (*After Salleras and Ortiz de Zárate*, 1950.)

External ophthalmoplegia has been distinguished from the *general fibrosis syndrome* of Brown, which typically gives bilateral ptosis, with the eyes fixed in a downward gaze and the head tilted backwards. The affection, due to fibrosis of all extra-ocular muscles and adhesions between the capsule of Tenon and the globe grossly limiting movement, has been recorded over four generations (Laughlin, 1956). It is not clear that it is an independent entity.

*Supranuclear disorders of the eye muscles*

Congenital disorders of lateral gaze movements and persistence of Bell's phenomenon, in addition to various palsies, have been noted in several families in whom inheritance was probably recessive (Stadlin and Klein, 1948).

*Paresis of the external rectus*

The affection is bilateral in 25 per cent of cases; in unilateral cases the left side is much more often affected than the right. Dominant inheritance is shown by Fig. 48 and many similar records. Nuclear aplasia has been established in some cases, but a myogenic defect is possible in others.

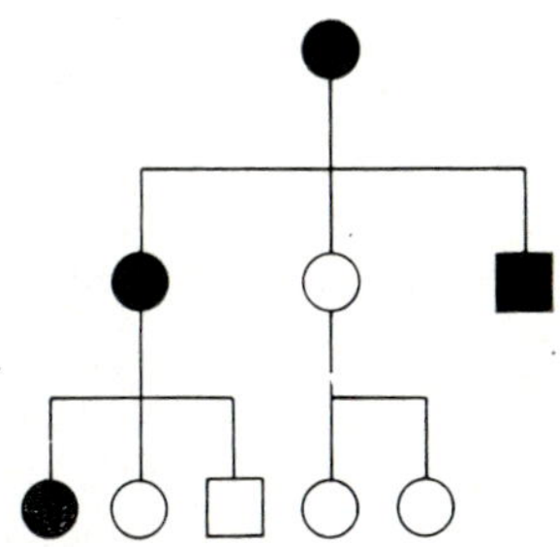

FIG. 48.—Congenital unilateral paralysis of the external rectus muscle. (*After François*, 1961.)

*Duane's phenomenon* (*Rectractio bulbi syndrome*)

This is frequently an association of congenital paresis of the external rectus. Laughlin (1937) has recorded the occurrence of the syndrome in some members of a family in which others showed the muscular palsy only. In this syndrome both concordance and discordance have been observed in univular twins. Out of a total of 277 cases culled from the literature, Danis (1948) found a family history in 32 cases concentrated in 12 families with dominant inheritance. In a personal series François found 15 out of his 22 cases concentrated in 3 families and as can be seen from Fig. 49 penetrance was not always complete and abortive cases were not uncommon. The status of the more common apparently sporadic cases still needs elucidation.

**The late developing varieties**

*Uncomplicated ophthalmoplegia*

The age of onset in this dominant affection varies with different families. The affection generally sets in in childhood but occasionally not until middle-age; and though remissions may occur, the affection is progressive and frequently the course is of unequal severity in the two eyes, but ultimately there is complete immobility of the two globes. An associated ptosis is not uncommon, whilst facial palsy and paralysis of accommodation have been observed. Originally regarded as nuclear in origin, it is now clear that the disorder is a muscle dystrophy of the myasthenia gravis type, as evidenced by the histological appearances and the

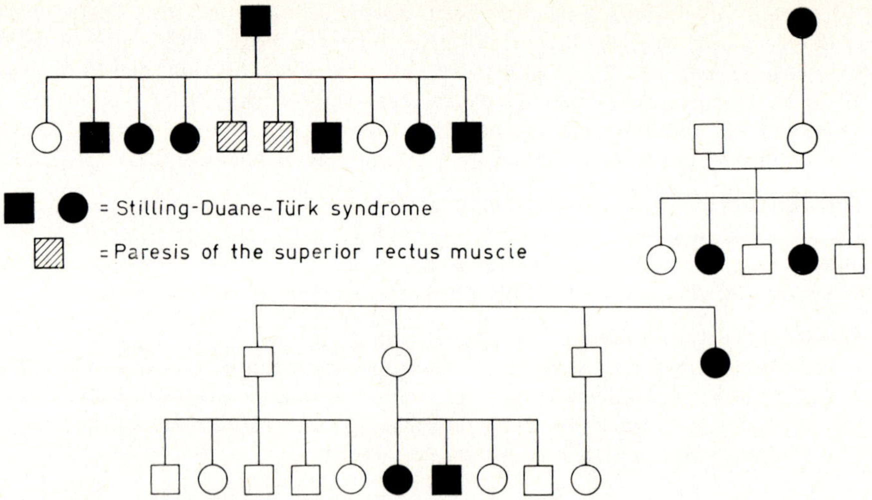


FIG. 49.—Duane's phenomenon. Pedigrees showing variable expression and penetrance. (*After François*, 1961.)

response to prostigmine. Fig. 50 is typical of many similar pedigrees. The purely ocular variety may constitute as much as 20 per cent of all cases of this affection.

*Ophthalmoplegia with retinal dystrophy*

A number of familial cases of an ill-defined retinal dystrophy associated with variable degrees of external ophthalmoplegia are available. They do not give a very consistent picture as to the mode of inheritance or the retinal lesion. Some of

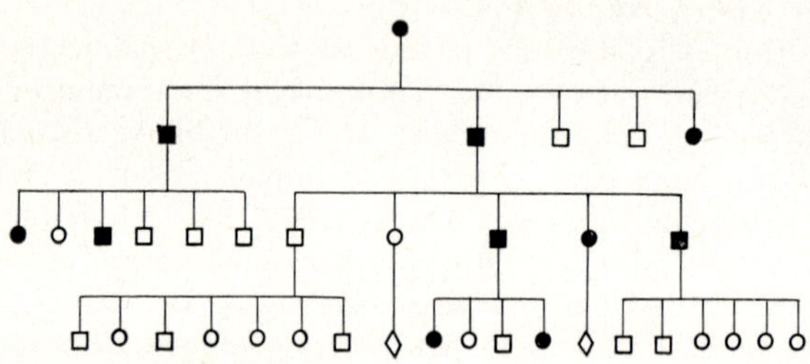

FIG. 50.—External ophthalmoplegia. Pedigree showing dominant inheritance in a family in which the affection appeared in adult life. Here ptosis was marked. (*After Beaumont*, 1900.)

these cases are not myogenic in origin as shown by the lack of response to prostigmine and by the fact that electromyography showed an intact nerve supply to the lateral muscles (Thorson and Bell, 1959; Davidson, 1960). It is possible that fuller investigation may link some of these cases with the hereditary ataxias and possibly also Refsum's disease.

## CONCOMITANT SQUINT

### Convergent squint

Secondary factors are presumably responsible for the occasional cases of convergent concomitant squint in children with a congenital structural anomaly in one or both eyes, or with such acquired lesions as a corneal opacity following ophthalmia neonatorum. In the bulk of cases, however, the eyes are structurally normal, except that undue degrees of hypermetropia are probably more common in squinting children than in the general child population. These cases are all genetically determined, even if environmental factors—such as debility after illness—may precipitate the squint.

The older literature contains a mass of statistics recording a high incidence of squint in the families of affected children. The incidence in different collections varies considerably, reaching over 50 per cent in some reports. More conclusive evidence than these figures and the mass of pedigrees on isolated families has come from studies on twins and unselected families.

*Twin material*

In collected material from the literature giving a total of 69 pairs of uniocular twins and 51 pairs of biocular twins, Waardenburg found concordance of 81·2 per cent and 8·9 per cent respectively. The contrast is less marked, however, in the four available unselected series recorded in Table IV.

TABLE IV

CONCORDANCE FOR CONCOMITANT CONVERGENT SQUINT IN UNSELECTED SERIES

| | *Uniocular twins* | | *Binocular twins* | |
|---|---|---|---|---|
| | *Concordant* | *Discordant* | *Concordant* | *Discordant* |
| Waardenburg | 11 | — | 4 | 13 |
| Weekers *et al.* | 3 | 4 | 6 | 2 |
| François | 2 | 4 | — | — |
| Richter | 11 | 1 | 7 | 20 |
| Total | 27 | 9 | 17 | 35 |

The low incidence of concordance in uniocular twins recorded by Weekers (and supported by the small series by François) is taken by Weekers as signifying that is is not the squint itself which is hereditary but the high hypermetropia which was present and showed marked concordance. This view is hardly valid, seeing that high hypermetropia is present only in a minority of cases of squint; furthermore the low concordance in his series is apparently exceptional.

*Pedigree material*

Czelliter, in a pioneer study in 1923, held that squint was inherited in a recessive manner. In his material (306 families with squint), there were 15 per cent affected and there was a high incidence of consanguinity (6 per cent). His rejection of dominant inheritance, however, is no longer accepted. What is true is that in families with the affection transmitted over two or more generations there is in fact a marked deficiency of cases, and this has been explained in general terms as due to incomplete penetrance. A more regular pattern of dominant transmission is obtained if cases of esophoria are regarded as incomplete forms of congenital squint; Fig. 35 *a* is illustrative but, even so, the theoretical values expected are not reached.

*Squint as a dominant polygenic affection.*—The significance of high hypermetropia in the genesis of squint would appear to be substantial in individual cases favourably influenced by a suitable correction, but in collected material its role is not outstanding, for it is far from constant and in squint families it may be inherited independently from the strabismus (Fig. 35 *b*).

Classically, amblyopia has been regarded as the consequence and not a causative factor in squint. The growing tendency to regard squint as primarily the result of faulty binocular vision, of which unilateral amblyopia is an extreme expression, helps to understand the mode of inheritance of squint, for the postulate that a number of factors have to be effective to produce a manifest squint would explain the irregularities in dominant transmission.

From a study on 697 children with squint, and 3,123 of their relatives, Susanne Richter (1967) concluded that squint is inherited in a polygenic manner; for squint to become manifest two independent dominant genes need to be expressed—one determining esophoria (motor anomaly) and the other an anomaly of binocular vision (sensory anomaly) ranging in severity from anomalous retinal correspondence to marked amblyopia. Both sensory anomalies and refraction anomalies can be present in families without manifest squint (Fig. 51) and different degrees

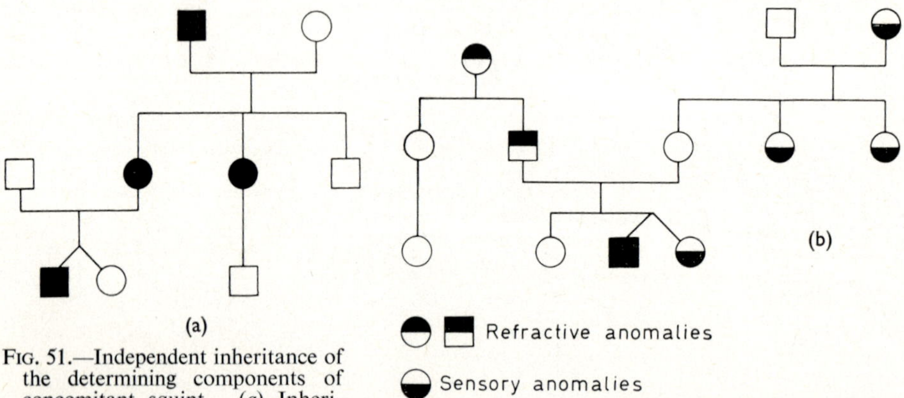


FIG. 51.—Independent inheritance of the determining components of concomitant squint. (*a*) Inheritance of sensory anomaly. (*b*) Inheritance of both sensory and refractive anomalies. (*After Richter*, 1967.)

of either of these anomalies and of heterophoria may be present in the relatives of squinters; Fig. 52 is illustrative of these findings. Richter also holds that squints manifest in the first year of life represent the most severe and least tractable degree of sensory anomalies.

### Divergent squint

Most divergent squints are probably non-genetic in origin. Adequate studies on twins and on families are lacking. The available data suggests irregular dominance in the hereditary forms; Fig. 53 illustrates the significance of exophoria as an incomplete manifestation of the affection.

### Alternating hyperphoria

Both concordance and discordance have been observed in twins, and irregular dominance has been recorded (Crone, 1952; Kubota, 1968).

## NYSTAGMUS

### Uncomplicated ocular nystagmus

Nystagmus occurs as a symptom of many hereditary ocular affections, such as

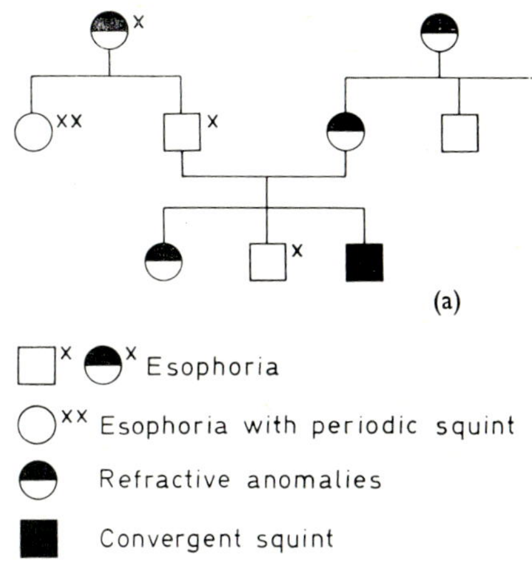


FIG. 52.—Inheritance of different degrees of refractive and of motor anomalies in relatives of patients with manifest concomitant squint. (*After Richter*, 1967.)

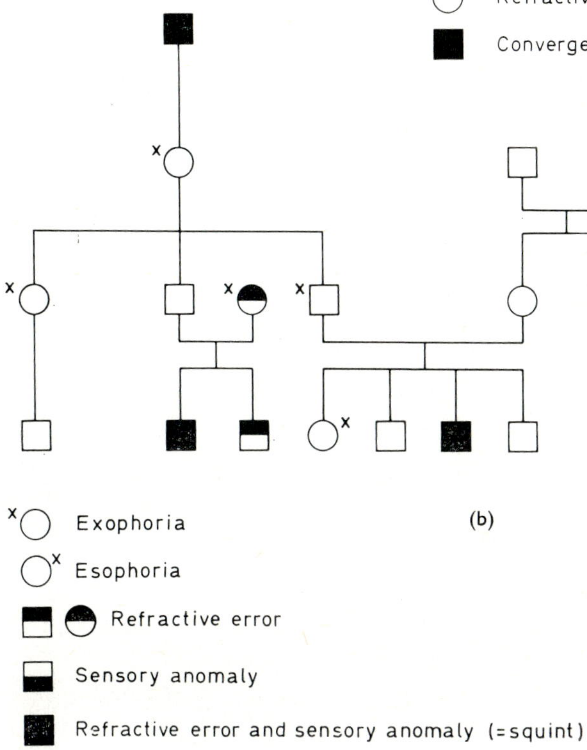


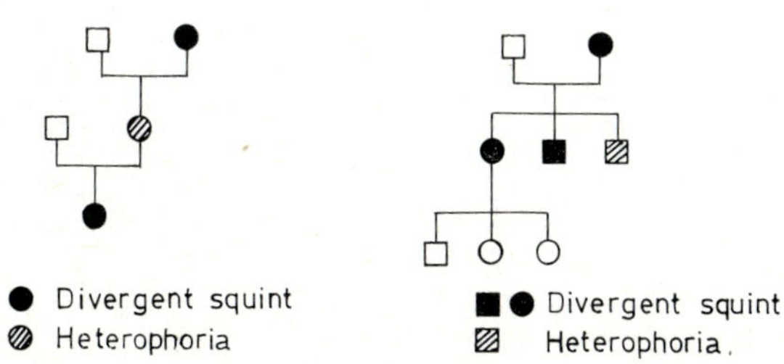


FIG. 53.—Divergent squint. Two pedigrees suggestive of dominant inheritance and showing heterophoria as the incomplete form of divergent squint. (*After Waardenburg*, 1948.)

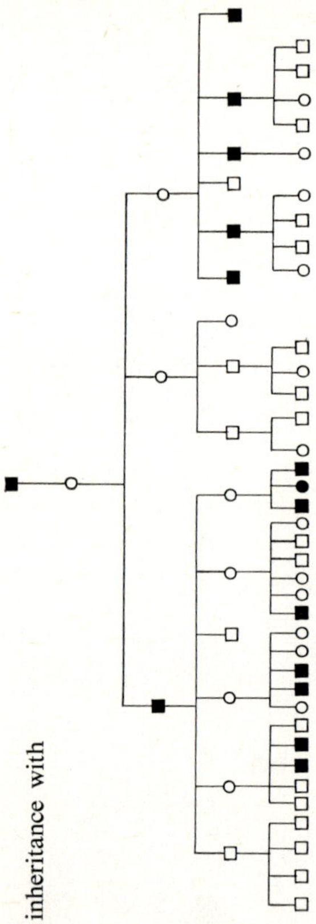

FIG. 54.—Nystagmus. Pedigree showing recessive sex-linked inheritance with manifestation in one woman. (*After Hemmes*, 1924.)

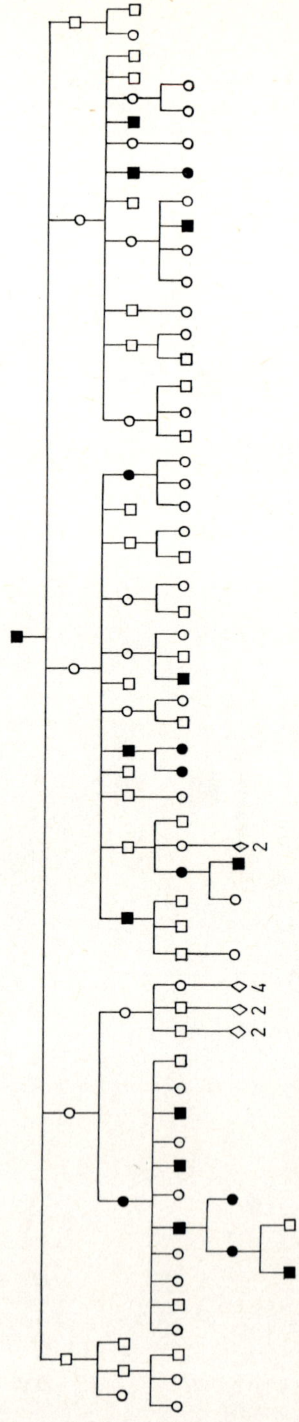


FIG. 55.—Nystagmus. A pedigree suggestive of dominant sex-linked inheritance with suppression of the manifestation in some one-third to one-half of the women carrying the gene. (*After Niccol*, 1915.)

albinism and total colour-blindness, apart from being a component of many hereditary affections of the central nervous system.

Congenital hereditary nystagmus may, however, occur in eyes that are apparently normal. In some cases there may be hypoplasia of the macula, and this is not easy to determine in the nystagmic eye. This explanation cannot always apply, for many patients with congenital hereditary nystagmus have good vision. In all cases a characteristic feature is the lack of subjective sensations of moving objects, so trying in acquired nystagmus. It would seem that the underlying cause of nystagmus may be anywhere in the central nervous system—the macula, the central connexions, and the labyrinthine apparatus.

*Modes of inheritance*

Uniovular twins show a high degree of concordance, and this is possibly less marked in uniovular twin girls. Both sex-linked and autosomal inheritance come into consideration.

*Sex-linked inheritance.*—Many pedigrees show only males affected. In some families affected women are also seen; such pedigrees are readily explained as showing recessive sex-linkage with occasional manifestation in carrier women; Fig. 54 is typical. Dominant sex-linkage is suggested by such pedigrees as that recorded in Fig. 55, but it is necessary to postulate suppression of the expected manifestation in some of the transmitting women.

*Autosomal inheritance.*—Recessive inheritance is rare; Fig. 56 is typical, whilst Fig. 57 is illustrative of the more common dominantly inherited variety. Pedigrees such as Fig. 55, given above as illustrative of dominant sex-linked inheritance, have been explained as showing irregular autosomal dominance. This is unlikely, however, because such pedigrees show a heavy excess of affected daughters and a frequent lack of affected sons amongst the offspring of affected men.

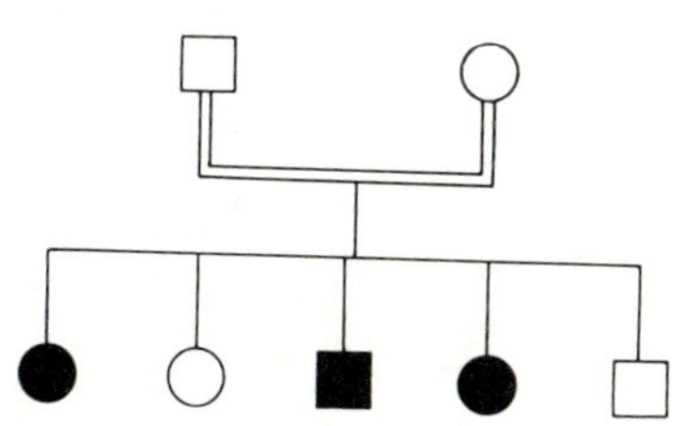

FIG. 56 (*right*).—Nystagmus: recessive inheritance. (*After Fukami*, 1924.)

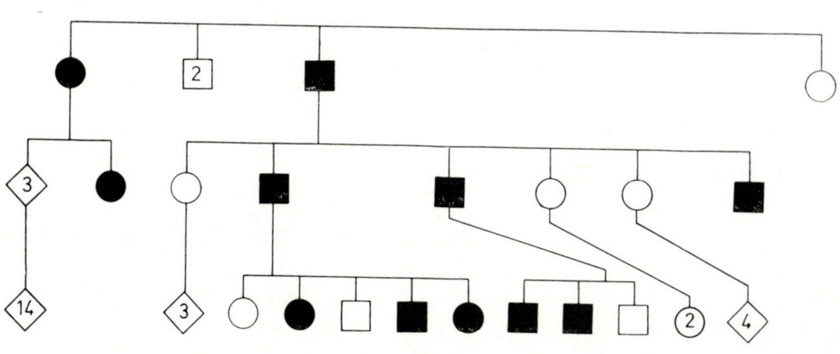


FIG. 57 (*below*).—Nystagmus: dominant inheritance. (*After Fattovich*, 1936.)

## Nystagmus with some unusual ocular associations

Nystagmus may be present independently as an inherited affection in families with hereditary disorders. It may occur in families with myopia and has been seen in a family with red-green blindness (Rucker, 1946, 1949). A more direct association is the nystagmus which is not infrequent in any of the severe congenital anomalies. In some of these cases it is symptomatic rather than an independent entity. There are, however, some ill-defined groups in which nystagmus is a significant aspect not overshadowed by gross ocular defects. Outstanding amongst these is nystagmus with myopia.

### *Nystagmus with myopia*

Sex-linked nystagmus, high myopia, night-blindness and concentric contraction of the field was recorded by von Hippel in 1934 and may possibly be a variant of sex-linked myopia with night-blindness. There is also on record a family with autosomal dominant nystagmus with high myopia and amblyopia (*see* Fig. 39); clinically but not genetically it resembles the family recorded by von Hippel.

## Some unusual forms of nystagmus

### *Latent nystagmus*

Dominant inheritance of latent nystagmus has been recorded by Waardenburg (Fig. 58); and Crone (1952) observed it as a concordant trait in a pair of uniovular twins. Various degrees of heterophoria or actual squint are common in latent nystagmus, and these, too, are probably hereditary rather than the result of cerebral damage in infants as is often suggested.

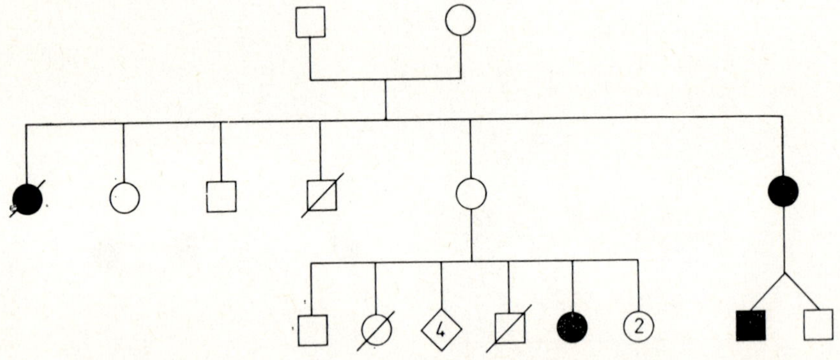


FIG. 58.—Latent nystagmus. (*After Waardenburg*, 1932.)

### *Myoclonic nystagmus*

This is probably another sex-linked affection, but it is likely that it is not a true nystagmus, but a rapid trembling of the eyes without two distinct phases, consequent on rhythmic irregular contractions of the eye muscles. Mild general disturbances are usually present and suggest that this is a neurological affection rather than an eye disorder (van Bogaert and de Savitsch, 1937).

## FOR FURTHER READING

**Ptosis**

Gutman, A. (1948–50). *Acta. genet. Statist. med.*, **1**, 295.
Usher, C. H. (1935). *Trans. Ophthal. Soc. U.K.*, **55**, 194, 241.

**Duane's Phenomenon**

François, J. (1961). *Heredity in Ophthalmology*, p. 247. St. Louis; Mosby.

**Squint**

François, J. (1961). *Heredity in Ophthalmology*, p. 257. St. Louis; Mosby.
Richler, S. (1967). "Untersuchungen ueber die Heredität des Utrabismus concomitans." *Abhandlungen aus dem Gebiete der Augenheilk*, Bd. 35, Ed. by K. Velhagen. Leipzig; Thieme.
Waardenburg, P. J. (1950). *Docum. Ophthal.*, **4**, 154.
— (1954). *Docum. Ophthal.*, **7**–**8**, 422.
Weekers, R., Moureau, P., Hacourt, J. and André A. (1956). *Bull. Soc. Belg. Ophtal.*, **112**, 146.

**Nystagmus**

Hemmes, G. D. (1924). *Over hereditare nystagmus*. Thesis; Utrecht.
Lenz, F. (1932). *Arch. Rass.-u. GesBiol.*, **26**, 194.
Nettleship, E. (1911). *Trans. Ophthal. Soc. U.K.*, **31**, 159.

# SECTION II

# INDIVIDUAL TISSUES

# CHAPTER 6

# THE CORNEA

## ANOMALIES IN SIZE AND SHAPE

### Normal measurements and their variation

*Diameters*

The actual distribution of measurements of the horizontal diameter of the cornea —as determined by Peter in 1,024 eyes of children aged from 5 to 16 years—is shown in Fig. 59. These observations agree with the classical findings of Priestley Smith, and do not differ markedly from much similar material. It would, therefore, appear that a cornea with a horizontal diameter of less than 10 millimetres or more than 13·5 millimetres must be regarded as falling outside the range of normal, and that the most frequent value is 11–12 millimetres. The most frequent value for the vertical diameter is rather less: from 10·5 to 11 millimetres.

*Refraction*

The significance of corneal refraction and of its normal variation in total refraction has been discussed in the section on refractive errors. Corneae with a refraction of less than 35 D and more than 50 D are outside physiological limits, i.e. the normal range of the radius of curvature appears to lie between 6·75 millimetres and 9·25 millimetres.

*Inheritance of normal corneal power.*—Corneal power is an inherited trait, as shown by studies on twins and on families (*see* Tables II and III, pp. 43–45). The coefficient of correlation in uniovular twins was 0·934 against 0·591 in binovular twins and 0·075 in control pairs. In families the coefficients for the parent/child correlation and for mid-parent/child correlation were close to the expected values of 0·50 and 0·71 respectively for inheritance of additive effects of a number of genes without dominance.

### Microcornea

Microcornea would appear to represent localized arrested development at five months in embryonic life. The smaller the diameter of the cornea, the greater is the corneal refraction. As most eyes with small corneae are not markedly ametropic it must be assumed that the axial length is probably small, and that the line of demarcation between microcornea and microphthalmos is fine. Uncomplicated microcornea is consistent with good vision. Glaucoma is said to be a complication in some 20 per cent of cases, but it is not clear that this applies to microcornea as distinct from microphthalmos.

Fig. 60 shows a pedigree recorded by Martin in 1888 as showing inheritance of microphthalmos; it is probably an example of the dominant transmission of microcornea, repeatedly recorded since. The range of dimensions of the cornea in one particular family of this dominant disorder is shown in Fig. 61, whilst Fig. 62 records a family in which microcornea was associated with congenital cataract.

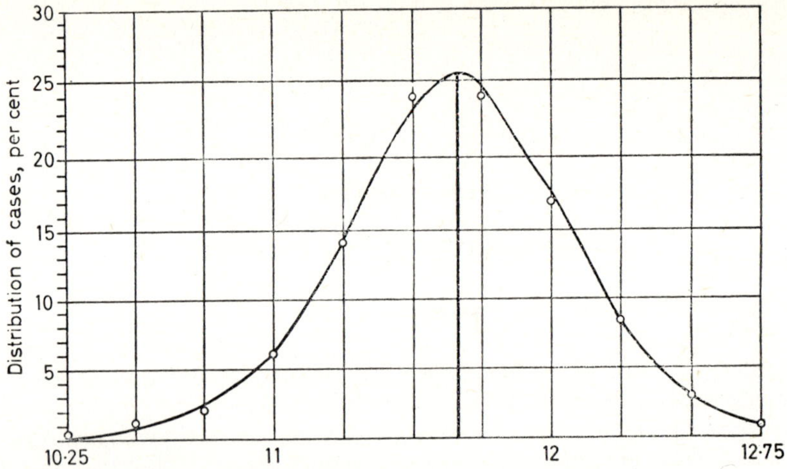


FIG. 59.—The frequency of distribution of the horizontal diameter of the cornea (in mm). (*After Rosa Peter*, 1925.)

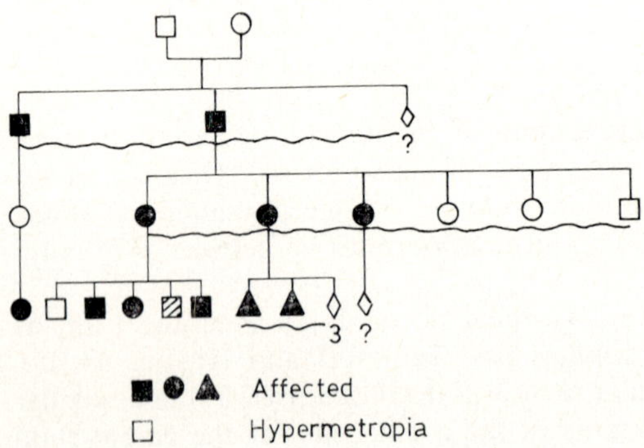


FIG. 60.—Microcornea. Inheritance over three generations. Recorded originally in 1888 as cases of microphthalmos. Vision appears to have been unaffected, and it is likely that this was a family with microcornea rather than microphthalmos. (*After Martin*, 1888.)

**Megalocornea**

The same difficulty as in demarcating microcornea from microphthalmos arises in distinguishing between megalocornea and buphthalmos. Here, however, the line of demarcation is more definite. Megalocornea is seen almost exclusively in males, is always bilateral, vision is generally good and demarcation from the sclera is as well defined as in the normal eye. With the slit-lamp increased relucency is seen at the limbus. Occasionally, changes in the anterior segment of the eye may be present, making differential diagnosis from buphthalmos difficult. In buphthalmos the cornea is generally abnormal in other ways than mere enlargement, for opacities and rupture of Descemet's membrane are frequent. The line of demarcation from the sclera is not always well defined, and a thin bluish sclera is generally evident. When changes are present in the anterior segment in megalocornea, the anterior chamber is deep, the iris may be tremulous, and the lens though normal in early life frequently becomes opaque later on. In buphthalmos the anterior chamber is either normal or shallow, and only occasionally deep, iridodonesis is rare, and secondary cataract is common in severe cases. Megalocornea is a non-progressive anomaly, buphthalmos a progressive affection.

In modes of inheritance the two conditions are sharply contrasted. Buphthalmos is in all probability an autosomal recessive, megalocornea on the other hand is a sex-linked recessive in most cases (Fig. 63 *a* and *b*) and less commonly an autosomal dominant (Fig. 64). Megalocornea may be an aspect of the Marfan syndrome—a dominant affection—and has been observed as possibly recessive in association with ectopia lentis et pupillae.

Like the curvature of the normal cornea, the two major anomalies of cornea curvature are genetically determined.

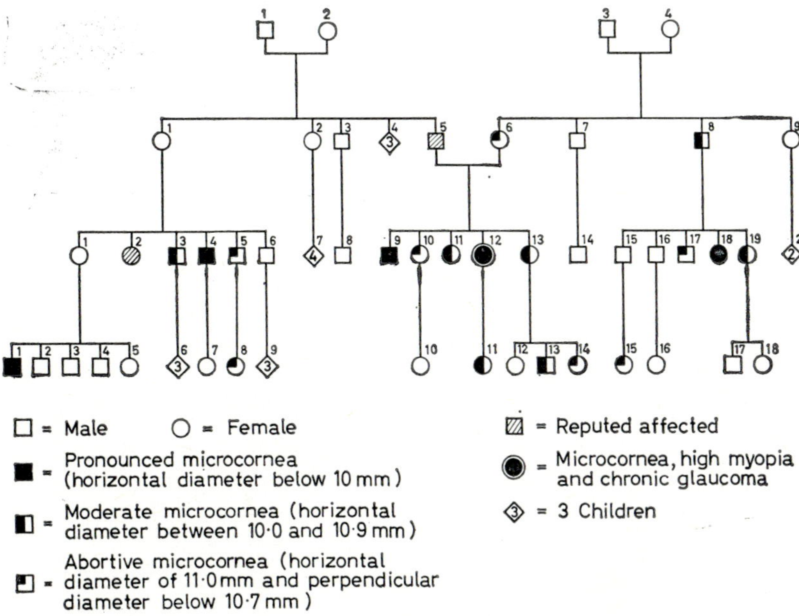


FIG. 61.—Pedigree of microcornea. Dominant inheritance over three generations. (*After Gatterbauer*, 1943.)

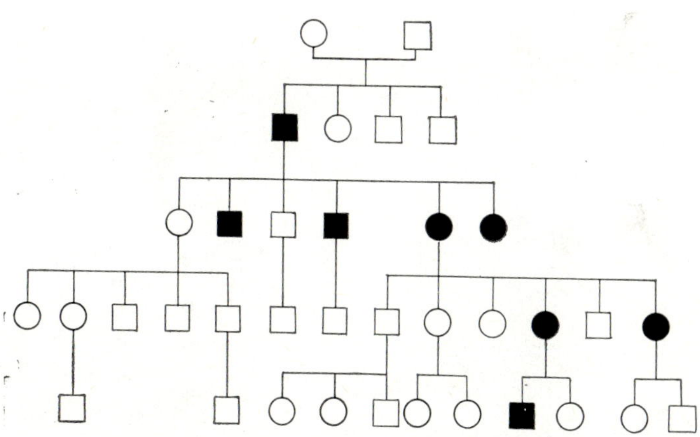

FIG. 62.—Pedigree of a family in which microcornea was associated with cataract. (*After Friedman and Wright*, 1952.)

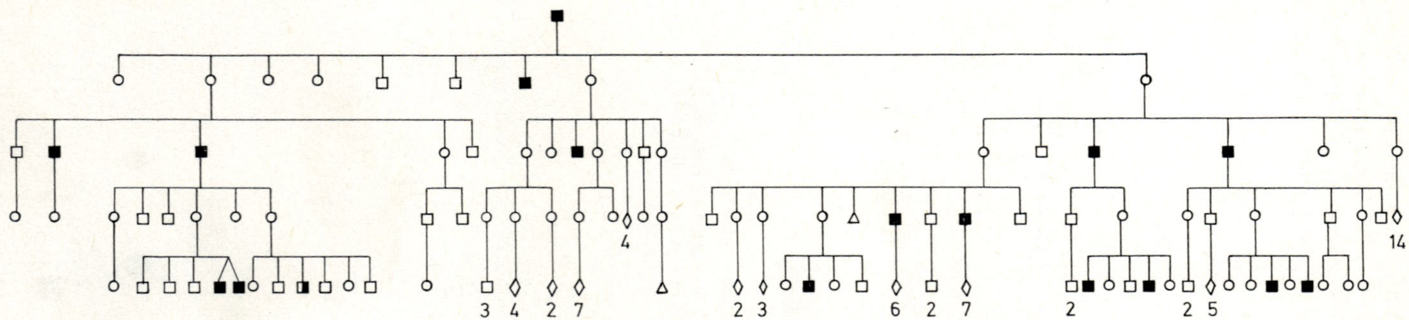


(a)

■ Bilateral
◨ Unilateral

FIG. 63.—Megalocornea. Recessive sex-linked inheritance. (*a*) A pedigree over five generations showing recessive sex-linkage. (*After Kayser*, 1914 *and* 1919.)

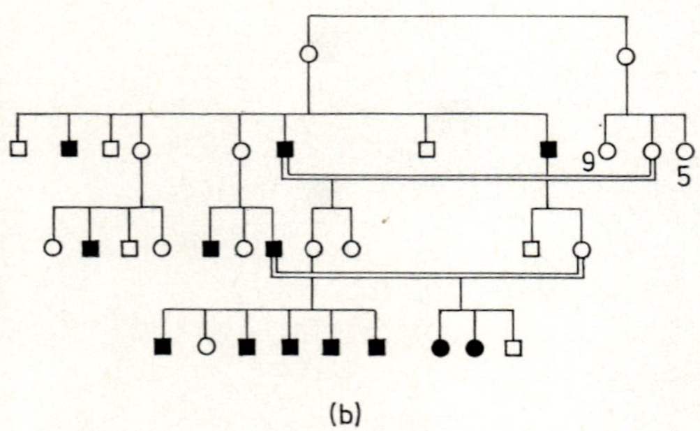


FIG. 63.—(*b*) A pedigree showing two affected women in the last generation. It may be assumed that they received an X chromosome with a pathogenic gene from each of their parents. (*After Grönholm*, 1921.)

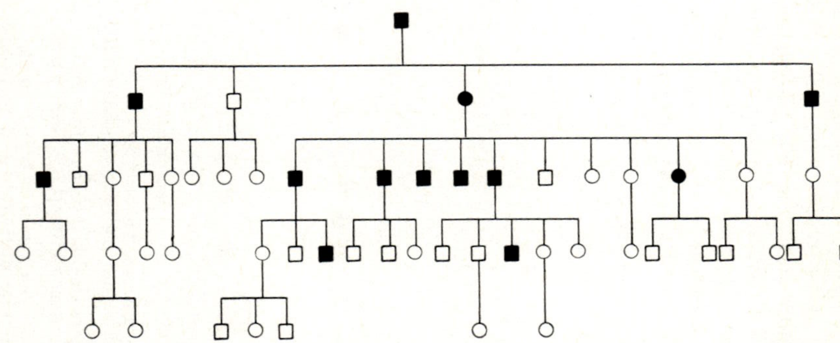

FIG. 64.—Megalocornea. A unique pedigree suggestive of autosomal dominance. (*After Gredig*, 1926.)

## Cornea plana

The cornea may be small with a horizontal diameter of 8–10 millimetres or of normal dimensions. The abnormal flatness may produce a corneal refraction as low as 20–30 D, although sometimes the refraction is still within normal limits. The line of demarcation with the sclera is ill-defined, and the transparent part of the cornea tends to be horizontally oval. Frequently there are associated ocular anomalies, so that vision is poor. Cornea plana is probably inherited in a dominant manner (Fig. 65 *a*), though some pedigrees suggest a recessive mode of inheritance (Fig. 65 *b*). Cornea plana together with bluish coloration of the sclera and xerosis of the conjunctiva has been observed once over two generations.

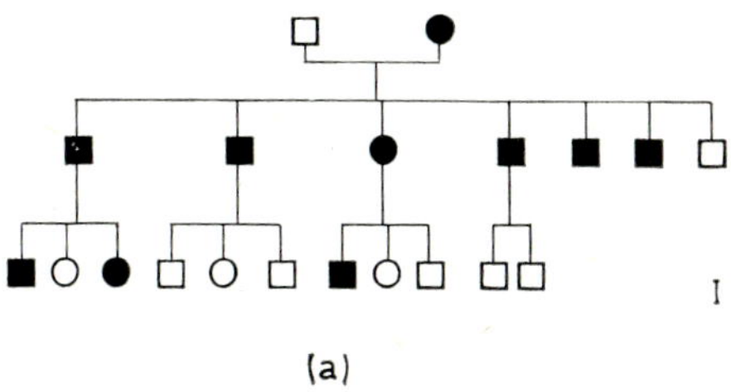


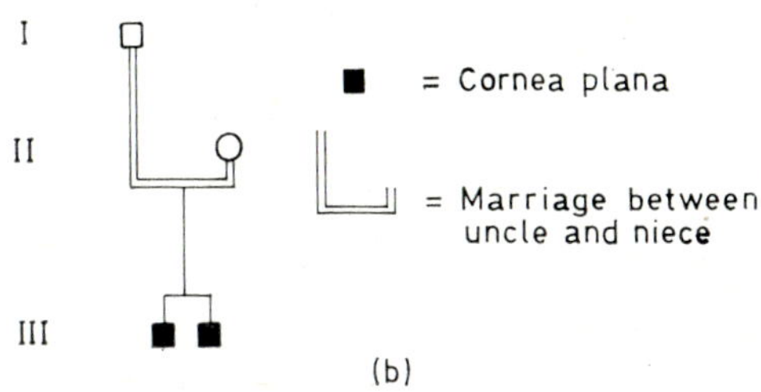


FIG. 65.—Cornea plana: (*a*) Pedigree showing dominant inheritance. (*After Larsen and Eriksen*, 1949.) (*b*) Pedigree suggesting recessive mode of inheritance. (*After Felix*, 1925.)

## Keratoconus

In some pedigrees (Fig. 66 *a*) keratoconus and severe corneal astigmatism appear as alternative forms within the same family. Frequently, too, when there is keratoconus in one eye there is a high degree of astigmatism in the other. This would suggest that high degrees of astigmatism are abortive forms of keratoconus, and there is evidence that some, at any rate, tend to evolve into the fully developed type. The majority of records concern sibships only and would suggest recessive inheritance but there are a substantial number of cases observed over two generations, and even three (Fig. 66 *b*). The interpretation of these pedigrees depends largely upon the significance attached to astigmatism as an abortive form of keratoconus.

FIG. 66.—Keratoconus. (*a*) Pedigree over two generations showing keratoconus and severe astigmatism as alternative forms. (*After Rumpf*, 1937.) (*b*) Pedigree suggestive of dominant inheritance. (*After Stähli*, 1925.)

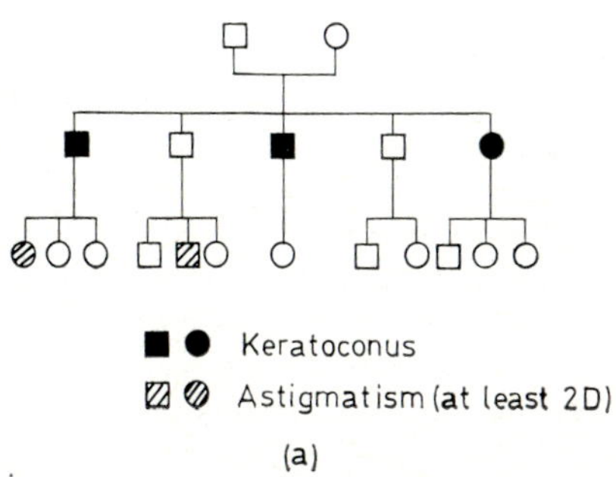


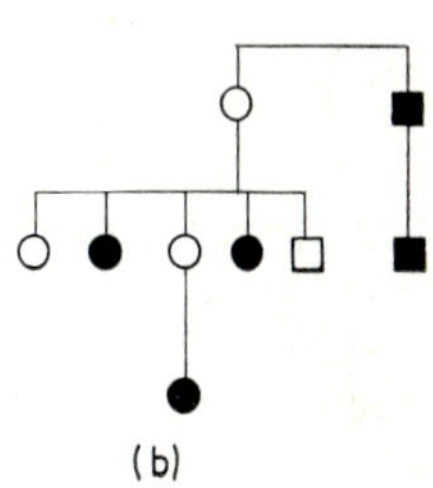

**Posterior conical cornea**

This is not related to classical keratoconus. Though occasionally traumatic in origin, it is usually congenital and may be associated with other congenital anomalies. It has been seen in sibs and over two generations (Jacobs, 1957; Haney and Falls, 1961; Collier, 1962).

## OPACITIES AND PIGMENT ANOMALIES

### Congenital Opacification of the Cornea

Congenital opacification of the cornea presents considerable complexities.

**Clinical aspects**

Clinically, three distinct types may be recognized, each sharing several subsidiary forms some of which are probably aspects of the anterior chamber cleavage anomaly.

*Cornea with diffuse haze*

(1) Diffuse haze of the cornea seen in severe buphthalmos present at birth.

(2) Diffuse haze seen in such metabolic disorders as gargoylism. Here the associated general disturbances are pathognomonic, although not necessarily obvious at birth. This also applies to cystinosis.

(3) Diffuse haze with otherwise normal eyes and normal body, but mental retardation. The nature of this disturbance is unknown.

(4) Diffuse haze with "nodules" in the stroma (Fig. 67). The general and slit-lamp appearances are those seen in established cases of recessive macular dystrophy, but the affection is present at birth and apparently only slowly progressive. It has been designated congenital parenchymatous corneal dystrophy.

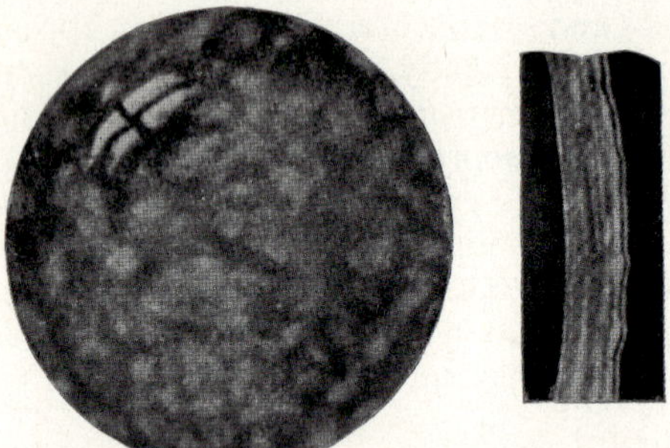

Fig. 67.—Congenital corneal lesion showing diffuse haze with "nodules" in the stroma. (*After Franceschetti and Klein*, 1961.)

*Cornea with gross opacities*

(1) Localized congenital opacity of the leucoma type. These opacities are bilateral and are situated deeply in the stroma centrally or paracentrally; they are sometimes sharply delineated, dense, opaque, and white, and sometimes greyish, semi-translucent and with hazy margins (Fig. 68). The depth at which it is placed suggests a defect in Descemet's membrane as the starting point, but the opacity may extend well forward towards Bowman's membrane, and may become ectatic and even perforate, but vascularization with some tendency towards healing may occur. The opacity may be the only anomaly, but often other defects are also present: iris adhesions, shallow anterior chamber, persistent pupillary membranes,

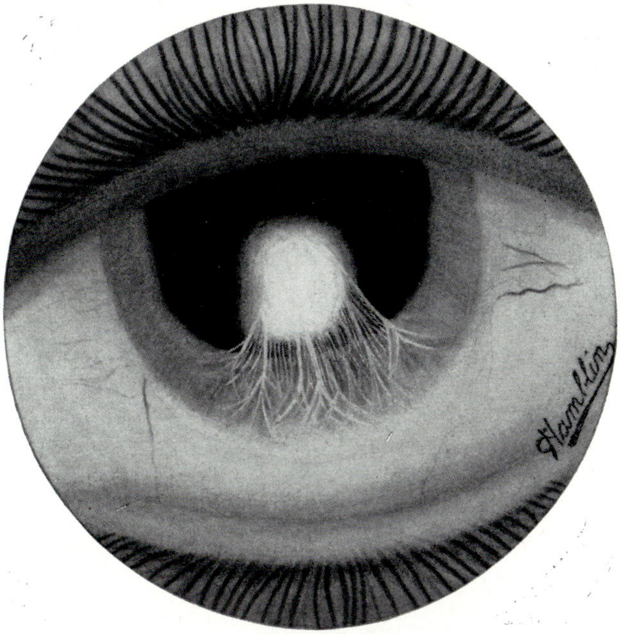


FIG. 68.—Localized congenital corneal opacity of the leucoma type. (*After Batten, in Hamblin's collection*)

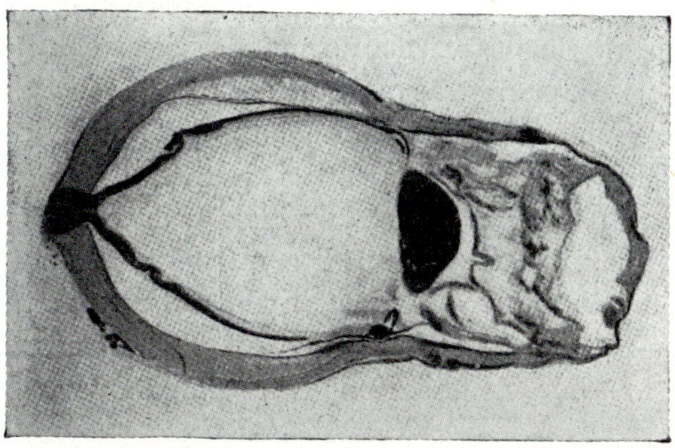

FIG. 69.—Congenital anterior staphyloma. Sagittal section × 2. The left eye of a child aged 3 days; the right eye was normal. An only sib and the parents were also normal. (*After Parsons*, 1904.)

various iris anomalies and even microphthalmos with or without colobomatous defects; occasionally a secondary buphthalmos may develop. The two eyes are not always affected in the same way, for a much more severe lesion may be present in one eye, the whole cornea being opaque (congenital total opacity of the cornea), and even staphylomatous (congenital anterior staphyloma). Such cases are clearly instances of the anterior chamber cleavage anomaly.

(2) Congenital total opacity of the cornea. Both corneae show a varying degree of white total opacification. Here buphthalmos, which is generally regarded as secondary in character, may supervene later. In other cases microphthalmos is present. Some of these might also be instances of the cleavage anomaly.

(3) Congenital anterior staphyloma (Fig. 69). This may be bilateral or unilateral; in unilateral cases the other eye may be entirely normal or show some degree of congenital leucoma or total opacification. Histologically there are gross anomalies

throughout the whole of the anterior segment of the globe, the normal differentiation into iris, ciliary body and lens being obscured—once more recalling the cleavage anomaly.

*Cornea with embryotoxon anomalies*

*Arcus juvenalis* (*anterior embryotoxon*).—The arcus normally present in the embryo may persist as arcus juvenalis. A layer of clear cornea separates it from the limbus.

*Posterior embryotoxon*.—In its mildest form there is an arcus caused by a marginal defect in Descemet's membrane; there is no clear corneal tissue separating it from the sclera. Generally the anomaly is more extensive (*see* Fig. 13 *c–e*). There may be whitish, glassy striae extending into the anterior chamber towards the angle: these are regarded as due to hypertrophy of Schwalbe's ring; sometimes a hyaline membrane extends from the back of the cornea on to the iris. In other cases there are opacities extending into the cornea and these may dominate the picture. More frequently there are various associated defects in the iris, mostly hypoplastic changes in the mesoderm; these are clearly cases of the anterior chamber cleavage anomaly.

**Heredity**

Genetically these anomalies are no less complex.

*Cornea with diffuse haze*

The genetic aspects of buphthalmos, gargoylism and cystinosis are discussed elsewhere. The association of corneal haze with mental deficiency and no other disturbance is not well established as a clinical entity. Fig. 70 shows its occurrence

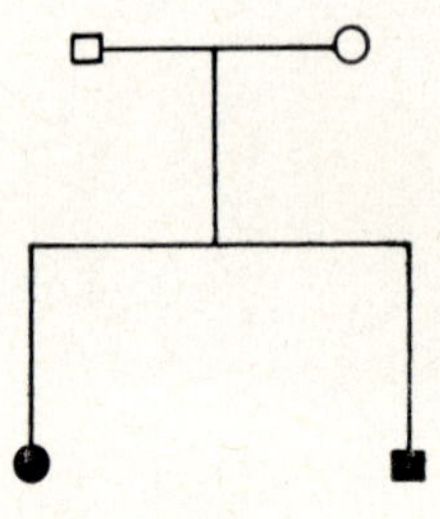

FIG. 70.—Pedigree showing the occurrence of corneal haze and mental deficiency in the two children of normal non-consanguineous parents. (*Personal observation.*)

in two sibs. Corneal haze with "nodular" reactions of the recessive macular type as a congenital defect has been recorded in a dominant form (Fig. 71) but also less commonly in a recessive form. It is possible that there is also an X-chromosomal type, and that the dominant type tends to be associated with ocular anomalies.

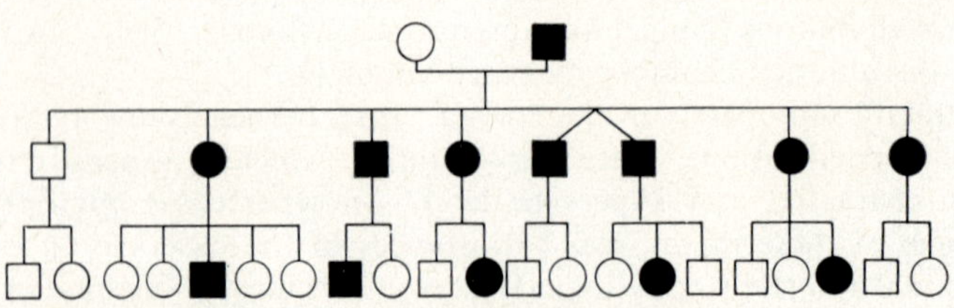

FIG. 71.—Congenital parenchymatous dystrophy of the cornea with dominant heredity. (*After Desvignes and Vigo*, 1955.)

*Cornea with gross opacities and with embryotoxon anomalies*

Many, and perhaps most, of these opacities are aspects of the anterior chamber cleavage complex. Critical genetic studies are still needed, although the many reports on posterior embryotoxon suggest that dominant inheritance is common.

In contrast, recessive inheritance is likely in cases with total opacification of the cornea and anterior staphyloma; this is suggested by older literature with its reports of isolated cases, affected sibs (and the assumption of "intra-uterine inflammation" as the cause); presumably the parents were normal.

## VORTEX-LIKE VEIL ("VORTEX DYSTROPHY", CORNEA VERTICILLATA)

Vortex-like veil is a non-progressive lesion without effect on vision (Fig. 72). The illustration suggests that the affection is inherited in a dominant manner, but it is

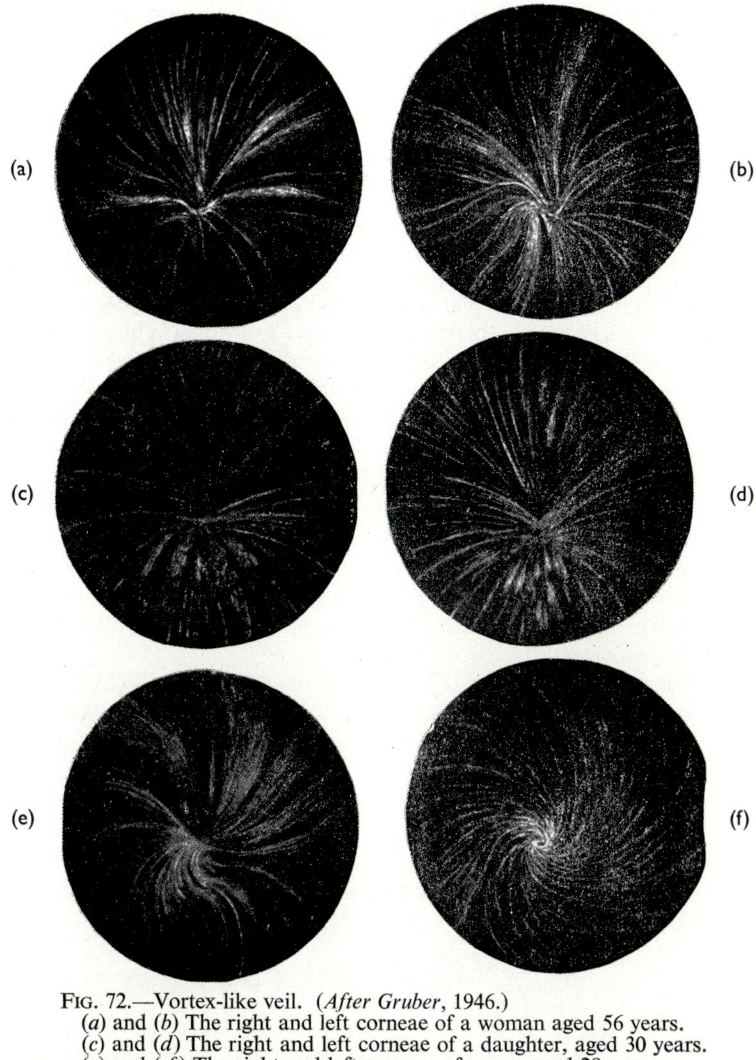


FIG. 72.—Vortex-like veil. (*After Gruber*, 1946.)
(*a*) and (*b*) The right and left corneae of a woman aged 56 years.
(*c*) and (*d*) The right and left corneae of a daughter, aged 30 years.
(*e*) and (*f*) The right and left corneae of a son, aged 28 years.

also likely that cornea verticillata in women is indicative of the carrier state of Fabry's disease (*see* p. 201)—a sex-linked disorder.

### Limbal Pigment Ring

Limbal pigment ring is a normal feature in some of the dark-coloured races. Waardenburg has observed it over three generations in the offspring of marriages between Caucasians and Malays.

### Krukenberg's Spindle

Krukenberg's spindle has been observed in megalocornea which is generally inherited in a recessive sex-linked manner. It is an important constituent of Sugar's pigmentary glaucoma which is probably also a recessive sex-linked affection. It has been recorded in two sisters who were uniovular twins (Vogt, 1938). In uncomplicated cases there is a marked female excess.

### Kayser-Fleischer Ring

This ocular sign of hepato-lenticular degeneration—occasionally a pointing sign in this recessive affection—is generally observed in all the affected sibs of a family.

## CORNEAL DYSTROPHIES

The reactions seen in the corneal dystrophies show a wide range. At the one extreme, seen in early cases, there may be merely minimal changes recognizable only with the slit-lamp and taking the form of infiltrates or of apparently enlarged nerve-endings. At the other extreme there are gross changes to be seen in the terminal stages of the different forms: discrete hard chalky foci, sited in otherwise clear cornea (seen in granular dystrophy), and extensive opacification of the cornea (present in macular dystrophy or in lattice-like dystrophy). Inflammatory reactions are not uncommon and complicate the appearances, but it should generally be fairly easy to recognize these secondary effects.

Considerable clarification has been achieved as a result of the stress laid by Kraupa on the different reactions shown by the different layers of the cornea, and of the work of Bücklers and of Saebø on the mode of inheritance of the classical forms of corneal dystrophy.

Kraupa stressed the secondary involvement of the epithelium in primary endothelial dystrophies, and isolated a juvenile form of presumably primary endothelial dystrophy with epithelial involvement. Bücklers in 1938 and Saebø in 1939 showed that most of the recorded cases of corneal dystrophy fell into three well defined clinical and genetic entities. It has become clear, however, that there are many more forms of corneal dystrophy. A combination of slit-lamp examination and genetic investigation has produced rapid advances in the recognition of these affections, whilst the increasing practice of keratoplasty has made available ample histological material.

### Essentially Parenchymatous Dystrophies

The three classical forms of corneal dystrophy—the recessive macular type, the dominant granular and the dominant lattice-like types—belong to this group. All three forms are localized centrally and even in the late stages the periphery of the cornea tends to remain clear. There is a striking lack of inflammatory reactions; vascularization is exceptional and generally occurs as a secondary feature to erosions of the epithelial surface which may develop. Whilst the reactions are essentially parenchymatous, both the epithelium and endothelium become involved, although the deeper layers of the parenchyma remain relatively uninvolved. In two of the three clearly defined types recognized "acute attacks" with severe symptoms but without any tangible structural changes are fairly frequent. The essential features of these dystrophies are summarized in Table V.

**Recessive macular dystrophy**

The earliest changes appear in the first decade of life as a delicate diffuse opacity of the whole corneal surface with thicker patches here and there. In the second decade the opacities become more marked, so that at puberty vision is already affected and the fundus is not easily seen. Increasing changes ultimately produce a characteristic corneal picture in which ill-defined opacities stand out in a diffusely cloudy cornea (Fig. 73). There is no actual loss of epithelial substance, but there is an increasing loss of corneal sensation. By the age of 30 years, most patients are practically blind. The mode of inheritance is clearly recessive (Fig. 74).

**Dominant granular dystrophy**

This affection begins at about the age of 5 years as a disturbance in the centre of the cornea, and progresses very slowly. From initial fine interstitial dots fine lines radiate out in all directions, and ultimately the greater part of the cornea is studded with white chalky interstitial opacities (Fig. 75). Vision is not severely affected, and sometimes not at all. Frequently the finding is incidental in the course of a routine examination.

As can be seen from the pedigree shown in Fig. 76, the condition is clearly dominant.

**Dominant lattice-like (or reticular) dystrophy**

This is a rare form of corneal dystrophy. It begins at puberty or earlier and may present difficulty in diagnosis owing to a spurious appearance of nodules where two of the characteristic lattice lines cross (Fig. 77). The condition is generally steadily progressive and vision becomes severely affected. With the slit-lamp the linear opacities show double-contoured outlines, and are seen to be delicate clefts of the anterior layers of the parenchyma. Histologically the stromal lesions show amyloid reactions (Smith and Zimmerman, 1968). As can be seen from Fig. 78, the condition shows typical dominant transmission.

**Other forms**

Two less well established varieties of parenchymatous dystrophy have been described.

*Disciform crystalline dystrophy (Schnyder)*

An accumulation of needle-like crystals axially in the superficial layer of the parenchyma, with white dots in the adjacent stroma (Fig. 79) has been recorded as a dominant affection (Fig. 80). Onset is early in life, progress is slow and largely asymptomatic, with steadily declining vision (Schnyder, 1939; Forni, 1951).

*Asymptomatic speckled dystrophy (François and Neetens)*

Small, isolated, semi-opaque dots of variable size and shape (some are round, others oval or irregular) are found on slit-lamp examination throughout the

TABLE V

ESSENTIALLY PARENCHYMATOUS CORNEAL DYSTROPHIES—CLASSICAL VARIETIES

TABULATION OF THE SIGNIFICANT CHARACTERISTICS

| *Features* | *Dominant granular dystrophy* | *Recessive macular dystrophy* | *Dominant lattice-like dystrophy* |
|---|---|---|---|
| Age of onset | At about 5 years | The first decade of life | Occasionally in infancy. More frequently in the second decade of life |
| Earliest signs | Small white dots in centre of cornea, some superficial, some fairly deep<br>May take the form of radiating lines from the centre | A thin superficial corneal veil seen with the loupe or slit-lamp. In this fine diffuse haze, isolated ill-defined subepithelial opacities occur. | A cobweb of delicate lines which frequently ramify and produce a lattice-like pattern when the lines cross each other. Here and there the crossings produce the illusion of a nodular reaction. The lines in the superficial layers of the parenchyma tend to raise the epithelium. The corneal tissue tends to be diffusely clouded. Though most marked at the centre of the cornea, the periphery is also involved |
| Course | The dots increase in size and number, and lose the radial arrangement sometimes seen in the early stages<br>The centre of the cornea is now studded with patterned figures of irregular shape and size. They are "hard", white, chalky and well defined | Increasing haziness of the central part of the cornea with an increasing number of isolated opacities which tend to become larger. At about puberty the corneal surface may be uneven and the fundus no longer clearly seen ophthalmoscopically. These changes become more intense so that the picture is one of largish, ill-defined opacities against a hazy background. The changes are most marked centrally but spread towards the periphery. By about the age of 30 years vision is grossly damaged. The further course is one of increasing opacification of the cornea, especially centrally | Increase in the number and thickness of line, "nodules" and general diffuseness of the affected cornea. Sometimes at 20 years of age, and sometimes not until 40 years or so, the centre of the cornea has become an irregular ill-defined opacity with raised epithelium |

| *Features* | *Dominant granular dystrophy* | *Recessive macular dystrophy* | *Dominant lattice-like dystrophy* |
|---|---|---|---|
| End-stage | By about the age of 50 years the opacities are sufficiently well marked to be visible with the naked eye. Until then the presence of this anomaly is frequently an incidental finding. At this stage the cornea loses some of its superficial lustre, and subsequently small localized elevations of the epithelium may occur | Late in life, corneal opacification is such that it may not be possible to see the pupil. The corneal epithelium remains intact until almost the end, though small localized epithelial projections may occur relatively early | Towards the end all evidence of the lattice-like appearance disappears in the diffuse opacification. At the extreme periphery of the cornea the lattice-like lines may still be seen |
| Corneal sensitivity | Only slightly, or not affected until late in life | This is diminished early and there is increasing loss of sensitivity | Affected early and diminishes progressively |
| "Acute attacks" | Absent, or possibly rare | Frequent. The symptoms are out of proportion to the physical signs. There is much photophobia and lacrimation. Vascularization is absent. These attacks are of short duration | Frequent. Epithelial erosions may occur |
| Slit-lamp appearance | Essentially an interstitial reaction<br>Most marked in the intermediate and deepest layers | The earliest opacities are at the level of Bowman's membrane. Later there may be epithelial projections over these opacities and considerable diffuse opacification throughout the parenchyma | The lines are seen to be obliquely running spaces, doubly contoured<br>The intervening parenchyma is hazy<br>The whole depth of the parenchyma is involved |
| Symptoms | Largely asymptomatic. Many patients remain unaware of the existence of the lesion | Declining vision, "acute attacks" and relatively early onset of blindness | As for recessive macular dystrophy, though perhaps not so severe |
| Effect on vision | Frequently none, and generally not severe, even late in life | Severe | Some cases run a mild course. In most, severe visual disturbances are present by the age of 30 years or earlier. The end-result is not infrequently only less severe than with recessive macular dystrophy |

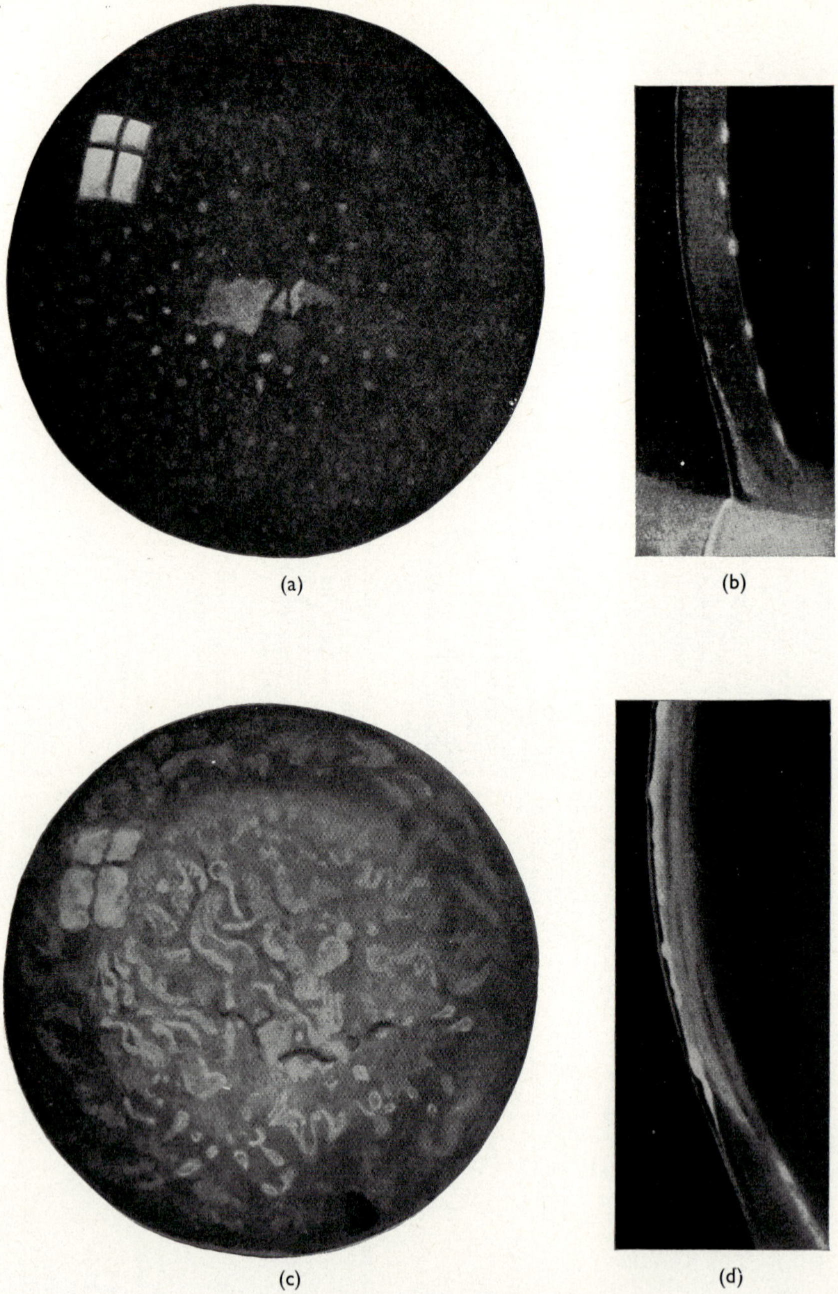


FIG. 73.—Recessive macular dystrophy of the cornea. Face views and optical sections respectively: (*a*) and (*b*) appearances in a man aged 28 years; (*c*) and (*d*) appearances in a woman aged 69 years. (*After Bücklers*, 1938.)

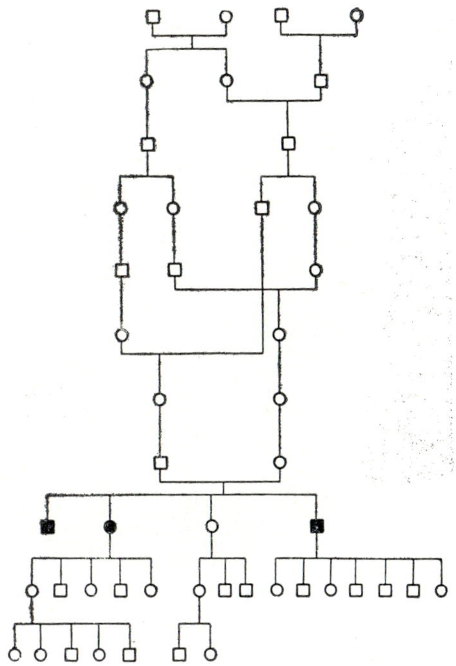

FIG. 74.—Macular dystrophy of cornea. Pedigree showing recessive inheritance. (*After Bücklers and Gilch*, 1938.)

parenchyma, both centrally and peripherally (Fig. 81). The condition does not affect vision, even when in some cases it appears to be progressive. The affection is dominant (Fig. 82).

Both these affections are strictly parenchymatous and have been observed in young children. It is possible that these disorders are congenital in type. Table VI summarizes the essential findings.

TABLE VI

ESSENTIALLY PARENCHYMATOUS CORNEAL DYSTROPHIES: RARE FORMS

TABULATION OF THE SIGNIFICANT CHARACTERISTICS

| *Condition* | *Clinical features* | *Mode of inheritance* |
|---|---|---|
| Disciform crystalline dystrophy (Schnyder) | Onset early in life. Progress is slow and asymptomatic with steadily declining vision. Needle-like crystals are deposited axially in the superficial layers of the parenchyma. There are white dots in the adjacent stroma, readily seen | Dominant |
| Asymptomatic speckled dystrophy (François) | Onset early in life. Progress is slow and asymptomatic without effect on vision. Small isolated semi-opaque dots of variable shape seen in parenchyma on slit-lamp examination | Dominant |

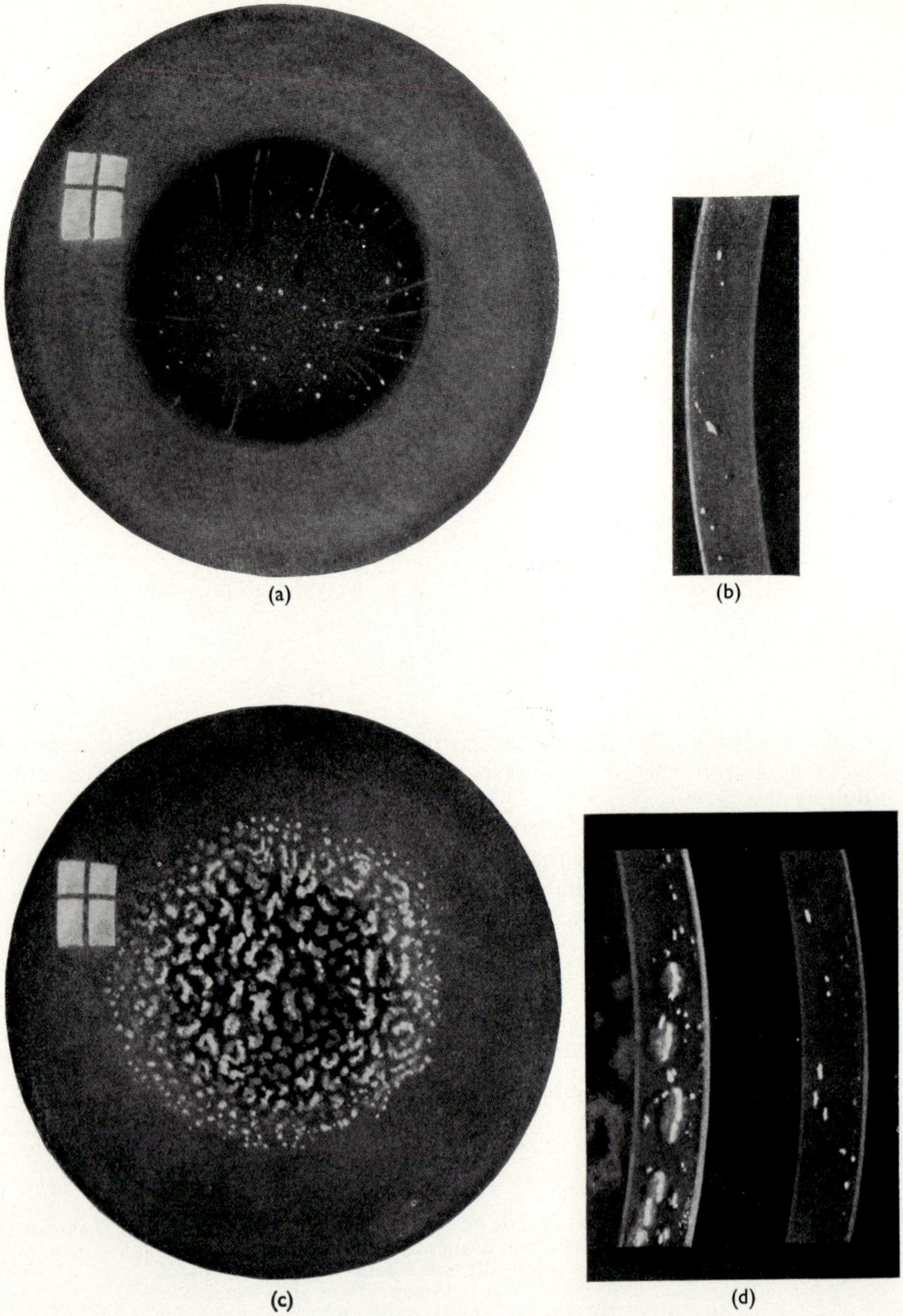


FIG. 75.—Dominant granular dystrophy of the cornea: (*a*) and (*b*) appearances in a boy aged 12 years—face view and optical section respectively; (*c*) and (*d*) appearances in a woman of the same family, aged 52—face view and optical section respectively. (*After Bücklers*, 1938.)

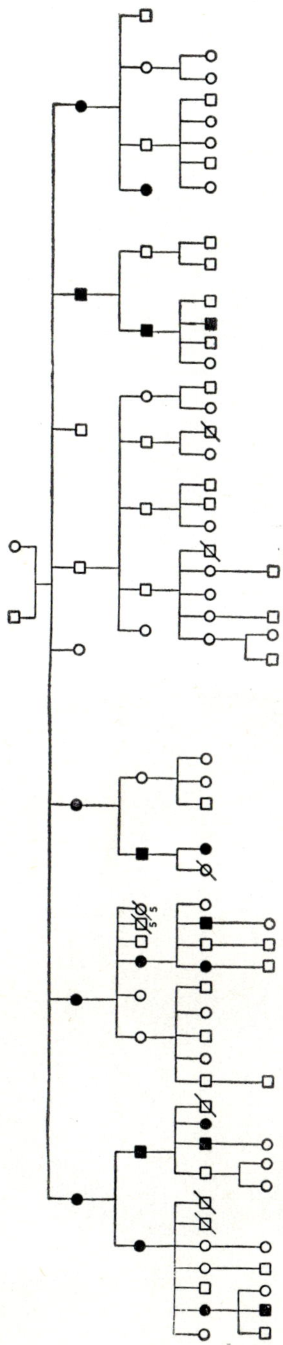

FIG. 76.—Granular dystrophy of the cornea. Pedigree showing dominant inheritance over four generations. (*After Gilch*, 1937.)

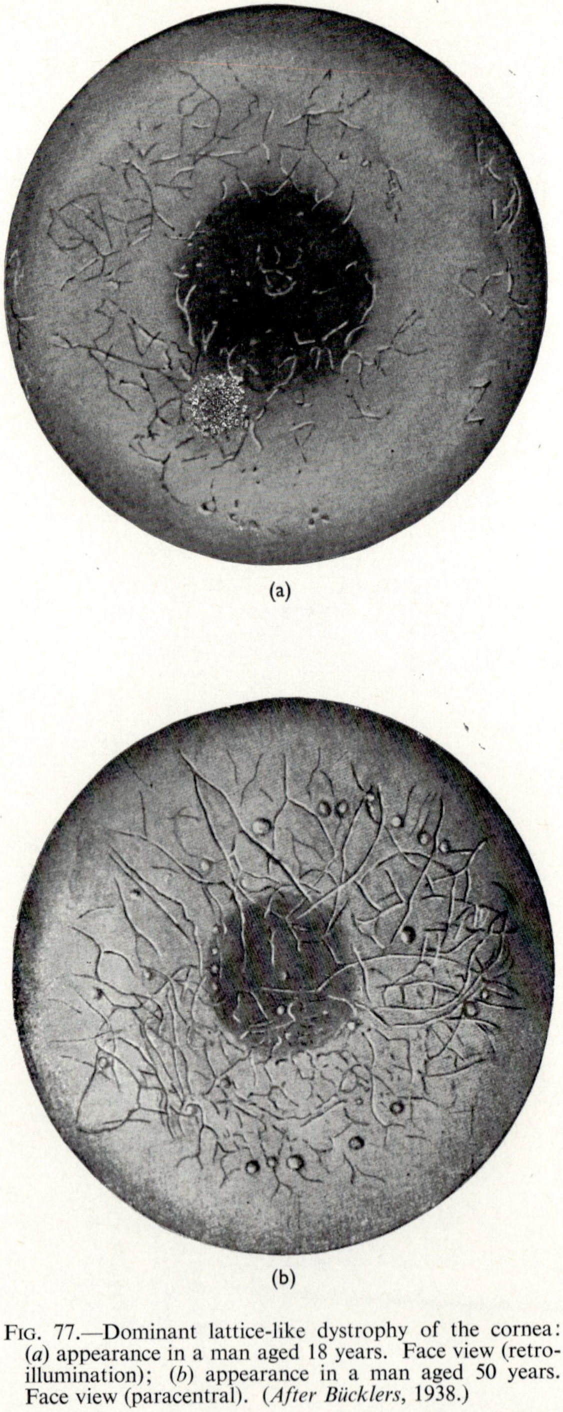


FIG. 77.—Dominant lattice-like dystrophy of the cornea: (*a*) appearance in a man aged 18 years. Face view (retro-illumination); (*b*) appearance in a man aged 50 years. Face view (paracentral). (*After Bücklers*, 1938.)

FIG. 77 (*continued*).—Dominant lattice-like dystrophy of the cornea: (*c*) appearances in a man aged 50 years. Optical sections (more peripheral). (*After Bücklers*, 1938.)

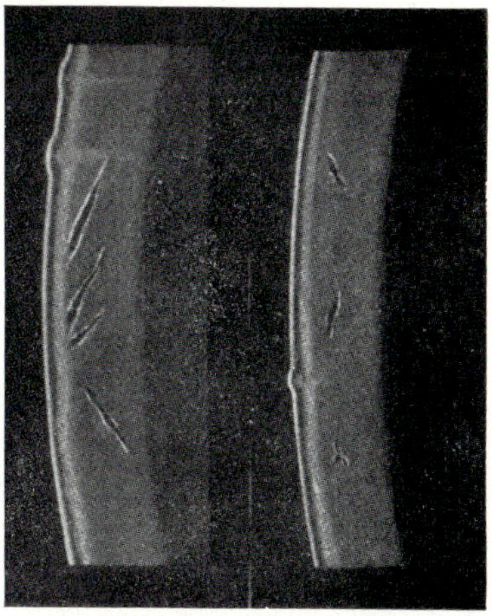


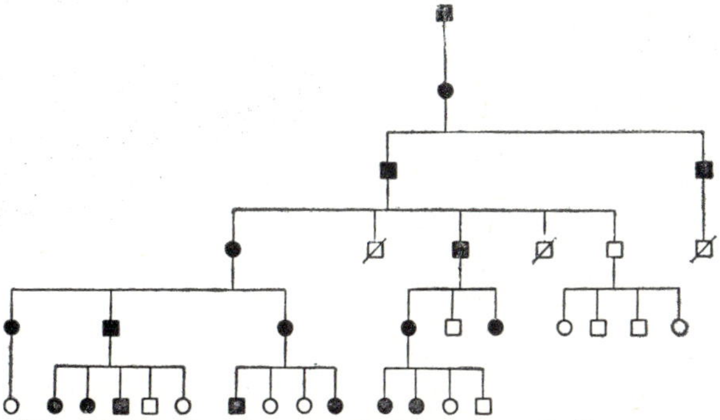

FIG. 78.—Lattice-like corneal dystrophy. Pedigree over six generations showing dominant inheritance. (*After Frykholm*, 1935.)

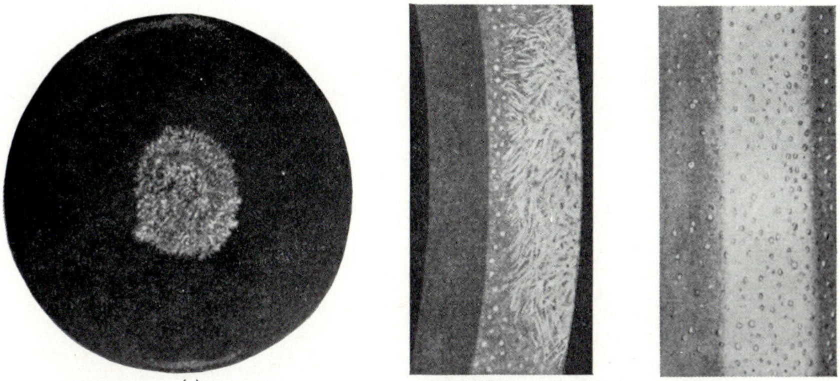


FIG. 79.—Disciform crystalline dystrophy of the cornea: (*a*) face aspect of right cornea showing central deposition of crystals; (*b*) optical section through central area showing central deposition of needle-like crystals with punctate opacities in the adjacent stroma; (*c*) the parenchyma as seen in retro-illumination. The punctate opacities appear like drops. (*After Schnyder*, 1939.)

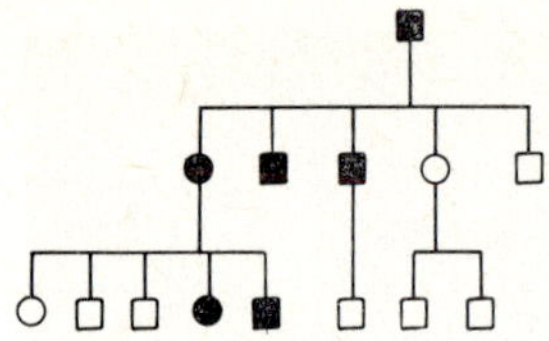

FIG. 80.—Disciform crystalline dystrophy of the cornea. Pedigree showing dominant inheritance. (*After Schnyder*, 1939.)

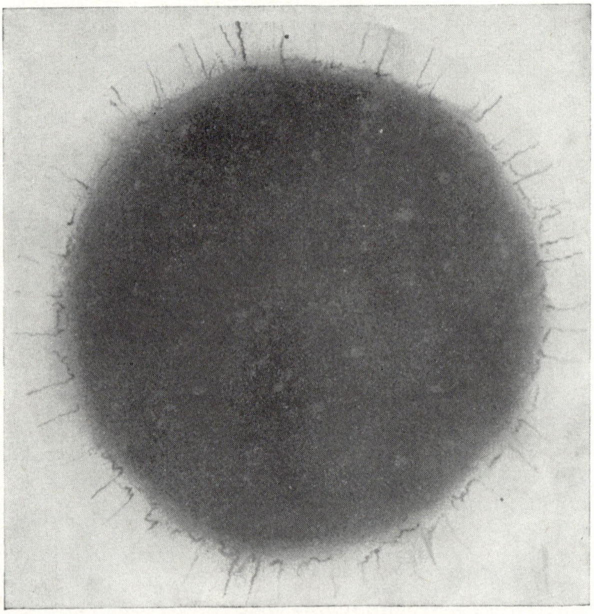

(a)

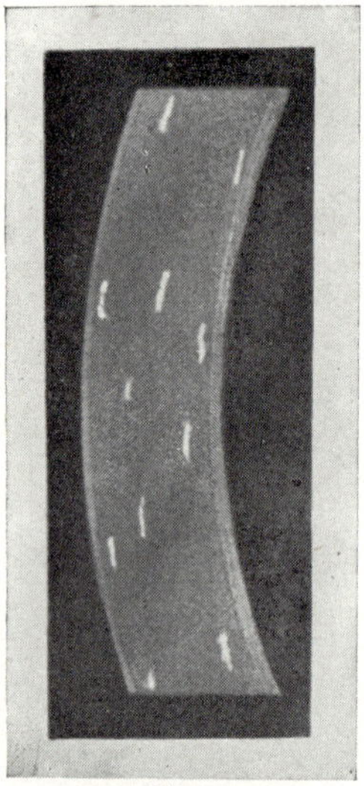

(b)

FIG. 81.—Asymptomatic speckled corneal dystrophy (François and Neetens): (*a*) face view; (*b*) slit-lamp section. (*After François and Neetens*, 1956.)

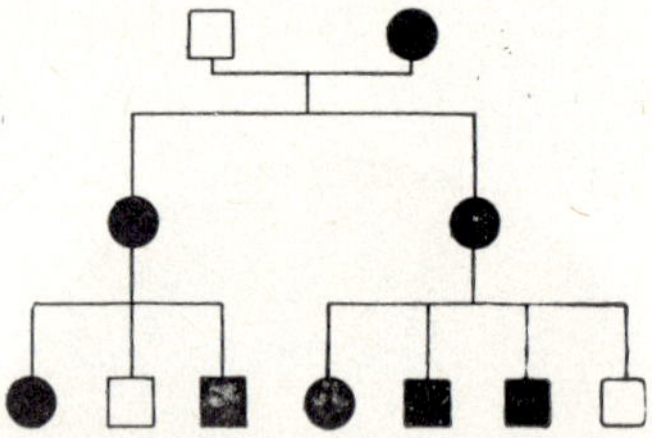

FIG. 82.—Asymptomatic speckled corneal dystrophy (François and Neetens). Pedigree showing dominant inheritance. (*After François and Neetens*, 1956.)

## ESSENTIALLY NON-PARENCHYMATOUS DYSTROPHIES

This group of dystrophies still requires considerable clarification, both as to clinical features and modes of inheritance (Table VII).

### Epithelial dystrophies

*Recurrent corneal erosion*

In a well-worked-out pedigree Franceschetti has recorded this affection as a dominant over six generations. In the affected members there was always reduced corneal sensitivity, which he regarded as the underlying condition. Recurrences were frequent, and tended to subside at about the age of 50 years (Fig. 83).

*Diffuse epithelial dystrophy*

Diffuse corneal dystrophy limited to the epithelium and involving Bowman's membrane in the late stages, is a progressive affection beginning in infancy. Repeated "acute attacks" lead to scar formation with reduction in vision. The

TABLE VII

ESSENTIALLY NON-PARENCHYMATOUS CORNEAL DYSTROPHIES

TABULATION OF THE SIGNIFICANT CHARACTERISTICS

| *Condition* | *Clinical features* | *Mode of inheritance* |
|---|---|---|
| | *Epithelial* | |
| Recurrent corneal erosion | Onset early in life. Reduced corneal sensation. Frequent relapses. Tendency to quiescence after 50 years of age | Dominant |
| Diffuse epithelial dystrophy | Onset in infancy. Repeated "acute attacks". Appearances of superficial punctate keratitis or herpes corneae. In late stages Bowman's membrane is involved. Ultimately there develops scar formation especially in the exposed interpalpebral area of the cornea | Dominant |
| | *Endothelial* | |
| Cornea guttata | Onset early in life. Possibly congenital. In late stages overlying parenchyma involved | Dominant |
| Polymorphous endothelial dystrophy | Excrescences, vesicles and polymorphic opacities | Dominant |
| | *Compound Endothelial and Epithelial* | |
| Senile epithelial dystrophy (Fuchs') | Develops after the age of 50 years; endothelial changes develop first. Subsequently there are progressive changes in the epithelium. Primary chronic oedema of the cornea may be an early stage | ? |
| Juvenile epithelial dystrophy (Kraupa's) | Onset early in life. Possibly congenital and related to congenital opacification of the cornea | ? Dominant |
| | Parenchyma as well as epithelium tends to become involved | ? Recessive |
| | *Dystrophies of Bowman's Membrane* | |
| Ring-like dystrophy | Onset in childhood with frequent "acute attacks". The earliest changes are in Bowman's membrane, but there are secondary epithelial defects. Corneal sensation is reduced, recovery from acute attacks is slow, recalling neuro-paralytic keratitis (except that the lesion is bilateral). The confluence of many ring-like epithelial and sub-epithelial lesions gives a map-like appearance in late stages. Vision is grossly affected | Dominant |
| Calcareous band shaped dystrophy | Bowman's membrane is probably involved primarily. Sibships with a lesion in childhood, or late in life are recorded | ? |

interpalpebral exposed cornea is most severely affected. In the early stages the appearance of superficial punctate keratitis, or of herpes cornea is seen. The scarring in the late stages may take on a striking yellow colour (Fig. 84). The affection is dominant (Fig. 85).

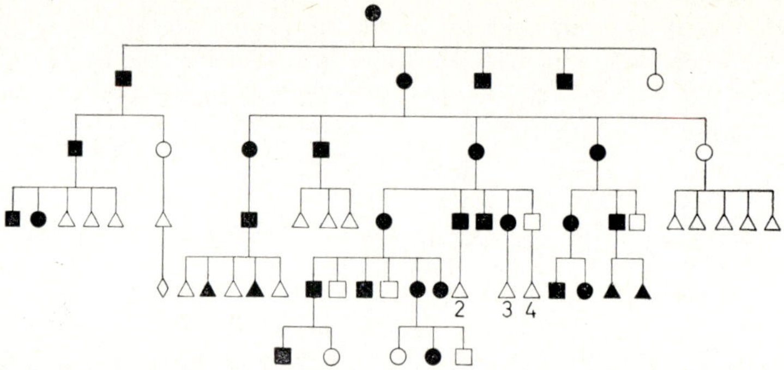


FIG. 83.—Recurrent corneal erosion. Dominant inheritance. (*After Franceschetti*, 1930.)

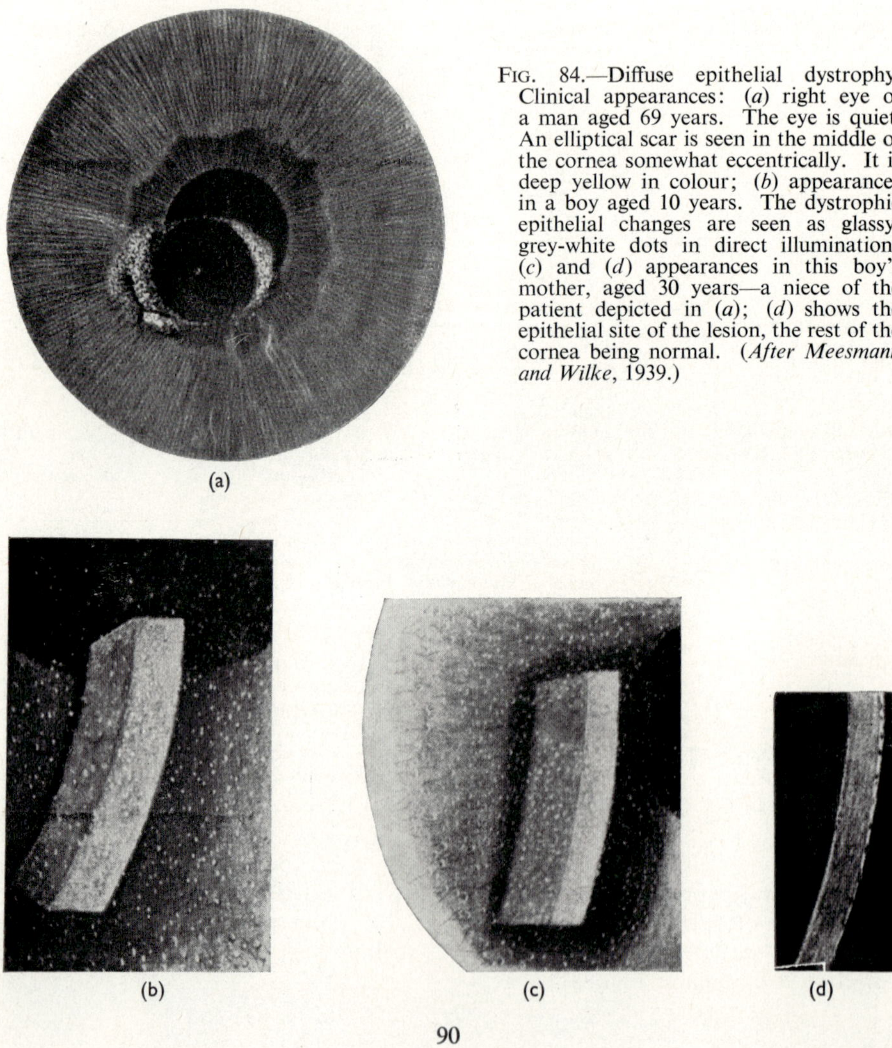

FIG. 84.—Diffuse epithelial dystrophy. Clinical appearances: (*a*) right eye of a man aged 69 years. The eye is quiet. An elliptical scar is seen in the middle of the cornea somewhat eccentrically. It is deep yellow in colour; (*b*) appearances in a boy aged 10 years. The dystrophic epithelial changes are seen as glassy, grey-white dots in direct illumination; (*c*) and (*d*) appearances in this boy's mother, aged 30 years—a niece of the patient depicted in (*a*); (*d*) shows the epithelial site of the lesion, the rest of the cornea being normal. (*After Meesmann and Wilke*, 1939.)

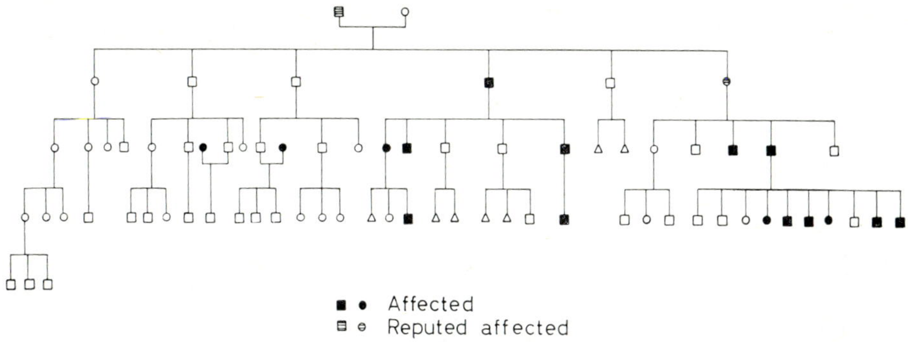


FIG. 85.—Diffuse epithelial dystrophy. Pedigree showing dominant inheritance. (*After Meesmann and Wilke*, 1939.)

## Endothelial dystrophies

### *Cornea guttata*

This is generally regarded as a common non-pathological change that develops with increasing age. The occurrence of these changes over three generations has been observed repeatedly, suggesting that there is a variety that occurs early in life. It is not clear whether in these families the course is free from pathological sequels.

### *Polymorphous endothelial dystrophy*

Changes more extensive than cornea guttata, taking the form of slight concavities, vesicles and polymorphic opacities (Fig. 86) have been reported, in several instances over two generations and over three generations (Fig. 87). Its course and complications are not too well established.

## Compound endothelial and epithelial dystrophies

Two types of compound endothelial and epithelial dystrophies may be distinguished. It is not known whether they are in fact different aspects of one and the same entity.

### "*Senile epithelial dystrophy*" (*Fuchs*)

The appearances are characteristic (Fig. 88) and the compound nature of this affection is well established. Small vesicles, which may coalesce to form bullae, appear in the epithelium, whilst the parenchyma becomes thickened and turbid, especially in the centre. Descemet's membrane and the endothelium show the appearances of cornea guttata to an exaggerated extent and vision is greatly reduced. It is generally accepted that the endothelial changes are primary. The possibility that this affection is genetically determined is supported by case records of the affection in sibships. The fact that the affection is only noted late in life (it is not often seen under 50 years) may account for the difficulty in obtaining adequate pedigrees. It is said to be more common in women. "Intermittent primary chronic oedema of the cornea" is an anomaly which affects the central part of the cornea mainly and is generally more marked in the mornings on waking. It is uncertain whether it is an independent and possibly genetic affection, or the early stages of Fuchs' dystrophy.

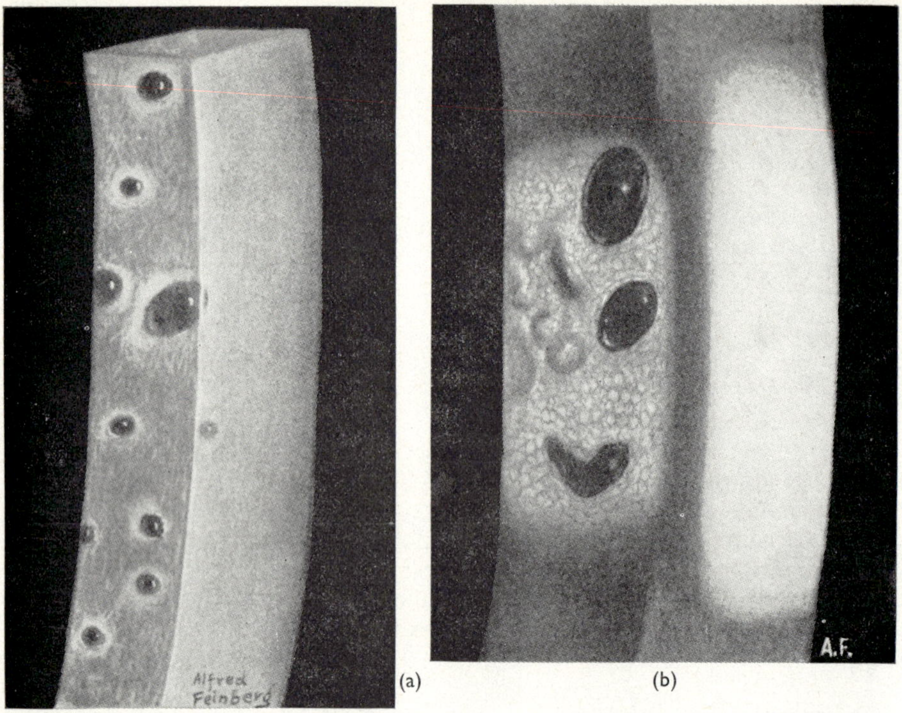


FIG. 86.—Endothelial dystrophy of the cornea. Slit-lamp appearances in a girl aged 18 years. (Magnification: × 16 and × 31 respectively.) (*After Theodore*, 1939.)

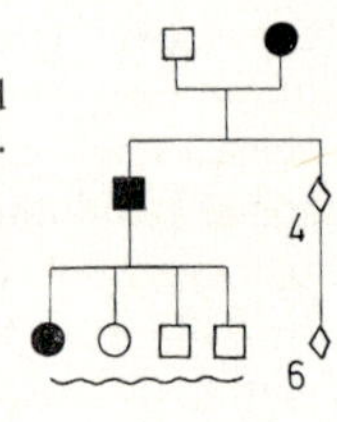


FIG. 87.—Endothelial dystrophy of the cornea. Pedigree of patient illustrated in Fig. 86. Observed occurrences of the lesion over three generations. (*After Theodore*, 1939.)

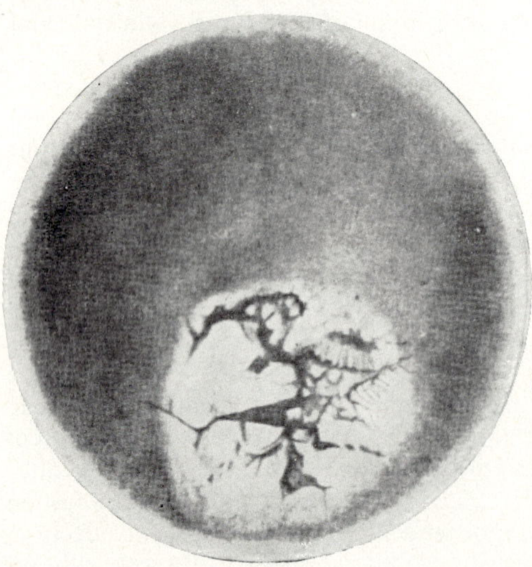

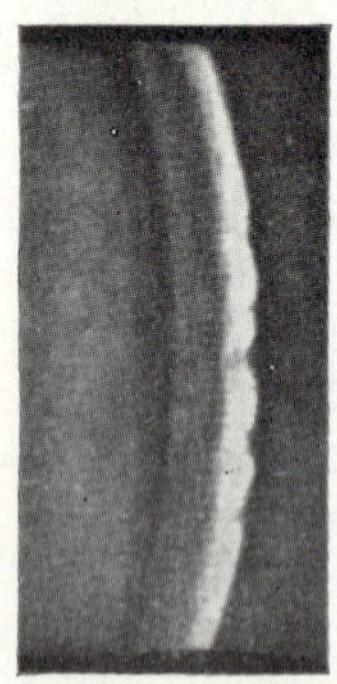

FIG. 88.—Compound endothelial and epithelial dystrophies. Clinical appearances of the senile type. (Senile epithelial dystrophy (Fuchs').) (*After Doggart*, 1948.) The appearances in the juvenile type, described by Kraupa, tend to be more acute and more marked, and include considerable milky haziness of the parenchyma.

*Juvenile epithelial dystrophy* (*Kraupa*)

Fine epithelial vesicles produce corneal haze; the parenchyma tends to be involved to a slight extent. It is possible that the condition is congenital and related to congenital opacification of the cornea. It would appear that there are both dominant and recessive varieties.

**Dystrophies of Bowman's membrane**

*Ring-like dystrophy* (*dystrophia annularis*)

Under this designation, Bücklers has described an apparently dominant affection characterized by early onset, frequent "acute attacks", superficial epithelial defects, which on healing leave opacities suggestive of the macular type of dystrophy, but, different from these in being located almost entirely in Bowman's membrane with secondary epithelial and apparently no parenchymatous involvement (Fig. 89). The markedly reduced sensation and slow recovery from acute attacks may suggest neuro-paralytic keratitis, except for the bilateral involvement. The confluence of many ring-like epithelial and subepithelial lesions gives a map-like appearance in late stages. Vision becomes grossly affected relatively early. A pedigree is shown in Fig. 90.

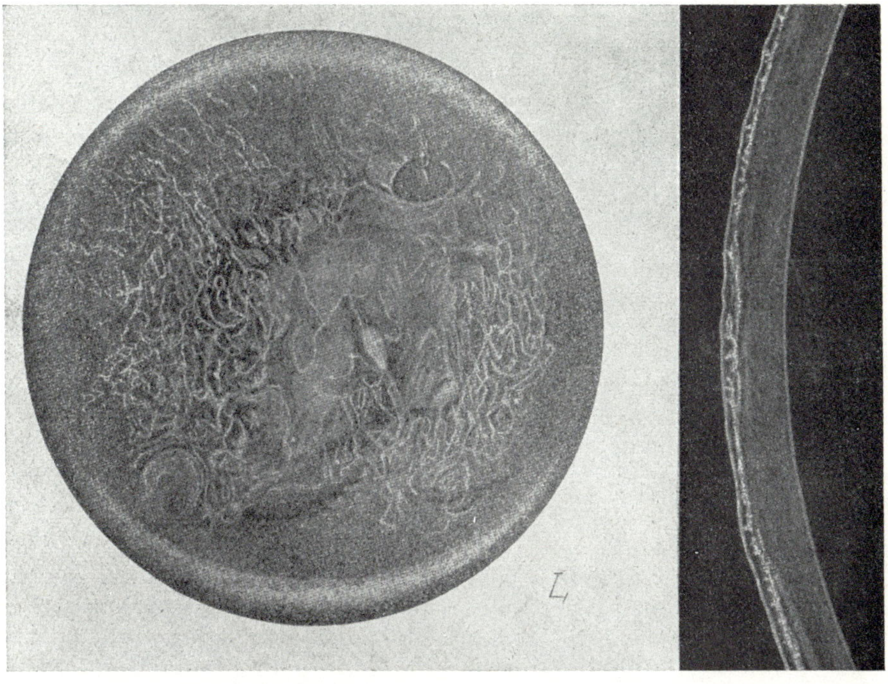

FIG. 89.—Ring-like dystrophy of cornea. (*left*) Appearances in a woman aged 50 years. Irregular heaping-up of narrow lines, arcs and rings. Radial distribution up and in. Cloudy opacification in the pupil area. A thin pigment line below. (*right*) Optical section of the same cornea. Note wave-like superficial surface, thickened epithelium, and marked changes in Bowman's membrane. The stroma is practically clear. (*After Bücklers*, 1949.)

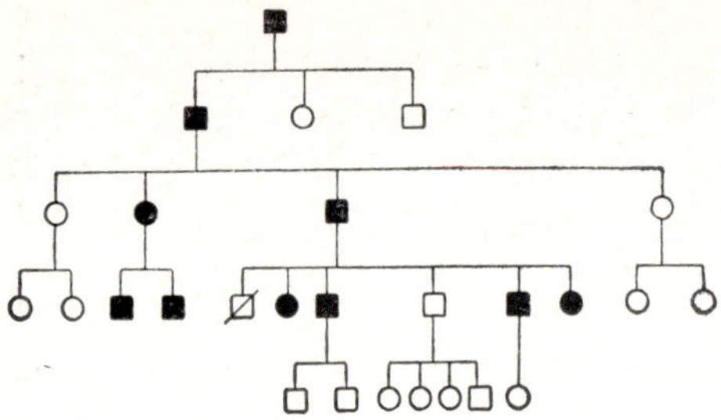

FIG. 90.—Ring-like dystrophy. Pedigree showing dominant inheritance. (*After Bücklers*, 1949.)

FIG. 91.—Calcareous band degeneration. Pedigrees showing three cases in a sibship. (*After Streiff and Zwahlen*, 1946.)

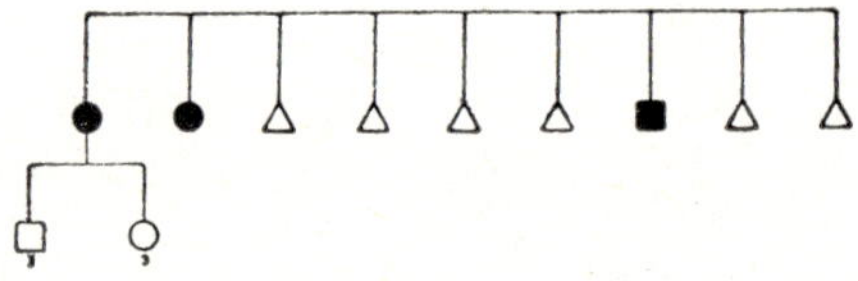

*Calcareous band-shaped dystrophy*

A genetic basis for primary calcareous band degeneration is suggested by several pedigrees, one example being shown in Fig. 91. Histologically, the disturbance is essentially in Bowman's membrane.

## DYSTROPHIES OF UNCERTAIN STATUS

**The marginal dystrophies**

The best established form—a bilateral marginal thinning of the cornea in youngish patients in whom it leads to groove formation and finally a transparent peripheral ectasia with the central cornea distorted to simulate a keratoconus, the cornea ultimately rupturing spontaneously or on slight trauma—is not known as an hereditary disturbance. Marginal anomalies from lipoid infiltration are likewise not known as genetically determined, nor is the deposition of whitish opacities ("white limbus girdle"). Crystalline deposits at the corneal periphery have been seen in two brothers affected with retinitis punctata albescens (Bietti, 1937).

**"Neuroparalytic keratitis"**

Fig. 92 shows the pedigree of a family with neurological disorders in which several members showed disturbances in sensation along the sensory branch of the fifth cranial nerve and the development of torpid corneal ulcers with scarring.

## DIFFICULTIES OF CLASSIFICATION

Although of considerable help clinically, the classification of corneal dystrophies into two main groups—those essentially parenchymatous and those largely non-parenchymatous and mainly limited to one or other layer—is essentially artificial. Few of the dystrophies are entirely confined to one layer only and it does not follow that even these few would be found to be so limited, if more extensive investigations were available. The classification given here is largely in deference to traditional teaching, in that the three classical forms of dystrophy are described as dystrophies involving mainly parenchyma of the cornea. There is no logical reason for not describing, say, recessive macular dystrophy as a lesion of Bowman's

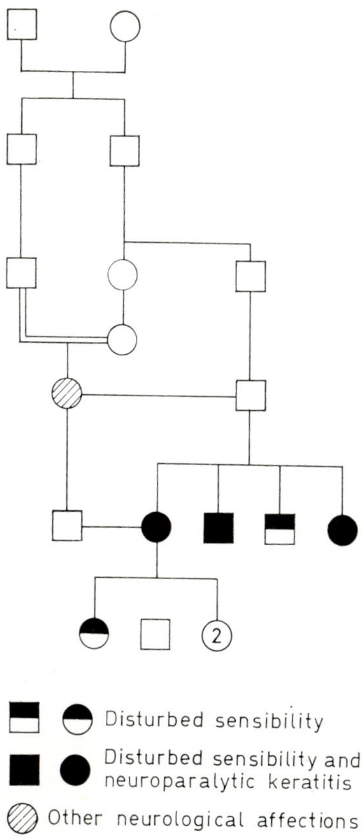


FIG. 92.—Neuroparalytic keratitis. (*After Verrey and Jécquier*, 1949.)

membrane with secondary involvement of the parenchyma. In contrast there is no logical reason for not describing endothelial dystrophy as a parenchymatous lesion with the earliest changes in the endothelium. In stressing these difficulties, it is not suggested that the different corneal dystrophies are not individualized entities with characteristic courses of their own. Such a reading would be as unhelpful as it is unwarranted. There is, however, room for more detailed studies than are as yet available. Such studies may well modify the present classification in important respects.

## FOR FURTHER READING

**Anomalies in Size and Shape**

*Microcornea*

François, J. and Neetens, A. (1955). *Acta Genet. med. Gemell.*, **4**, 217.
Friedman, M. W. and Wright, E. S. (1952). *Am. J. Ophthal.*, **35**, 1017.

*Megalocornea*

Bell, Julia (1933). In *The Treasury of Human Inheritance*, Ed. by K. Pearson, Vol. II, Pt. V. London; Cambridge University Press.
Gredig, C. (1926). *Arch. Klaus-Stift. Vererb. Forsch.*, **2**, 79.
Grönholm, V. (1921). *Klin. Mbl. Augenheilk.*, **67**, 1.
Kayser, B. (1914). *Klin. Mbl. Augenheilk.*, **52**, 226.

*Cornea Plana*
Barkan, H. and Borley, W. E. (1936). *Am. J. Ophthal.*, **19**, 307.
Forsius, H. and Lehmann, W. (1962). *Acta genet. Statist. med.*, **12**, 230.
Larsen, V. and Eriksen, A. (1949). *Acta ophthal.*, **27**, 275.

*Keratoconus*
Amsler, M. (1946). *Ophthalmologica*, **111**, 96.
— (1951). *Bull. Soc. franç. Ophtal.*, **64**, 272.
Rados, A. (1948). *Archs Ophthal.*, **40**, 454.
Rumpf, J. (1937). *Contribution á l'etude de l'hérédite de Keratocône.* Lausanne; Thesis.

*Krukenberg's Spindle*
Evans, W. H., Odom, R. E. and Wenaas, E. J. (1941). *Archs Ophthal.*, **26**, 1023.

*Cornea Verticillata*
Denden, A. (1963). *Ber. dt. ophthal. Ges.*, **65**, 125.
François, J. (1967). *Ann. mèd. Nancy*, **6**, 382.
Gruber, M. (1946). *Ophthalmologica*, **112**, 88.

**Corneal Dystrophies**
*Essentially Parenchymatous*
Bücklers, M. (1938). *Die erblichen Hornhautdystrophien* (*Klin. Monatsbl. f. Augenheilk.*, Suppl. 3). Stuttgart; Enke.
Franceschetti, A. and Klein, D. (1963). In *Genetics and Ophthalmology*, Ed. by P. J. Waardenburg, A. Franceschetti and D. Klein, Vol I, pp. 456–498. Oxford; Blackwell.
Saebø, J. (1939). *Skr. norske vid. Akad. Oslo*, No. 3.

*Essentially Non-parenchymatous*
*Epithelial*
Burki, E. (1946). *Ophthalmologica*, **111**, 134.
Meesmann, A. and Wilke, F. (1939). *Klin. Mbl. Augenheilk.*, **103**, 361.

*Endothelial*
McGee, H. B. and Falls, H. (1953). *Archs Ophthal.*, **50**, 462.
Theodore, F. H. (1939). *Archs Ophthal.*, **21**, 626.

*Compound endothelial and epithelial*
El-Arabi, M. E. (1953). *Bull. Ophthal. Soc. Egypt*, **46**, 223.
Guntz-Schussler, E. (1947). *Klin. Mbl. Augenheilk.*, **112**, 70.
Kraupa, E. (1934). *Z. Augenheilk.*, **83**, 179.

*Ring-like Dystrophy* (*of Bowman's Membrane*)
Bücklers, M. (1949). *Klin. Mbl. Augenheilk.*, **114**, 386.

*Calcareous Dystrophy*
Franceschetti, A. and Schlaeppi, V. (1957). *Dermatologica* (*Basle*), **115**, 217.
Streiff, E. B. and Zwahlen, P. (1946). *Ophthalmologica*, **111**, 129.

## CHAPTER 7

# THE LENS

## ANOMALIES IN SHAPE, SIZE AND SITE

### Congenital subluxation

Whilst the recognition of Marfan's syndrome goes back to 1896, recent years have brought two further syndromes in which anomalies of the shape, size and site of the lens are cardinal signs: the Marchesani syndrome recognized in 1939 and the homocystinuria defect in 1962. These syndromes are discussed elsewhere (pp. 209 and 238); their recognition raises the question of whether the older pedigrees recording inheritance of subluxation of the lens, coloboma of the lens and the spherophakia-microphakia defect are indeed incomplete records of these syndromes rather than of localized lens defects. Fig. 93 illustrates dominant inheritance of subluxation of the lens: in the first the affection was present at birth, and in the second it developed in middle life. Fig. 94 shows that coloboma of the lens is often an aspect of dominantly inherited subluxation. These and such like families do not appear to have been investigated for the possibility of the dominantly inherited Marfan's syndrome or its variants.

One form of subluxation of the lens—that associated with ectopic pupils—is regarded as inherited in a recessive manner and to constitute a distinct entity differing from the dominantly inherited anomalies. The many familial cases recorded and the high incidence of parental consanguinity in such cases support such a reading, but recent records, such as that in Fig. 95 have shown that some members of affected sibships may have the lens defect only, without the ectopic pupils. Fuller studies than are as yet available on any associated systemic anomalies in these cases should help to clarify their status.

### Delayed spontaneous subluxation

In some individuals subluxation of the lens, generally downwards, occurs without apparent cause in adult life at almost any age. A congenital abnormality of the zonule is assumed; the symptoms and complications are essentially those seen in the congenital variety of subluxation.

Fig. 96 shows an early pedigree recorded by Vogt in 1905 and 1931. This shows dominant inheritance and the pedigree has since been extended to cover four generations (Franceschetti and Klein, 1961). Irregular dominance has also been recorded (Waardenburg, 1938).

### Coloboma of the lens

This has been observed in typical colobomatous defects of the eye. It may, however, also occur as an aspect and possibly as a variant of subluxation of the lens (*see* Fig. 94).

### Microphakia or spherophakia

Occasionally the lens is both small and highly spherical; with a dilated pupil the margin of the lens can be seen clearly, and with the slit-lamp the zonule easily

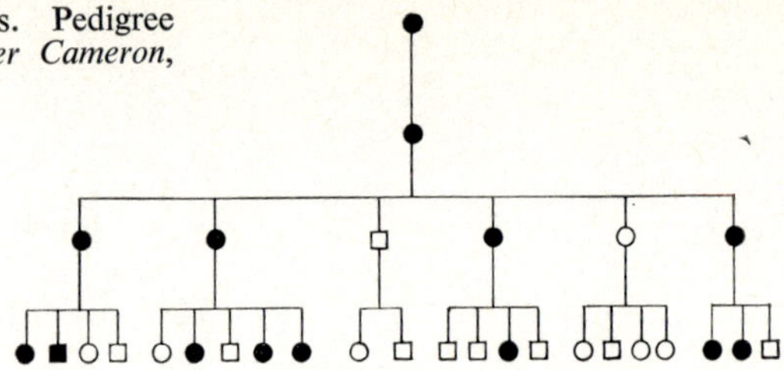

FIG. 93.—Congenital subluxation of lens. Pedigree showing dominant inheritance. (*After Cameron*, 1926.)

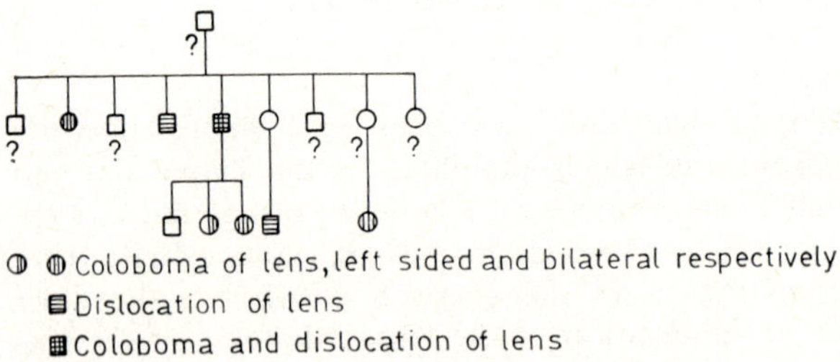


FIG. 94.—Coloboma of lens. Pedigree over two generations of a family, some members of which showed coloboma or dislocation of the lens only, and others both defects. (*After Clark*, 1919.)

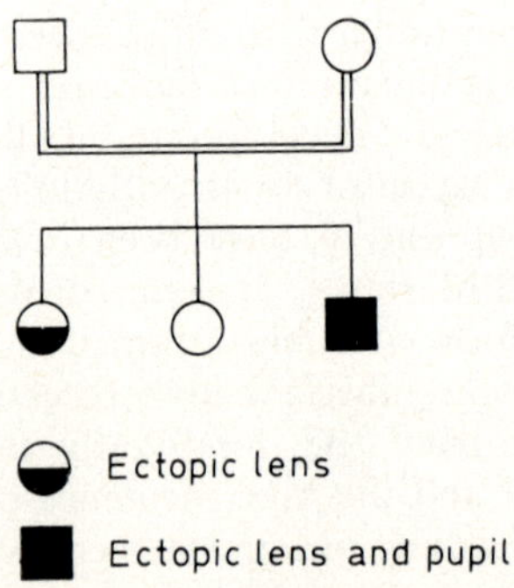


FIG. 95.—Ectopia lentis et pupillae. Incomplete penetrance. (*After Diethelm*, 1947.)

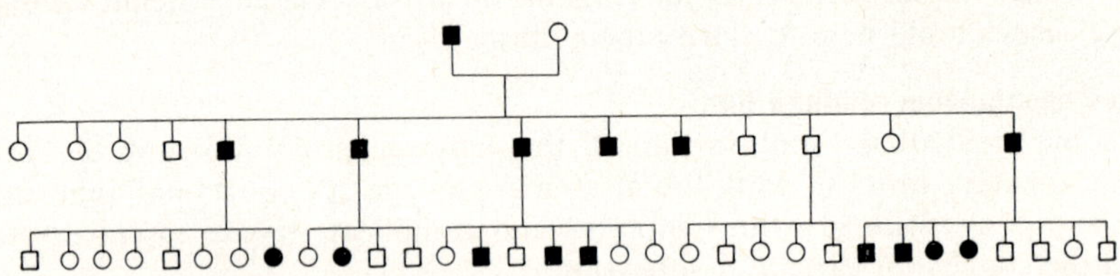

FIG. 96.—Delayed spontaneous dislocation of the lens. Pedigree showing dominant inheritance. (*After Vogt*, 1931.)

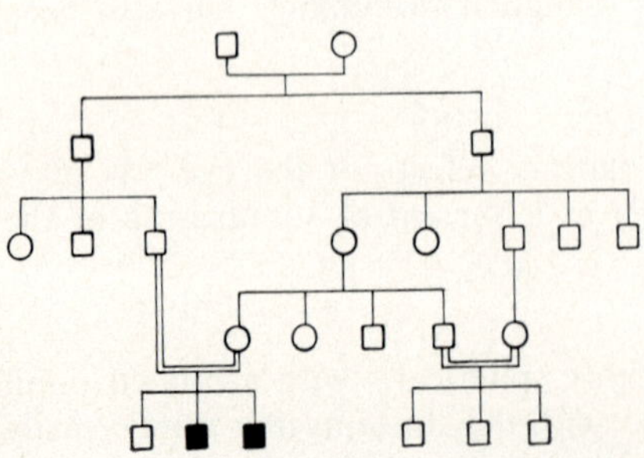

FIG. 97.—Microphakia and high myopia. Pedigree suggestive of recessive inheritance. (*After Waardenburg*, 1932.)

distinguished. A high degree of lenticular myopia is common, and subluxation and secondary glaucoma are not infrequent. Accommodation is affected.

The available evidence suggests that the affection is exclusively recessive (Fig. 97).

**Lenticonus**

Most cases are sporadic and unilateral. Recessive or possibly irregularly dominant inheritance may occur (Butler, 1938).

## CATARACT

The architecture of the lens, as revealed by the slit-lamp, enables a clear distinction to be made between congenital and post-natal cataract. Only nuclear or capsular cataract can be congenital, whilst a cortical cataract must be postnatal.

### Congenital Cataract

Cataract may occur as an aspect of other congenital and hereditary anomalies of the eye, as in microphthalmos, and aniridia, and presumably also in abiotrophic affections, as in some forms of retinitis pigmentosa. Frequently, however, cataract is the only, or the outstanding, abnormality.

FIG. 98.—Congenital cataract. Pedigree showing recessive inheritance—apparently unusual in congenital cataract. (*After Saebø*, 1949.)

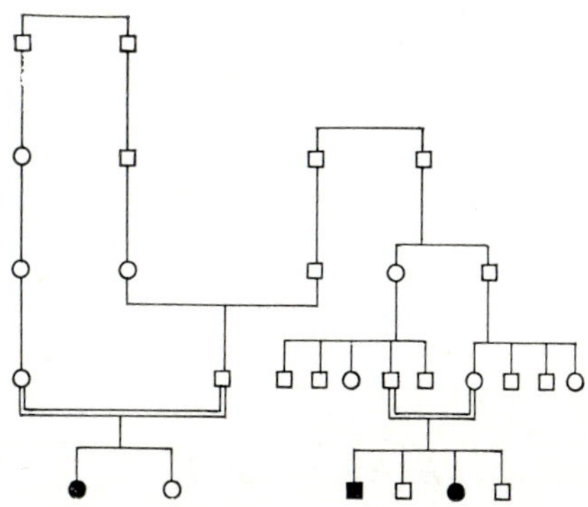

The older literature has established that hereditary congenital cataract is usually transmitted in a dominant manner, and although this holds good for the individual types that have become clearly defined with the advent of slit-lamp microscopy, recessive inheritance in some families is no longer regarded as very exceptional. This is shown by Fig. 98, which is one of 17 consecutive pedigrees in which consanguinity could be established in 9 families, whilst in no family was there any evidence of dominance. A few pedigrees—such as that shown in Fig. 99—suggest the possibility of sex-linked inheritance.

**Total cataract**

Total congenital cataract may be part of various developmental anomalies, including those caused by maternal rubella, and those seen in infants with very

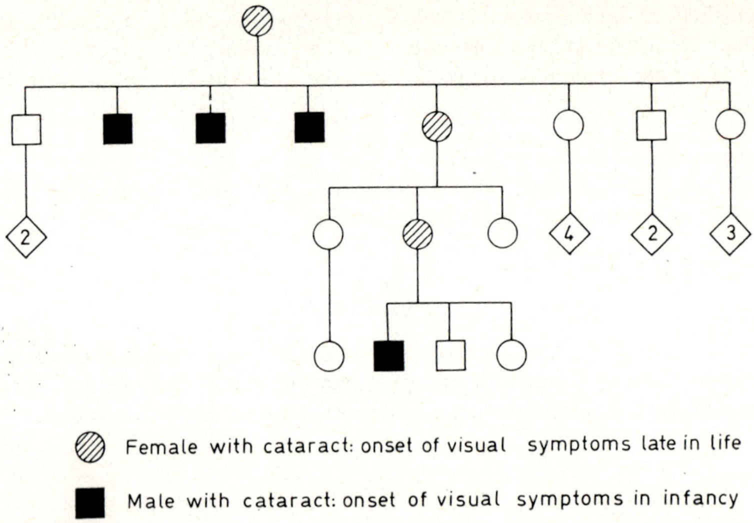


FIG. 99.—Cataract: possibly sex-linked inheritance. (*After Fraser and Friedmann*, 1967.)

low birth weights. In the genetic forms inheritance appears to be dominant (Fig. 100).

These cataracts are frequently fibrous, and do not respond well to needling. The presence of nystagmus in many of the children may be secondary, but may also presumably arise from foveal hypoplasia—an assumption supported by the fact that the results of successful surgical treatment are not too good; the resultant vision is generally of the order of 6/60 to 6/36.

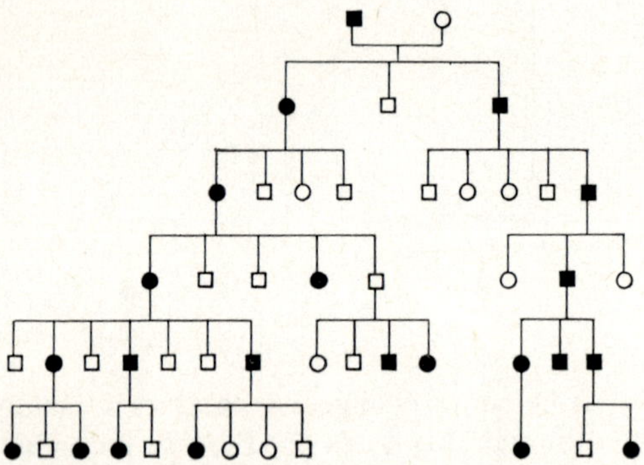

FIG. 100.—Total congenital cataract. Pedigree showing dominant inheritance. (*After Meissner*, 1933.)

**Lamellar cataract**

This is a composite entity, and some forms at least are due to nutritional disturbances in the mother. Dominant inheritance has been observed repeatedly (Fig. 101 *a*); irregular dominance also occurs. A possibly recessive mode of inheritance is suggested by Fig. 101 *b*.

**Nuclear cataract**

This is not always easy to distinguish from lamellar cataract, as many nuclear cataracts have outlying riders. There are at least three distinct types. (1) In one form the opacity is dense or patterned, with severe visual disturbances (Fig. 102 *a* and *b*). (2) There is a less severe form, which may be observable only by slit-lamp examination—the so-called cataracta pulverulenta, of which the Coppock cataract is a specially marked variety (Fig. 102 *c*, *d* and *e*). (3) Disc-shaped (ring) cataract. In this anomaly the lens is dumb-bell shaped with the centre being fibrous (Fig. 102 *f*). Clinically there is a central opacity at a distinctly deeper level than the rest of the surface of the lens, with other irregular opacities. With a small pupil

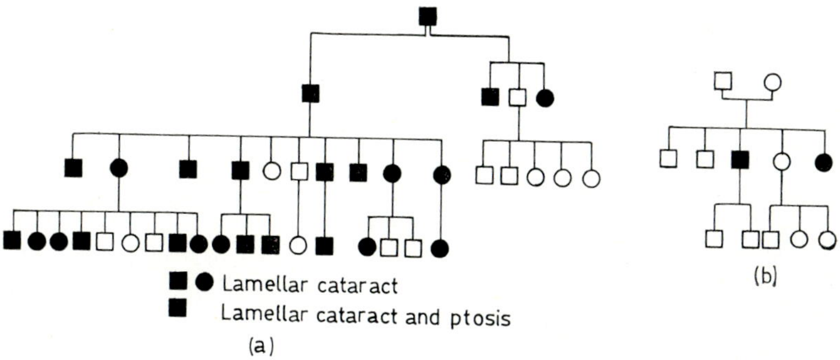


FIG. 101.—Lamellar cataract. (*a*) Pedigree showing dominant inheritance. (*After Nettleship*, 1909.) (*b*) Pedigree suggestive of recessive inheritance. (*After Saebø*, 1949.)

the central opacity may fill the entire pupillary area; with a dilated pupil a peripheral clear zone can be seen. The lens as a whole is the shape of a ring-like life-belt. Subluxation of the lens is a frequent, and possibly a constant concomitant.

Inheritance of all these forms of central cataract would appear to be dominant (Fig. 103 *a*, *b*, *c* and *d*). In the Coppock family originally studied by Nettleship, the locus for the pulverulent cataract has been found closely linked with that for the Duffy blood group (Renwick and Lawler, 1963).

## Other forms

### *Anterior and posterior polar cataracts*

*Anterior polar cataracts* may be minimal without any visual disturbance, or may take the variant form of pyramidal cataract with considerable visual disturbance; it may also be an aspect of other forms of congenital cataract, such as lamellar cataract. Fig. 104 shows dominant inheritance.

In *posterior polar cataract*, too, there is a considerable range in manifestation. Dominant inheritance is shown in Fig. 105.

### *Suture cataract*

Anterior axial embryonal cataract hardly falls within the pathological range. It has been observed over four generations (Schmid, 1924). Stellate cataract, involving both Y sutures, is also of no great clinical significance. It has been observed over three generations (Jordan, 1955).

### *Crystalline cataract*

Three forms of cataract show crystal formation (Fig. 106). They are apparently independent entities with the same dominant mode of inheritance. Fig. 107 *a*, *b* and *c*, show pedigrees of coralliform, spear-like, and floriform cataract respectively.

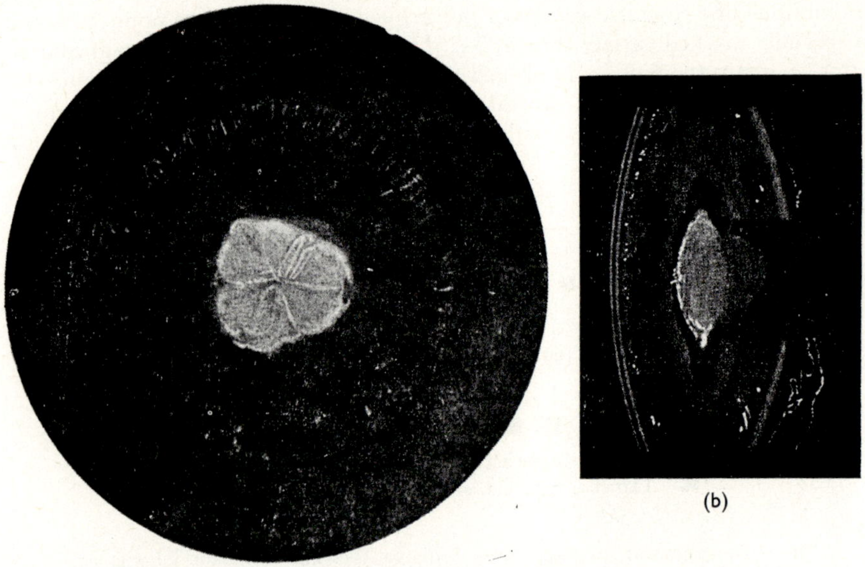

(b)

(a)

FIG. 102.—The clinical forms of central cataract. (*a–e after Bücklers*, 1938.)
(*a*) and (*b*) Central cataract. Face view and optical section respectively in a woman, aged 29 years.

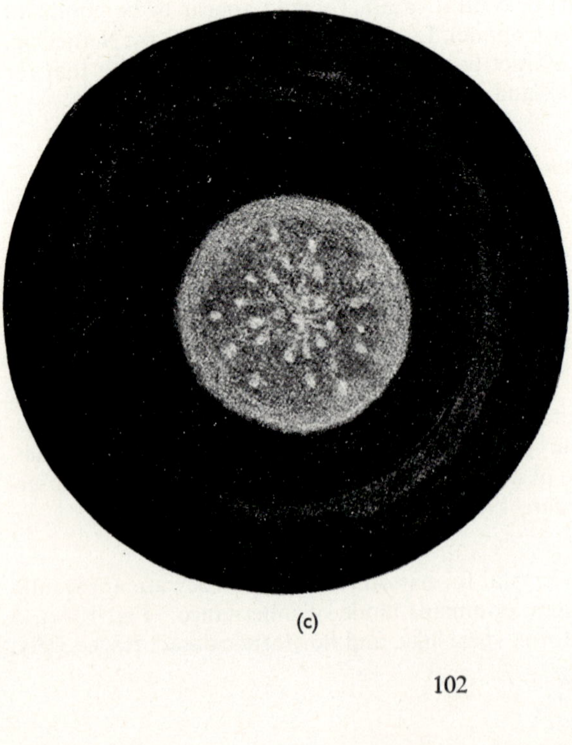

(c)

FIG. 102 (*cont.*).—(*c*) Pulverulent cataract; moderately developed. Face view in a boy aged 12 years.

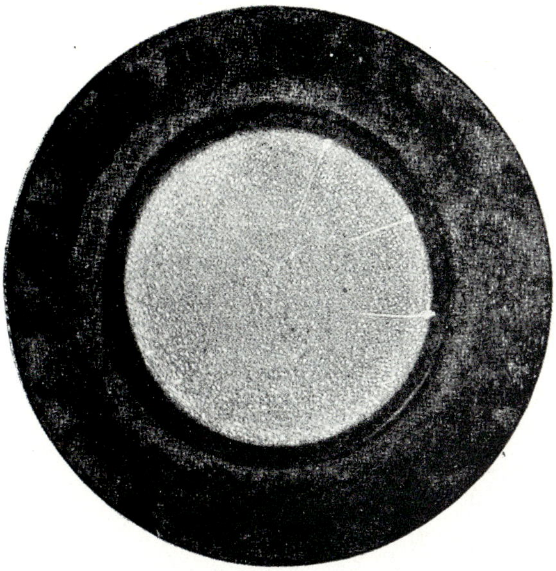

(d)

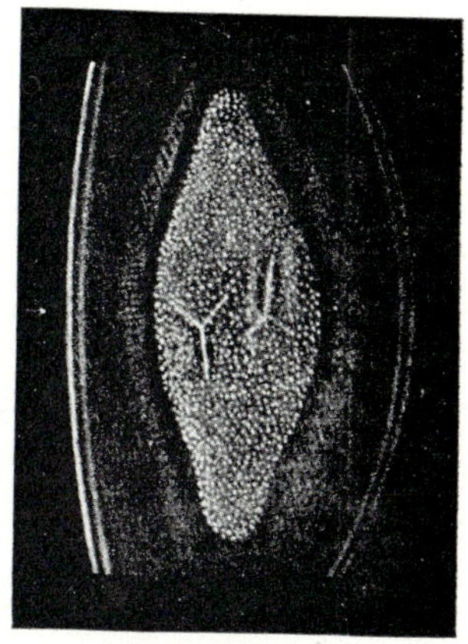

(e)

FIG. 102 (*cont.*).—(*d* and *e*) Pulverulent cataract. Face view and optical section respectively of a well-developed pulverulent cataract in a man aged 37 years.

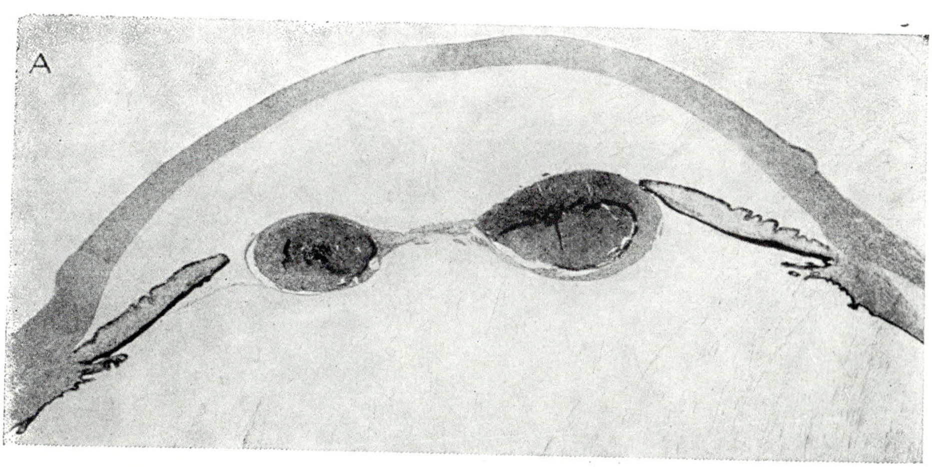


(f)

FIG. 102 (*cont.*).—(*f*) Disc-shaped cataract. Anatomical section of an eye in a girl aged 5 years. (*After Haro*, 1946.)

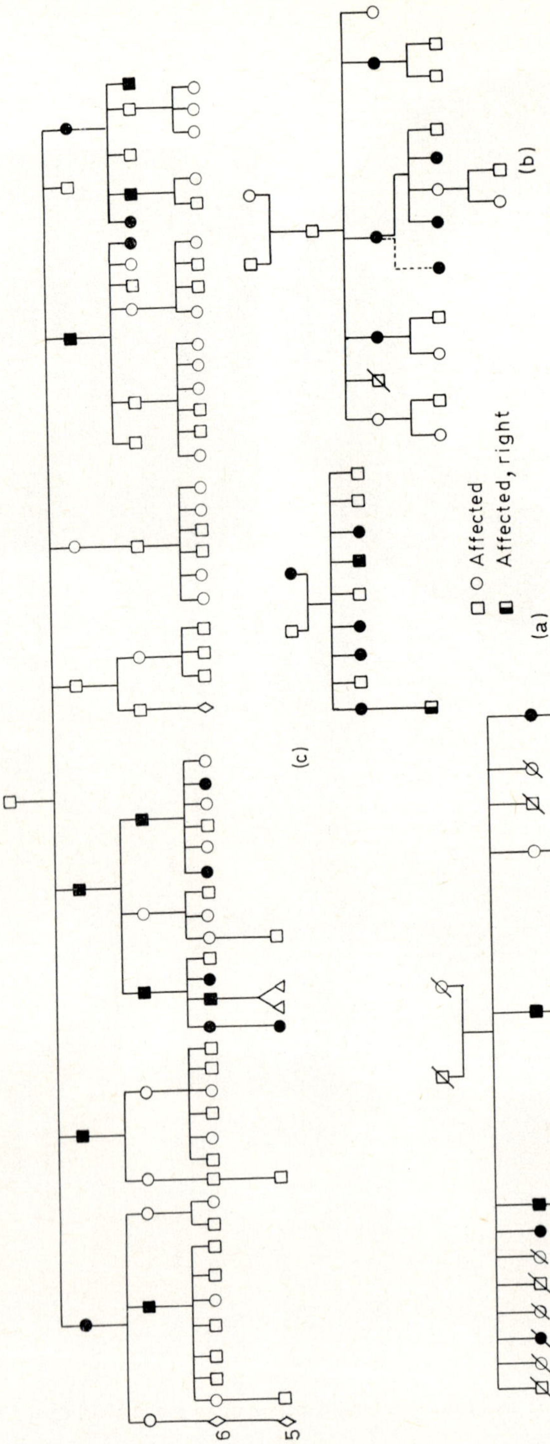


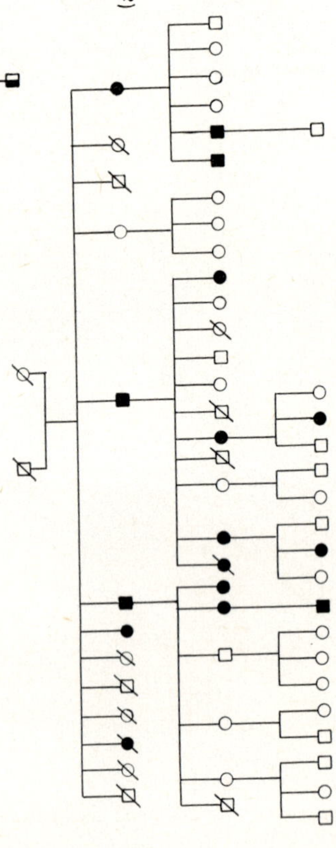


FIG. 103.—Central cataract. Pedigrees. (*a*) Inheritance of central cataract over three generations. (*After Bücklers*, 1938.) (*b*) Pulverulent cataract. Inheritance over two generations. (*After Vogt*, 1931.) (*c*) "Coppock" cataract. Dominant inheritance. (*After Nettleship and Ogilvie*, 1906.) (*d*) Disc-shaped "ring" cataract. Dominant inheritance. (*After Haro*, 1946.)

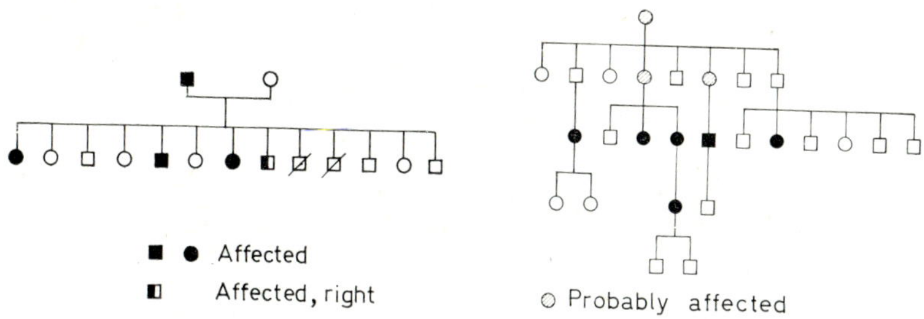


FIG. 104.—Anterior polar cataract. Pedigrees suggestive of dominant inheritance. (*After Vogt*, 1931, *and Dohlman*, 1951.)

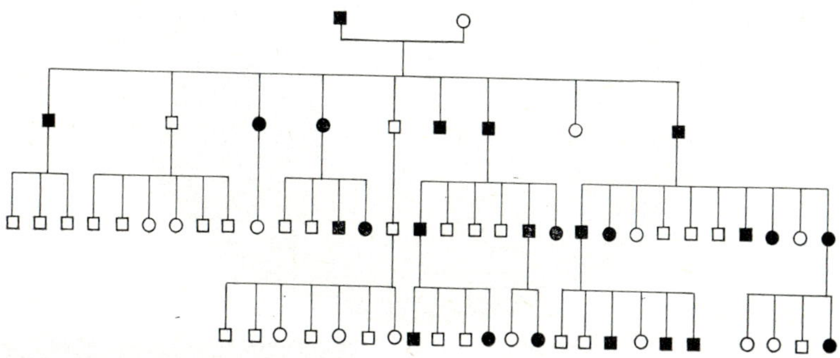

FIG. 105.—Posterior polar cataract. Pedigree showing dominant inheritance. (*After Ziegler and Griscom*, 1915.)

*Lentoid formation.*—Occasionally lens fibres may regenerate from capsular remains after needling operations. Genetically determined formation of multiple lentoid structures resulting in bizarre bodies in front of or behind the iris has been observed in a family with needled congenital cataract, "perinuclear" in type and dominant in inheritance (Fig. 108).

## POST-NATAL CATARACT

Evidence of the genetic character of post-natal cataract is readily available for the cataracts occurring early in life. For the primary cataract late in life there are no adequate pedigrees, probably owing to the difficulty in obtaining satisfactory information.

### Coronary cataract

In this form, adequately described by the synonyms coronary cataract, blue dot cataract and punctate cataract, changes first appear at about puberty and are confined to the periphery of the lens, covered by the contracted pupil. As these changes are common, their inheritance must be held as unproved until there is more information than is at present available.

### Pre-senile cataract of the adult nucleus

This is a well defined type with dominant inheritance. Fig. 109 *a* illustrates a pedigree in which coronary cataract, nuclear and perinuclear opacities occurred in the same family. Whether these were interchangeable, or an accidental

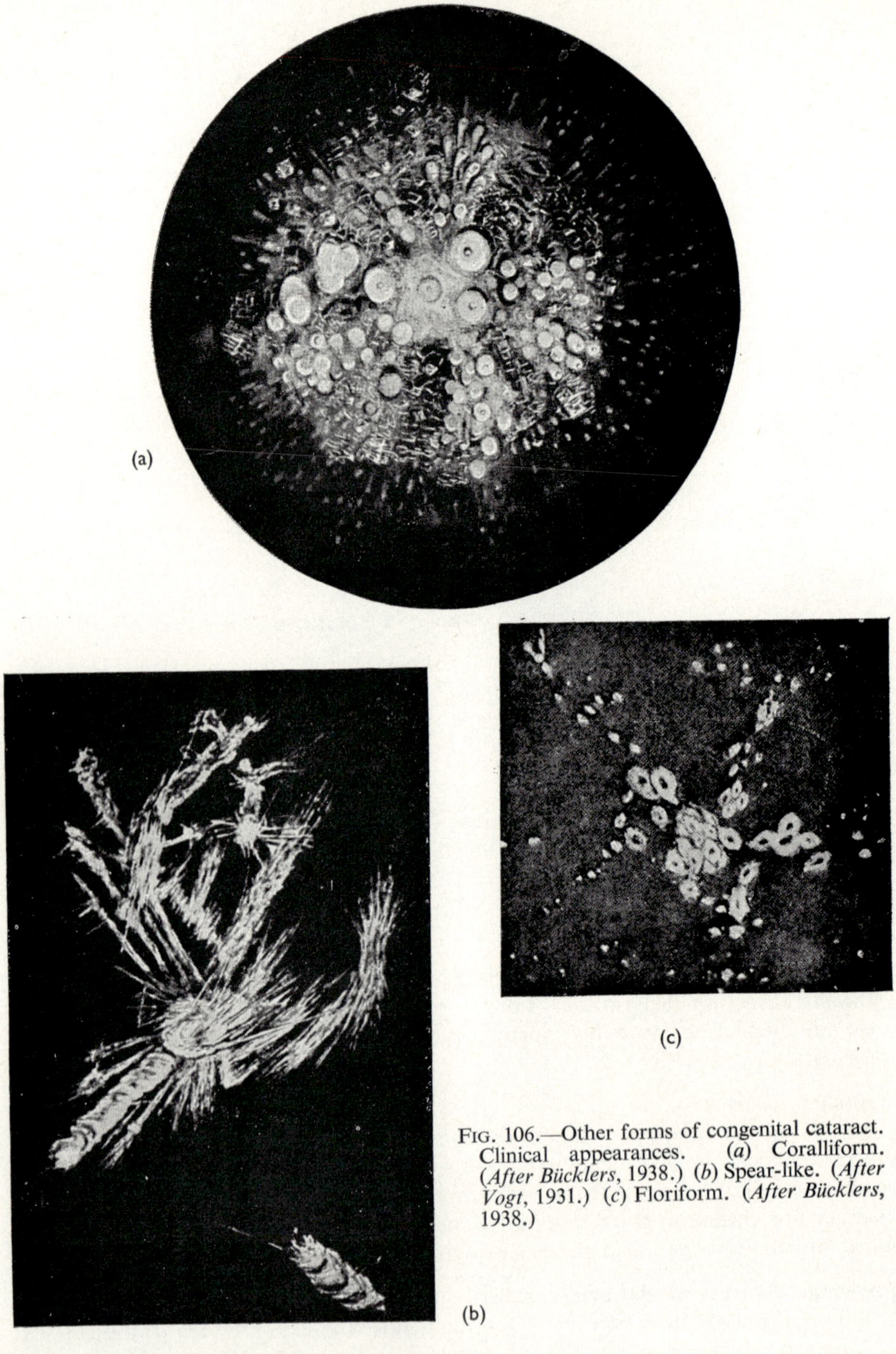

FIG. 106.—Other forms of congenital cataract. Clinical appearances. (*a*) Coralliform. (*After Bücklers*, 1938.) (*b*) Spear-like. (*After Vogt*, 1931.) (*c*) Floriform. (*After Bücklers*, 1938.)

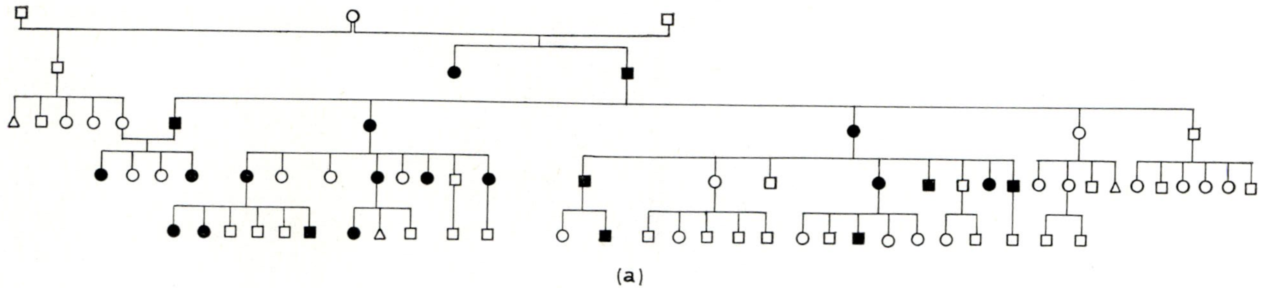


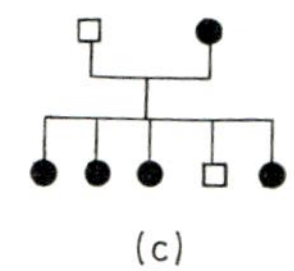


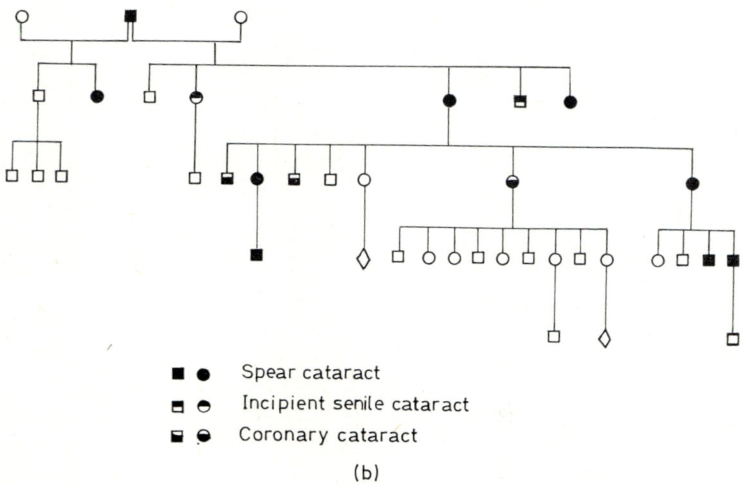


FIG. 107.—Other forms of congenital cataract. Pedigrees. (*a*) Coralliform cataract. Pedigree showing dominant inheritance. (*After Nettleship*, 1909.) (*b*) Spear-like cataract. Pedigree showing dominant inheritance. (*After Romer*, 1926.) (*c*) Floriform cataract. Pedigree showing inheritance over two generations. (*After Koby*, 1923.)

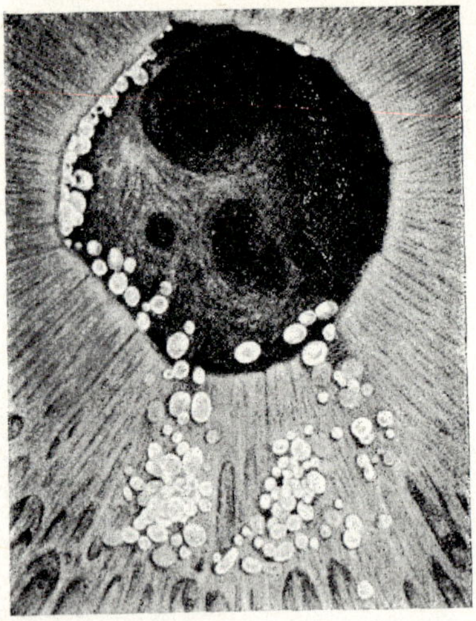

FIG. 108.—Lentoid formation. Observed in different members of a family after needling for congenital dominant "perinuclear" cataract. (*After Riedl*, 1939.)

combination of two genetic anomalies within the same family, is not known. Fig. 109 *b* illustrates dominant inheritance of changes in the cortex.

A pedigree in which different members were affected by opacities in the axial region of the anterior adult nucleus, and others by opacities in the foetal nucleus is shown in Fig. 109 *c*. The pedigree of a family in which some members had pre-senile cataract and others total cataract present at birth or developing in infancy is recorded in Fig. 109 *d*.

**Pre-senile posterior cortical cataract**

This has been observed in several members of the same sibship. Its mode of inheritance is uncertain (Schnyder, 1926, 1927; Alajmo and Rubino, 1935).

TABLE VIII

SYSTEMIC DISORDERS IN WHICH CONGENITAL CATARACT IS SEEN

| | |
|---|---|
| Metabolic disorders | Galactosaemia<br>Lowe's syndrome |
| Syndermatotic cataract | Rothmund's syndrome<br>Werner's syndrome<br>Congenital ichthyosis<br>Incontinenti pigmenti |
| Muscle affections | Myotonia dystrophica |
| Neurological disorders | Sjögren's syndrome of mental deficiency with cataract<br>Marinesco–Sjögren syndrome with the additional feature of spinocerebellar ataxia<br>Sjögren–Larsson syndrome<br>Down's syndrome<br>Cockayne's syndrome |
| Bony disorders | Contradi's syndrome<br>Mandibulo-facial dysostosis |

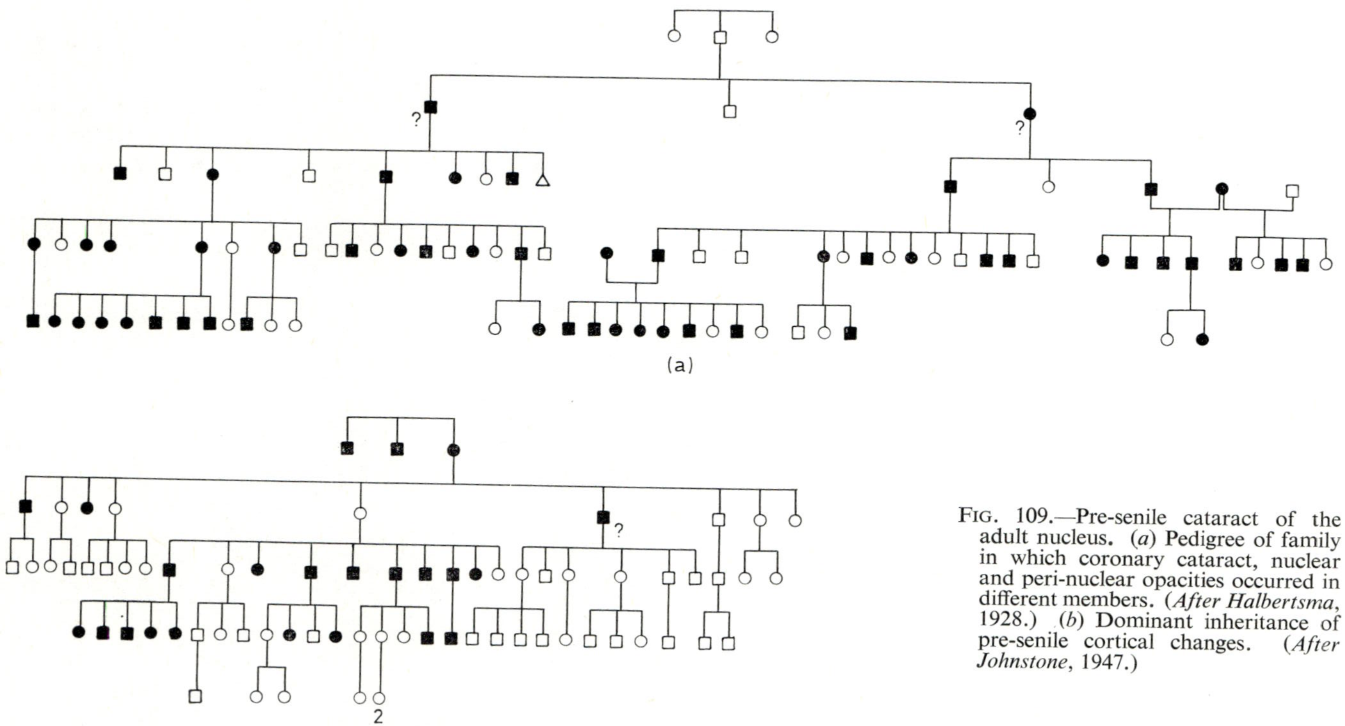


FIG. 109.—Pre-senile cataract of the adult nucleus. (*a*) Pedigree of family in which coronary cataract, nuclear and peri-nuclear opacities occurred in different members. (*After Halbertsma*, 1928.) (*b*) Dominant inheritance of pre-senile cortical changes. (*After Johnstone*, 1947.)

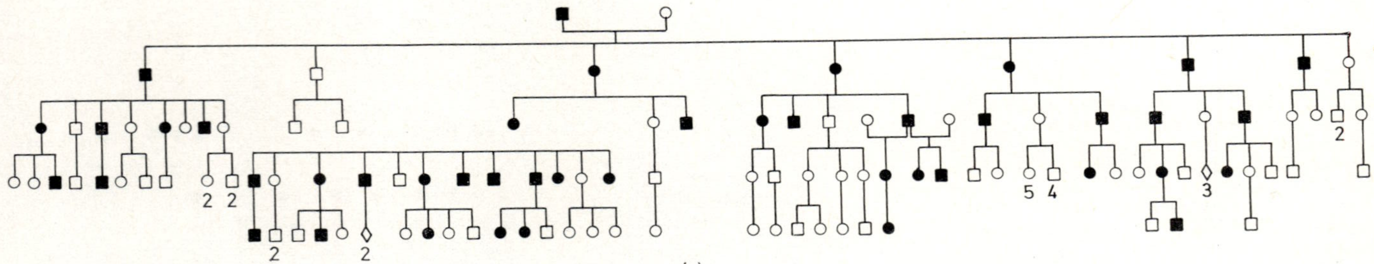

(c)

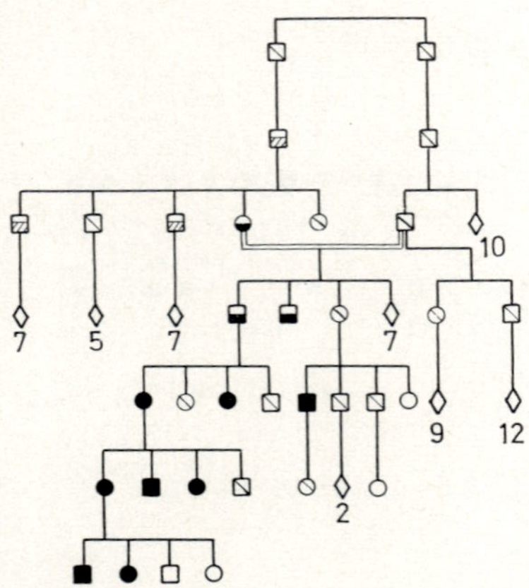


(d)

FIG. 109 (*cont.*).—(*c*) Pedigree of a family in which opacities of either adult or foetal nucleus occurred. (*After Lutman and Neel*, 1945.) (*d*) Pedigree of a family in which pre-senile cataract occurred in some members and total congenital or infantile cataract in others. (*After Redl*, 1949.)

- Reputed affected with pre-senile cataract
- Observed as affected with pre-senile cataract
- Observed as affected with congenital or infantile total cataract
- Reputed normal
- Observed as normal

### Senile cataract

The best evidence as yet available as to the genetic basis of senile cataract is derived from the work of Vogt on the frequency of senile cataract in both members of a pair of uniovular twins late in life. Concordance in such cases extends to the details observed during the development of the cataract (Vogt and colleagues, 1939).

## Further Considerations

### Relationship of the different forms of cataract to each other

Early pedigrees recorded by Nettleship, and such pedigrees as those shown in Fig. 109 *a*, *c* and *d*, suggest that whilst it is true that within given families the same type of cataract tends to appear, different clinical types tend to overlap. On balance it is unlikely that different members of such families carry genes for different types of cataract. Further clinical observations are required to determine the nature and significance of these morphological variations.

### Cataract as an associated condition

Cataract—usually of the congenital type—is an important aspect of many hereditary systemic disorders. They are considered elsewhere. Table VIII lists the more significant of these disorders.

## FOR FURTHER READING

**Congenital Subluxation**

Cotterman, C. W. and Falls, H. F. (1944). *Ann. Eugen.*, **12**, 158.
Falls, H. F. and Cotterman, C. W. (1943). *Archs Ophthal.*, **30**, 610.

**Congenital Cataract**

François, J. (1959). *Les cataractes congenitales.* Paris; Masson.
Harman, N. B. (1910). In *The Treasury of Human Inheritance*, Ed. by K. Pearson, Vol. 1, Pt. IV, p. 126. London; Cambridge University Press.

**Post-natal Cataract**

Johnstone, I. L. (1947). *Br. J. Ophthal.*, **31**, 385.
Lutman, F. C. and Neel, J. V. (1945). *Archs Ophthal.*, **33**, 341.
Marner, E. (1949). *Acta ophthal.* (*Kbh.*), **27**, 537.
Saebø, J. (1949). *Br. J. Ophthal.*, **33**, 601

## CHAPTER 8

# THE ANTERIOR UVEA

A large number of anomalies of the iris of no pathological significance are recognized. They appear to have a genetic basis, and some, at any rate, are aspects of the wider issue of colour of the iris. It is possible that some of the more marked physiological variants, such as some forms of hypoplasia of the mesodermal layers, are abortive forms of aniridia or of the anterior chamber cleavage syndrome.

## ANOMALIES IN IRIS STRUCTURE

### Atypical coloboma of the iris

Some forms of atypical coloboma of the iris are probably independent of aniridia. Fig. 110 shows the pedigree of a family in which atypical colobomas, unilateral, bilateral or merely minimally developed, occurred. Assuming that such pedigrees illustrate a variety of atypical colobomas independent of aniridia, a possible embryological explanation would lie with the non-closure of secondary fissures in the optic vesicle.

### Hyperplasia

Hyperplasia of the mesodermal layers, giving the appearance of doubling of the mesodermal part of the iris, has been recorded as dominant in inheritance (Pagenstecher, 1925). Hyperplasia of the ectodermal layer of the iris, taking the form of flocculi iridis, has likewise been observed in a dominant mode of inheritance (Fig. 111*a*). The relationship to congenital cyst of the iris—also recorded as dominant (Cowan, 1936)—is not clear.

### Hypoplasia

Hypoplasia of the ectodermal layers is probably part of the aniridia complex. It was seen in an eye which showed a translucent iris with intact stroma, the fellow eye showing aniridia. Hypoplasia of the mesodermal layers has also been observed as dominantly inherited (Hemmes, 1931). In one pedigree in which recessive sex-linkage was seen and was probably a case of the anterior chamber cleavage complex, secondary glaucoma appeared frequently (Fig. 111 *b*). Progressive atrophy of the iris is, however, a possible alternative reading in this family.

### Persistent pupillary membrane

This, too, may be part of the cleavage complex. It may also appear as an isolated hereditary anomaly.

## ANOMALIES IN PIGMENTATION OF THE IRIS

Hypo- and hyperpigmentation of the iris are relative terms and are usually only meaningful on comparing the two eyes. A piebald pattern resulting from unequal pigmentation of different sectors of the iris also occurs.

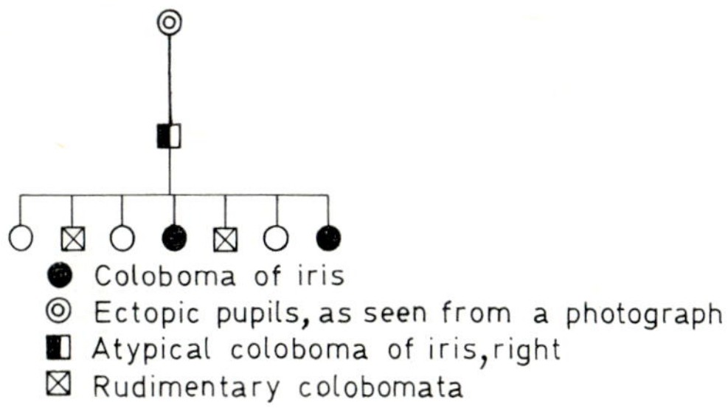


FIG. 110.—Atypical coloboma of the iris. Pedigree showing the range of defects—some minimal—observed in one family. (*After Halbertsma*, 1928.)

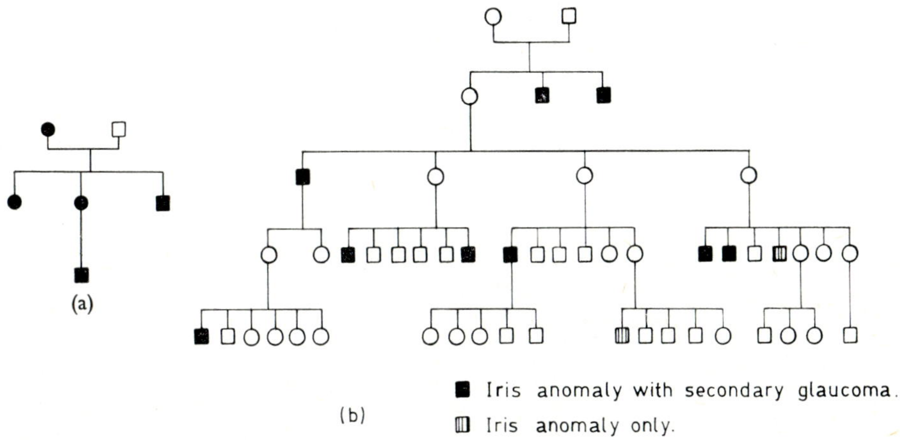


FIG. 111.—Anomalies in iris structure. (*a*) Pedigree showing dominant inheritance of flocculi iridis. (*After Fröhlich*, 1924.) (*b*) Pedigree showing sex-linked inheritance of hypoplasia of the iris complicated by secondary glaucoma. (*After Frank-Kamenetzki*, 1925.)

*Piebald pattern* (*partial heterochromia*)

This is generally in the nature of *iris bicolor*. Common in animals as a dominant feature, it is relatively rare and usually sporadic in man, but dominant inheritance has been observed.

*Heterochromia*

This has been observed in uniovular twins and as a dominant inherited feature (Fig. 112). It is also seen as part of the Klein–Waardenburg syndrome with its irregular dominance and of the regularly dominantly transmitted "wall eye with deafness" in cats and dogs.

*Heterochromia with the Horner syndrome*

There are several records of familial or apparently dominant transmission of this complex (Fig. 113).

*Heterochromic cyclitis*

Dominance or irregular dominance is suggested by several records (Fig. 114). It has been observed as a concordant feature in a pair of uniovular twins (Makley, 1956).

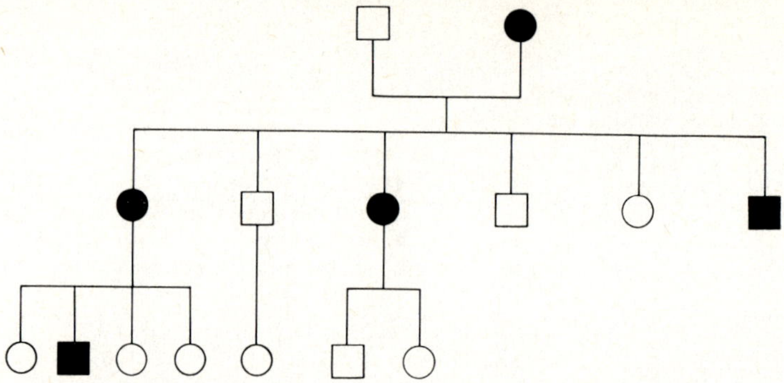

FIG. 112.—Simple heterochromia of the iris with dominant inheritance. (*After van den Breggen*, 1915.)

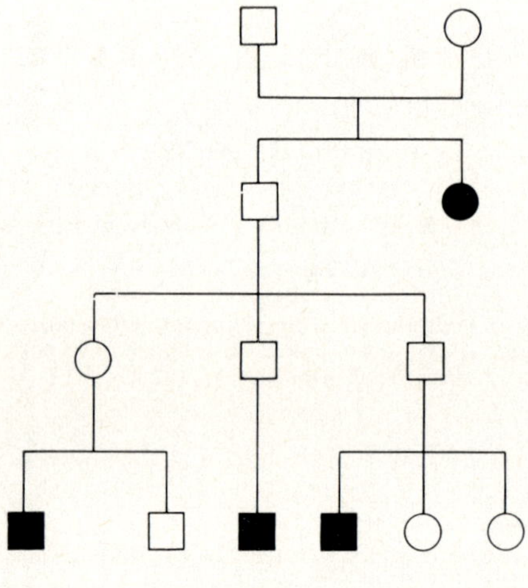

FIG. 113.—Sympathetic heterochromia of the iris with irregularly dominant transmission. (*After Calhoun*, 1919.)

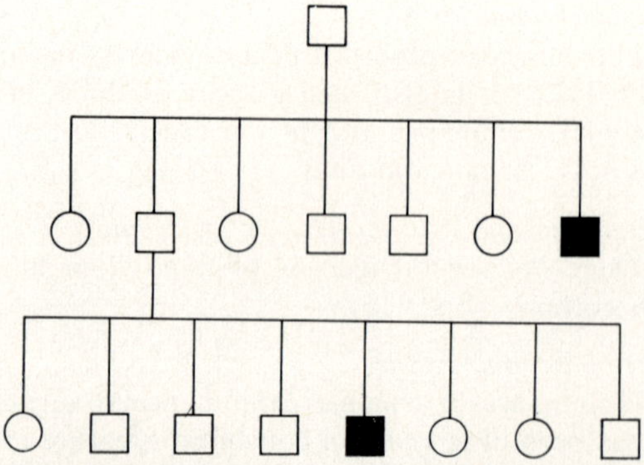

FIG. 114.—Fuchs' complicated heterochromia with dominant irregular inheritance. (*After Streiff*, 1947.)

## PUPIL ANOMALIES

*Polycoria*

This has been observed over two generations, probably as an aspect of hypoplasia of the mesodermal layers, or of atypical coloboma of the iris, or of aniridia, or of the anterior chamber cleavage syndrome. When such defects were observed towards the periphery of the iris they have been designated as congenital iridodialysis. The rare cases of true polycoria are probably always sporadic.

*Ectopic pupils*

This anomaly is generally seen in association with congenital dislocation of the lens. A dominant mode of inheritance for uncomplicated ectopic pupil has been recorded (Fig. 115). The extent of the deformity varies considerably in different

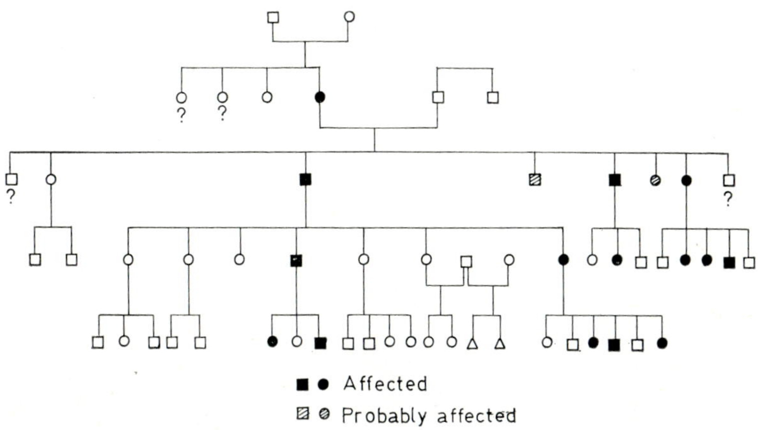


FIG. 115.—Ectopic pupils. Pedigree showing dominant inheritance. (*After Waardenburg*, 1932.)

members of the family. Ectopic pupils may be vertical in shape, simulating a cat's pupil.

*Anisocoria*

Several dominant pedigrees are on record (Berryman, 1953).

*Non-reacting pupils*

Miotic non-reacting pupils have been observed in a family with recessive total ophthalmoplegia (Waardenburg, 1924) and have also been seen in sibships without external ophthalmoplegia (Holth and Berner, 1923). Dominant inheritance has also been recorded (van Leeuwen, 1949). Non-reacting pupils without miosis have been observed in a sibship.

*Dilated pupils*

Dilated pupils incompletely reacting to light and accommodation have been seen in a pair of uniovular twins (White and Fulton, 1937).

## FOR FURTHER READING

**Anomalies of Pigmentation of the Iris**

Waardenburg, P. J. (1961). In *Genetics in Ophthalmology*, Ed. by P. J. Waardenburg, A. Franceschetti and D. Klein, pp. 693–714. Oxford; Blackwell.

**Ectopic Pupils**

Diethelm, W. (1947). *Ueber Ectopia lentis ohne Arachnodaktylie und ihre Beziehungen zur Ectopia lentis et pulillae*. Geneva; Thesis.

Usher, C. H. (1921). *Br. J. Ophthal.*, **5**, 289.

**Anisocoria**

Berryman, M. L. (1953). *L'Anisocorie congenitale familiale*. Geneva; Thesis.

# CHAPTER 9

# THE RETINA AND CHOROID

## CONGENITAL ANOMALIES

### Stationary Defects

**Atypical choroidal coloboma**

As distinct from anomalies seen with typical colobomatous defects involving the choroid, there is the relatively rare atypical choroidal coloboma—atypical in position rather than in form. These atypical colobomas have been observed in association with macular colobomas, and their status is obscure.

**Macular coloboma**

The term macular coloboma is descriptive of a variety of clinically distinct affections. Many, possibly most, macular colobomas are inflammatory in origin—heavy pigmentation being particularly suggestive—whilst associated calcified lesions towards the periphery of the fundus are characteristic of toxoplasmosis infection. The status of the rare non-pigmented ectatic coloboma is uncertain, but moderately pigmented macular colobomas are frequently hereditary in character. It has been observed in both members of a uniovular twin pair, several times over two generations (Fig. 116 *a*), and once (in association with apical dystrophy of the hands and feet) over three generations (*see* Fig. 116 *b*).

**Opaque nerve fibres**

Most cases are unilateral and appear to be sporadic. Opaque nerve fibres have been seen in monovular twins, in whom discordant findings have also been reported. There is considerable variation in expression of the gene. Fig. 117 suggests dominant inheritance. Pedigrees showing affected sibships only might possibly illustrate irregular dominance.

Many ocular and general abnormalities have been recorded in association with opaque nerve fibres. These are probably incidental; their relationship with high myopia, frequently unilateral, is more definite but requires further clarification.

**Asymptomatic macular defect**

Fig. 118 illustrates the dominant transmission of an apparently congenital macular lesion, which ophthalmoscopically (Fig. 119) could not be distinguished from the classical forms of macular dystrophy, but from which it differs in these two significant respects: (1) it is present early in life and is presumably congenital, and (2) in contrast to the macular dystrophies, there is no loss of central vision. These cases are probably rare, but they have to be borne in mind in the differential diagnosis of dominant macular dystrophy. Ophthalmoscopically the distinction may be impossible, whilst subjectively in the early stages of dominant macular dystrophy there is a macular lesion without substantial symptoms. At this stage the differential diagnosis can generally be established by the presence of anomalies

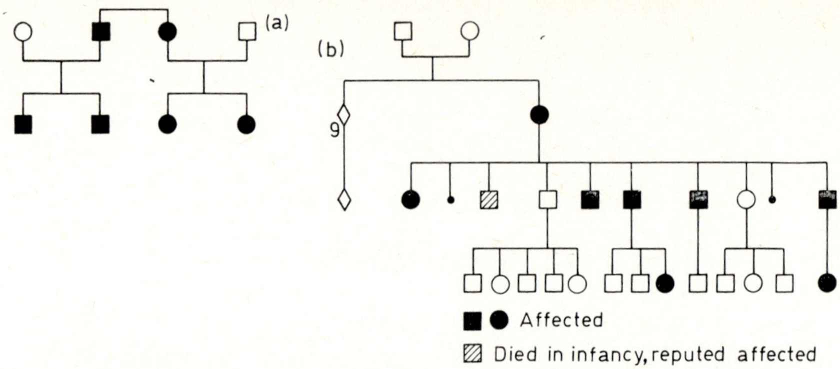


FIG. 116.—Macular coloboma. (*a*) Pedigree over two generations. (*After Clausen*, 1921 *and* 1928.) (*b*) Pedigree showing dominant inheritance (in this family there was an associated apical dystrophy of the hands and feet). (*After Sorsby*, 1935.)

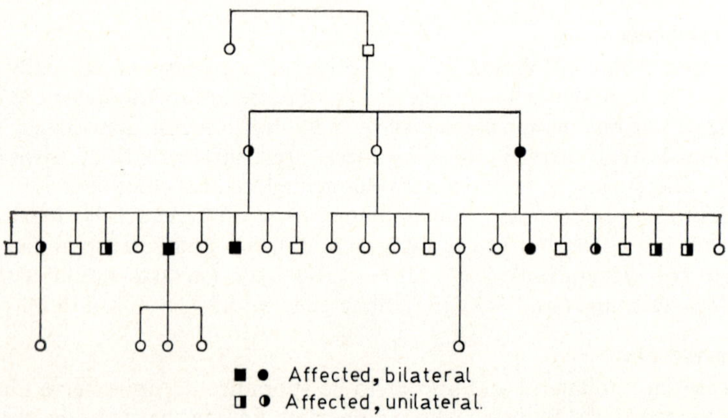


FIG. 117.—Opaque nerve fibres. Pedigree over two generations. (*After Cockayne*, 1936.)

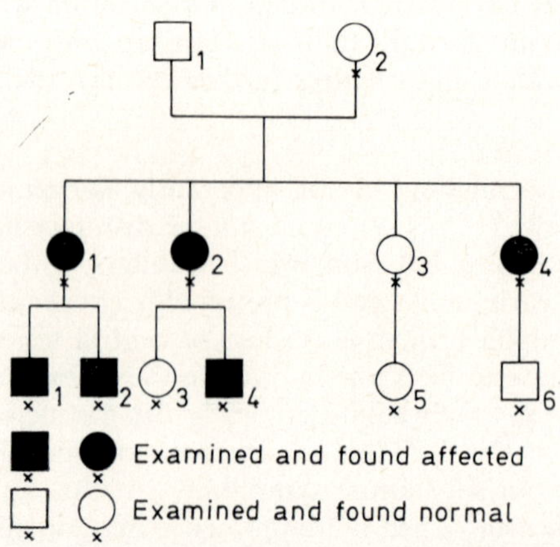


FIG. 118.—Asymptomatic macular defect. Pedigree showing dominant inheritance. (*After Sorsby and Wren*, 1960.)

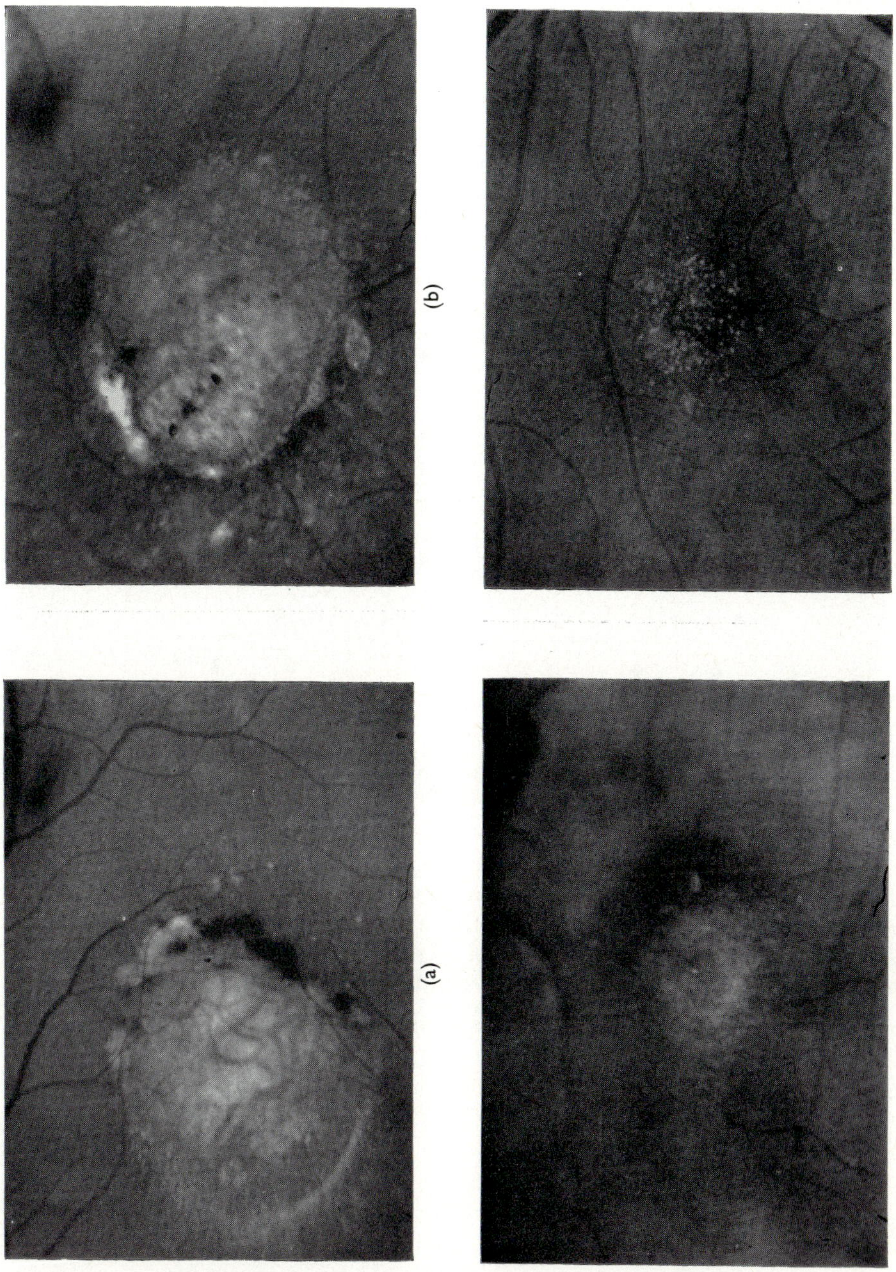

(a) (b) (c) (d)

FIG. 119.—Dominant asymptomatic macular defects. Appearances seen in two generations: *(a)* and *(b)* Marked atrophic changes in a son and his mother (III, 2) and (II, 1) in Fig. 118. *(c)* and *(d)* Milder lesions in a brother and in their mother's sister (III, 1, and II, 4) in the pedigree shown in Fig. 118.

of colour-vision in dominant macular dystrophy, but not in the asymptomatic lesion.

**Congenital stationary night-blindness**

*Uncomplicated night-blindness*

Congenital stationary night-blindness occupies a special place in human genetics because of the fact that it has contributed exceptionally well-worked-out pedigrees. In 1838, Cunier published an account of night-blindness in the offspring of one Jean Nougaret, born 1637 at Vendémian near Montpellier. Nettleship, in collaboration with Truc and with the help of a local clergyman, completed this pedigree in 1907. There were ten generations with 2,116 members, of whom 135 were known to have been night-blind. Fig. 120 is an extract from this pedigree. The dominant

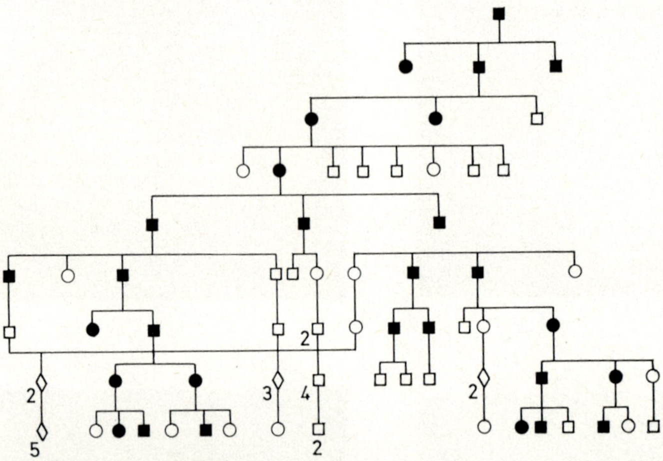


FIG. 120.—Dominant inheritance. Part of the Cunier-Truc-Nettleship pedigree of congenital stationary night-blindness. (*After Nettleship*, 1907, *and Bell*, 1933.)

mode of inheritance is obvious. A number of other pedigrees of dominant inheritance are available and they all conform to type (Fig. 121). There is no suggestion of irregular dominance in any of them, or of any ocular complications. There is no disability apart from the night-blindness.

Much has been written concerning the excess of unaffected over affected individuals in the Cunier-Truc-Nettleship pedigree. The expected ratio of 1 : 1 is not borne out by 134 affected to 255 normal in the affected branches of the family. As information on the earlier generations is largely from hearsay, it is of course possible that many affected members who died young were not reckoned amongst those affected. The rather complicated theoretical explanations which have been advanced seem unwarranted.

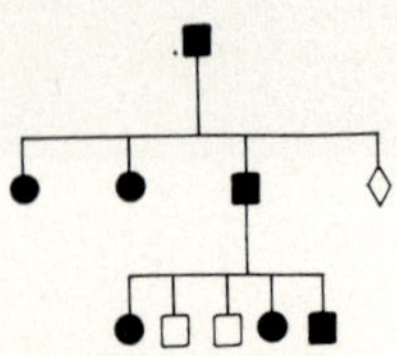

FIG. 121.—Uncomplicated night-blindness. Dominant inheritance. (*After Atwool*, 1895.)

*Night-blindness with myopia*

*Sex-linked recessive.*—Fig. 37 *a* (page 48) is taken from another famous pedigree, the Pfluger–Amman–Kleiner pedigree. The mode of inheritance is clearly that of recessive sex-linkage. A characteristic feature in this pedigree—and in some pedigrees recorded by Nettleship (Fig. 37 *b*)—was the presence of myopia ranging from 6 D to 11 D. Astigmatism was not uncommon, as also was some degree of visual defect. It is not unlikely that the pedigree of sex-linked recessive myopia recorded by Worth falls into this category. In one of Nettleship's pedigrees, an affected woman appeared.

*Autosomal recessive.*—Fig. 37 *c*, an extract from yet a third well-known pedigree (the Gassler pedigree), shows autosomal recessive inheritance. It is uncertain whether the myopia or the night-blindness differs from features as seen in sex-linked recessive inheritance. In the Gassler pedigree, the myopia varied between 9 D and 16 D and corrected vision varied between 6/60 and 6/18.

*Night-blindness with abnormal fundus coloration*

In Oguchi's disease there is a characteristic greyish reflex on ophthalmoscopic examination. After an hour or more in a dark room the normal fundus coloration appears—the Mizuo sign. Only a few cases have been recorded in Caucasians; the affection appears to be fairly prevalent amongst Japanese. The available pedigrees show a high rate of consanguinity and suggest recessive inheritance.

*Fundus albi punctatus*

Lauber in 1910 sought to differentiate between retinitis punctata albescens, which he regarded as a progressive affection of the retinitis pigmentosa group, and fundus albi punctatus, which he considered to be a congenital stationary affection with no complications beyond night-blindness. The disorder is recessive; phenoscopies are seen with vitamin A aldehyde deficiency (*see* p. 174).

## PROGRESSIVE AFFECTIONS

### Retinal aplasia

This affection, first clearly isolated by Alström and Olson in 1957 and recorded by them under the designation "heredo-retinopathia congenitalis monohybrida recessiva autosomalis" is now better known by the name of retinal aplasia. The designations of "amaurosis congenita (Leber)" or "Leber's congenital tapeto-retinal degeneration" commemorate one of several earlier and rather incomplete accounts of the affection. In fact, the literature contains a very large number of case records of "cortical blindness" in infants and of atypical retinitis pigmentosa, congenital or infantile chorioretinitis, and of congenital optic atrophy which might well be examples of this affection. Leber's studies have many noteworthy observations: he stressed the hereditary nature of a blinding affection seen in infants, and the fact that the blind infant may at first show an apparently normal fundus and that the fundus reactions may have intermediate forms with features reminiscent of classical retinitis pigmentosa.

*Alström and Olson's study.*—Alström and Olson's elucidation was based on a systematic study in the blind schools of Sweden. Since 1897 blind children in that country have been subject to compulsory education, and there is one central elementary school through which they all have to pass. In an investigation on the material from 1897 to 1948 they paid special attention to the cases recorded as congenital retino-choroiditis without known cause. It became clear that these cases were proband material leading to families, and altogether 105 families were isolated. The material was found to overlap with cases admitted as suffering from "congenital amaurosis" and from congenital optic atrophy of unknown origin. In all, 175 affected and 303 unaffected sibs were traced. Cases examined under the age of 15 years were found to consist of 61 per cent with "retinochoroiditis", 28 per cent with congenital amblyopia and 10 per cent with optic atrophy. Two cases had cataract on admission to the school. When the collected material was classified into three age-groups—under 15, 15 to 45 years of age, and over 45—the incidence and extent of retinochoroidal changes were found to increase progressively, while the incidence of congenital amblyopia without fundus lesions declined. The term "retinochoroidal changes" covers a wide range of lesions from minute round pale spots at the periphery, scarcely visible, to heavy irregular pigmentation scattered throughout the fundus. While some optic atrophy and a moderate degree of narrowing of the vessels were common, optic nerve lesions were not as conspicuous as in cases of retinitis pigmentosa with equally severe impairment of sight. Moreover, in the youngest age-group, total or subtotal blindness without any fundus changes was present in some 33 per cent of cases. Associated conditions were cataract and keratoconus, cataract being present in some 10 per cent of the youngest patients and increasingly in the higher age-groups, while keratoconus was present only exceptionally in young patients, but again increased with age. Different members of the same sibship showed the different components to a variable degree. Variations therefore occur not only with age, but as between families and between individuals within the same family. A striking aspect was the gross impairment of vision noted soon after birth or during the first year of life. Nystagmus was a common association, and the electroretinographic response was abolished in almost all cases. Genetic analysis showed the condition to be a monofactorial recessive affection widely scattered throughout Sweden, with a probable mutation rate of $2{\cdot}3\text{–}10^{-5}$. There was no significant excess of mental anomalies in this group. Alström and Olson regard the affection as responsible for about 10 per cent of all cases of blindness in Sweden.

*Other studies.*—Waardenburg in 1957 and Schappert-Kimmijser and her colleagues in 1959 studied the material in Holland, and it became clear that the affection is indeed not uncommon: in Holland it was responsible for some 18 per cent of all blindness in children. Neurological or psychiatric complications were present in 14 out of 56 children studied in detail. Many subsequent observations have confirmed the great frequency of this polymorphic affection.

### *Heredity*

The available material shows the affection to be recessive (Fig. 122 *a*). Exceptions, however, are accumulating. A family with dominant inheritance was recorded in London by Sorsby and Williams in 1960 (Fig. 122 *b*) and three more families with such mode of inheritance by François and De Roeck from Ghent (1960 and 1961). It is likely that the family recorded by Hoare in 1965 as showing an unusual form of retinal dystrophy is an example of retinal aplasia inherited in an intermediate sex-linked manner with occasional manifestation in carrier women (Fig. 123).

### *Clinical considerations*

The marked polymorphism of the fundus lesion is clearly seen when comparing the early stages with the end stages, and some of the changes are shown in Fig. 124. Progressive changes do, of course, occur with all abiotrophies, but generally, as in retinitis pigmentosa, the different stages are clearly recognizable as belonging to the same affection. Retinal aplasia falls within the small group of disorders in which the wide range of appearances during the course of the affection are such that they are not readily recognized as belonging to the same disorder. While

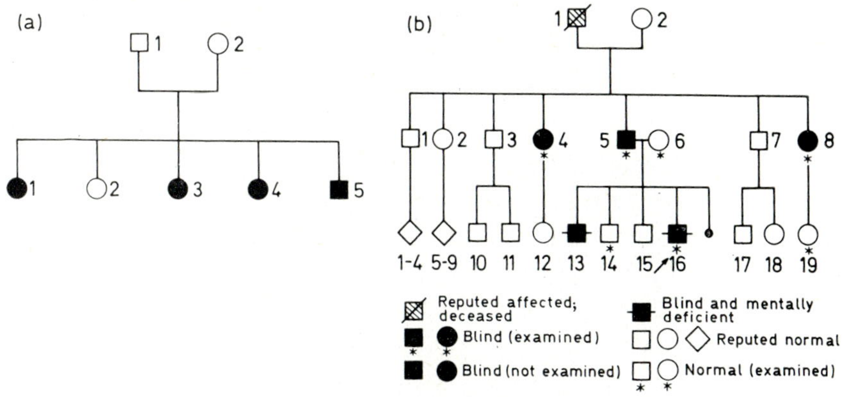


FIG. 122.—Retinal aplasia. (*a*) Pedigree showing the common recessive type. (*b*) Pedigree showing the uncommon dominant type. (*After Sorsby and Williams*, 1960.)

this makes diagnosis more complex, it helps in recognizing the significance of unusual fundus appearances. Retinal aplasia is in this respect as protean as choroideremia and generalized fundus dystrophy with their exceptionally wide range of intermediate stages. Fig. 123 illustrates the range seen in a family with intermediate sex-linkage.

The electroretinogram response is generally abolished or grossly abnormal. It is possible that only the most severe cases show blindness at birth, for the degree of retinal organization appears to vary considerably even within the same family. In one sibship personally observed, an infant was apparently totally blind, whilst an elder sib had vision of the order of 6/24. Similar observations are recorded by François in 1963. "Cortical blindness" in infants, therefore, is not the only form that the affection presents.

The frequency of mental deficiency, psychiatric disorders, neurological disturbances and skeletal anomalies varies with the source of the material. Retinal aplasia without complications is probably the commonest, but if—as discussed below—many of the cases of "atypical retinitis pigmentosa" seen in various congenital syndromes are indeed cases of retinal aplasia, this disorder is obviously an important component in children with multiple congenital defects.

*Differential diagnosis from congenital hereditary optic atrophy.*—Commonly, congenital optic atrophy shows deep atrophic cupping, and there is a relatively mild disturbance of vision with relatively slow progression of the defect. The total or subtotal blindness usual in retinal aplasia is, therefore, the significant point in the differential diagnosis of the two affections. Thus, the progressive course of congenital hereditary optic atrophy is shown by increasing failure of vision, whereas the progressive character of retinal aplasia is revealed, not so much by the increase of the blindness—which in most cases is total to begin with—but by the increasing pigmentary and atrophic changes in the retina. Furthermore, retinal aplasia is commonly recessive whilst congenital optic atrophy is more often dominant (when hereditary) and it is possible that much that passes in the literature as congenital recessive optic atrophy may have represented cases of retinal aplasia.

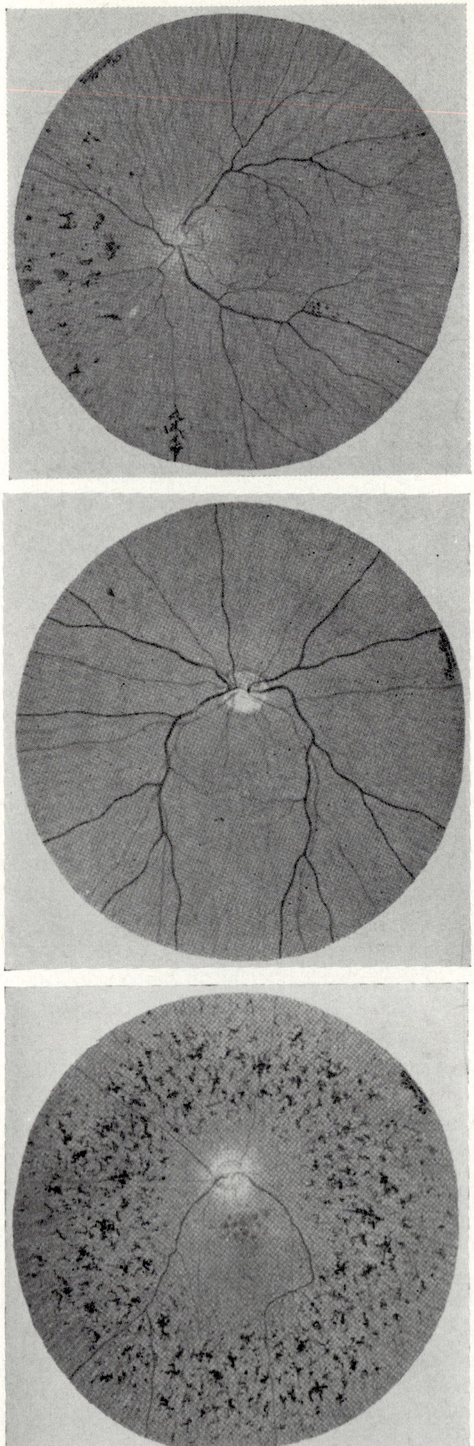

(a) (b) (c)

FIG. 123.—Intermediate sex-linked retinal dystrophy—probably retinal aplasia. (*a*) Appearances in a man aged 34. (*b*) Appearances in a boy aged four (the most marked lesion being pallor of the disc). (*c*) Appearances in a female carrier, aged about 60, the mother of the patient illustrated in (*a*). (*After Hoare*, 1965.)

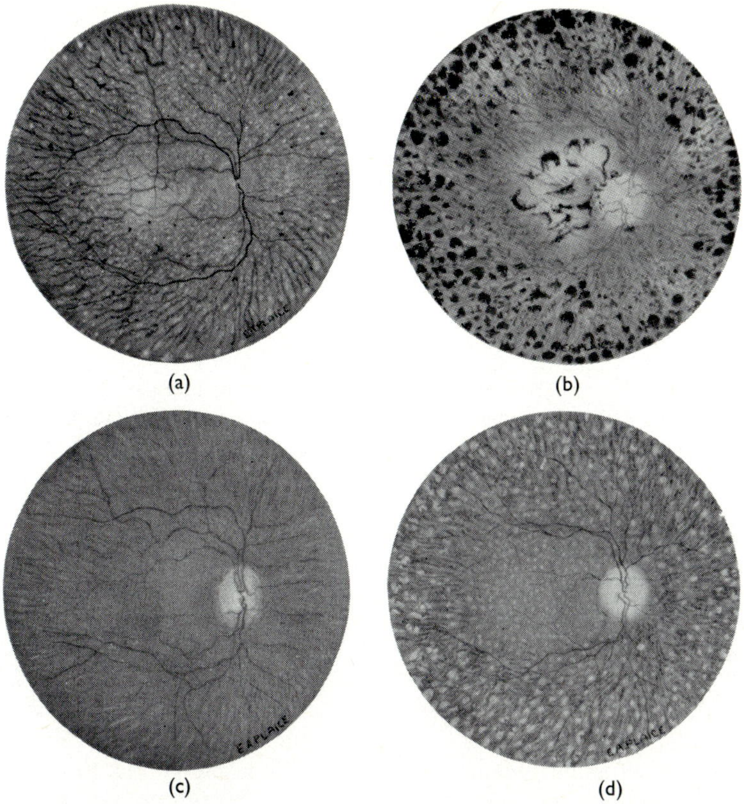


FIG. 124.—Retinal aplasia. (*a*) and (*b*) Appearances in a family showing the dominant form of the affection. (*a*) The right fundus in a boy aged 9 years. The disc is grey, the arteries and veins are narrow, and the fundus background shows diffuse mottling of a crude pepper-and-salt type. (*b*) The right fundus of a woman aged 40 years, an aunt of the boy shown in (*a*). In addition to advanced optic atrophy with marked narrowing of the retinal vessels, there is crude pigmentation scattered throughout the fundus with extensive areas of chorio-retinal atrophy. (*c*) and (*d*) Appearances in a family, with the recessive form of the affection. (*c*) The right fundus in a girl aged 19 years. There is marked optic atrophy, with fine pepper-and-salt changes throughout the fundus. (*d*) The right fundus in a younger sister of the patient shown in (*c*). The fundus background shows the same optic atrophy, and a considerably more obvious retinal atrophy is shown by the crude pepper-and-salt patterning with whitish exudate-like reactions predominating. Note the essential similarity ophthalmoscopically of the two genetic types. (*After Sorsby and Williams*, 1960.)

### *Classification*

The intensity of the lesion at birth—histologically various degrees of degeneration of the retinal neuroepithelium have been recorded—presupposes that the retina either had failed to develop into functioning layers or had developed normally only to degenerate before birth. It is tempting to draw a parallel with retinitis pigmentosa. We now know that in retinal dystrophy in the mouse, the Irish setter and the rat, where the ophthalmoscopic picture and clinical course are reminiscent of human retinitis pigmentosa, the affection is due to failure in the final differentiation in the rod layer (*see* p. 166). If human retinitis pigmentosa does represent a retina that has developed fully enough to function apparently normally (though presumably not so fully as to give a normal electroretinographic response nor normal dark-adaptation) then retinal aplasia might be considered as the counterpart of retinitis pigmentosa, in so far as the failure of development has occurred at an earlier stage, so that the retina has never reached functional maturity. On this reading, retinal aplasia and retinitis pigmentosa are in fact closely allied affections, aplasia representing an earlier and more severe failure in retinal development. Both affections have a considerable post-natal course. In retinal aplasia this is shown by degenerative changes visible ophthalmoscopically, and presumably histologically; in retinitis pigmentosa the post-natal changes are shown by the development of the typical ophthalmoscopic picture and the steady disintegration of visual functions.

*Relationship to "atypical retinitis pigmentosa"*.—It has already been stressed that in some families retinal aplasia does not always lead to blindness at birth in the affected members. Whilst fuller studies of such families are needed, it is likely that the milder cases of retinal aplasia constitute a substantial proportion of cases diagnosed as "atypical retinitis pigmentosa". This is a crucial issue with the various syndromes in which "atypical retinitis pigmentosa" is an essential component. In most of these syndromes blindness is exceptional at birth, but not later on. Yet the fundus anomaly is likely to be a congenital defect, judging by the multiple congenital defects seen in these syndromes. Such a reading helps to bridge the clinical gap between "typical" retinitis pigmentosa with its post-natal onset and "typical" retinal aplasia with its blindness at birth. It would seem that the concept of retinal aplasia needs to be expanded to include not only cortical blindness, some cases of congenital optic atrophy and of chorioretinitis, but also of atypical retinitis pigmentosa including "congenital retinitis pigmentosa". The ill-defined fundus changes seen in many of the syndromes would seem to fit best with the assumption that they represent variants of retinal aplasia, and Table IX summarizes the more significant syndromes—discussed elsewhere—to which this assumption applies.

**Dominant macular cyst**

In 1905 Best described a family with macular lesions apparently congenital, sometimes central, sometimes paracentral, and often with good vision. This family has been studied subsequently by Weisel in 1922 and Jung in 1937, and it is fairly definite that this is a congenital anomaly with variable degrees of visual defect. It is not clear from the accounts whether macular cysts were present in these cases and if so whether they had spurts later in life with deterioration in vision. Apart from the family recorded by Best in Germany, there is a study by Falls (1949) of an American family, but the diagnosis is not conclusive; whilst the family reported by Grimm and Tetford (1963) is clearly one showing dominant macular cyst.

Macular cysts have been recognized for many years as cysts or "holes" at the macula and differentiated from retinitis serosa centralis. It has also been known that vision can be good with a macular "hole". That the affection is hereditary and shows a progressive polymorphic course, beginning with a macular cyst and ending with a scar, has been recognized only recently (Sorsby and colleagues, 1956), and it is clear now that the affection includes several early records on unusual macular dystrophy and also the cases recorded by Best and his successors (Remky, Rix and Klier, 1965).

TABLE IX

SYNDROMES WITH RETINAL APLASIA ("ATYPICAL RETINITIS PIGMENTOSA")

| | *Laurence–Biedl* | *Alström* | *Hallgren* | *Refsum* | *Sjögren–Larsson* | *Cockayne* | *Bassen–Kornzweig* | *Senior–Friedmann–Braudo* |
|---|---|---|---|---|---|---|---|---|
| Retinal aplasia .. .. | + | + | + | + | + | + | + | + |
| Mental deficiency .. | + | | + | | + | + | | |
| Obesity and hypogenitalism | + | + | | | | | | |
| Deafness .. .. .. | ± | + | + | | | + | | |
| Cerebellar ataxia .. .. | | | + | + | | | + | |
| Spastic ataxia .. .. | | | | | + | + | | |
| Progressive polyneuritis .. | | | | + | | | | |
| Dwarfism .. .. .. | | | | | | + | | |
| Epiphysial anomalies .. | | | | + | | | | |
| Polydactyly .. .. | + | | | | | | | |
| Ichthyosis .. .. | | | | ± | + | | | |
| Diabetes .. .. .. | | + | | | | | | |
| Renal dysplasia .. .. | | | | | | | | + |
| Steatorrhoea .. .. | | | | | | | + | |
| Acanthosis .. .. .. | | | | | | | + | |
| Heart attacks .. .. | | | | + | | | | |
| Lipoid metabolism anomalies | | | | + | | | + | |
| Mode of inheritance .. .. | ← | | | Recessive | | → | ? Intermediate | |

*Ophthalmoscopic appearances*

Four phases have to be distinguished: (1) the quiescent cyst; (2) the cyst during an "acute attack"; (3) rupture of the cyst; and (4) degenerative changes following such rupture. Phases 1, 3 and 4 are illustrated in Fig. 125, and phase 2 in Fig. 126.

*The quiescent cyst.*—Typically the appearances are simulated by those of central serous retinopathy, except that the edges of the cyst are more defined. The cysts vary in size, being sometimes very much smaller than the disc, and they then often suggest a "hole" at the macula, or very much larger, up to 2 D in extent. Symmetry as between the two fundi is a striking feature in most cases. The degree of projection forward also varies considerably. In some cases the cyst comes well forward,

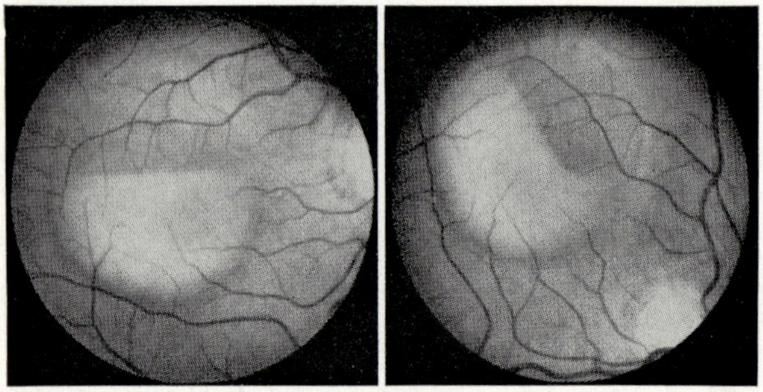

FIG. 126.—"Pseudohypopyon" in macular cyst. (*a*) Appearances on looking straight ahead. (*b*) Appearances after turning the head towards the left for three minutes. (*After Remky, Rix and Klier*, 1965.)

possibly as much as 3 D; in others the projection is barely perceptible. In consequence of these variations as to width and protrusion, some cysts are difficult to recognize as such. Within the same family the range of appearances may be considerable.

The cyst generally shows no special coloration: oedema is simulated rather than a coloured reaction. Some cases show the appearances, described by Riser in 1948 and more fully by Zanen and Rausin in 1950, suggestive of egg-yolk and designated as a disc-like vitelliform reaction. That this is not an independent entity but an aspect of macular cysts has been stressed by Remky, Rix and Klier (1965), who in an analysis of the literature have shown that the vitelliform reaction is seen in families in which other members show the more typical aspects of macular cysts, and that it appears to be most frequent in the younger members of affected families.

*The cyst during an "acute attack" and its aftermath.*—The exudative reactions, stressed by Huysmans and by Sorsby in 1940 in hereditary macular lesions, are now recognized as "hypopyon like" reactions within the cyst. These "pseudohypopyons" may even change in position with change of body-posture (Fig. 126). Exacerbation of these reactions is one of the causes of blurring of vision which persists for weeks. Fleck-like white exudates within the zone of the cyst may remain as tell-tale findings for many months. The reaction is often misdiagnosed as central choroiditis.

Acute attacks may also be precipitated by haemorrhage within a cyst. This

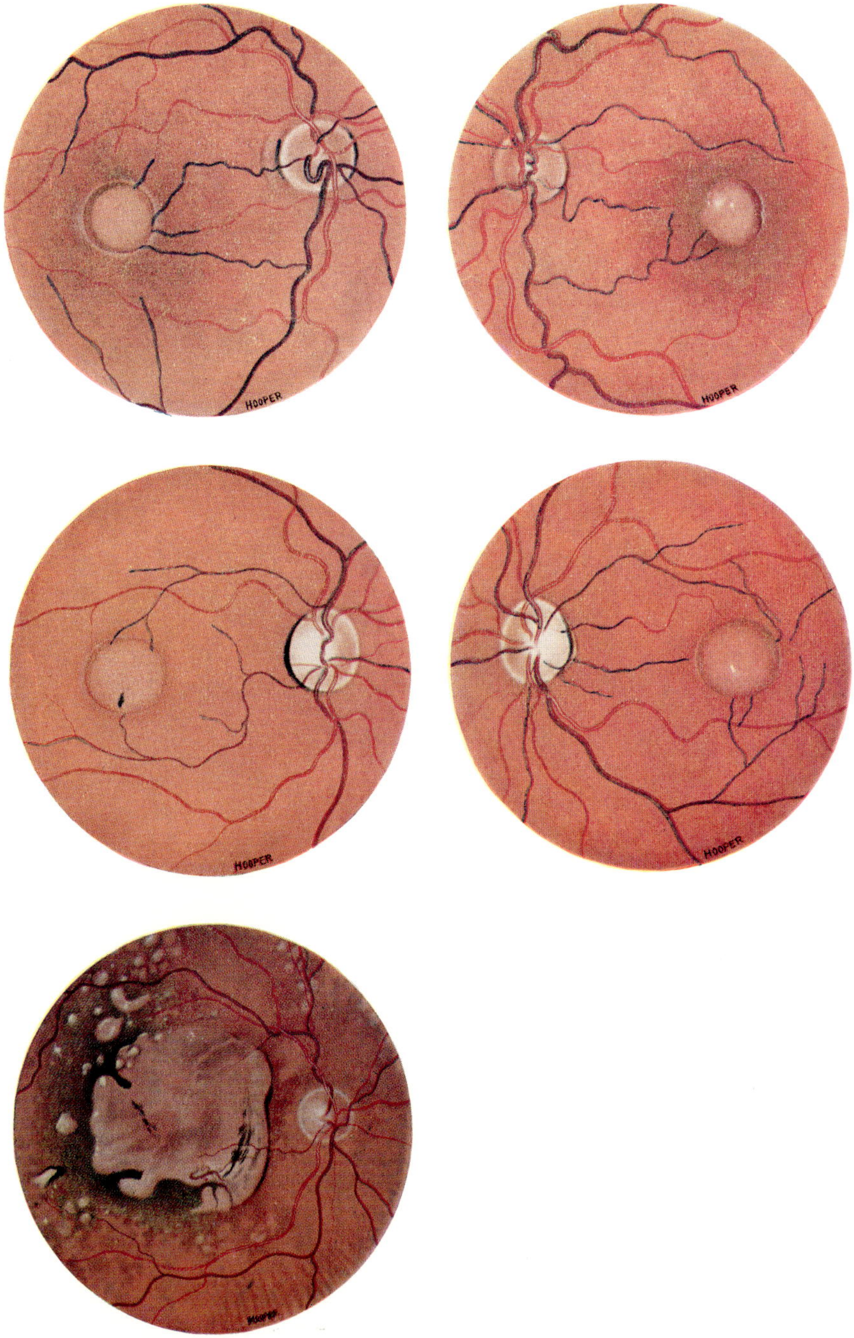


(a) (b)

(c) (d)

(e)

FIG. 125.—Dominant congenital cyst at macula. (*a*) and (*b*) Right and left fundi of a man aged 43 years (II, 3). Visual acuity: right 6/6, left 6/9 partly. Vision in the left eye had become blurred only lately. No central field defect, or marked anomaly in colour vision. Left cyst probably ruptured. (*c*) and (*d*) Right and left fundi of a younger sister aged 34 years (II, 7). Visual acuity: right 6/6, left 6/9 partly, recently complicated by distortion of objects. Cysts intact. (*e*) Right fundus of their father aged 79 years. Visual acuity 6/60 in each eye. (*After Sorsby, Savory, Davey and Fraser*, 1956.)

[*To face page 128*

may simulate a macular haemorrhage very closely. The vitreous may show opacities arising from these haemorrhages which have tracked forward.

*Rupture of the cyst.*—When this occurs, the torn roof may be recognized ophthalmoscopically or by slit-lamp fundus examination. Whether this serious development can occur in a symptomatically silent manner or always produces an "acute attack" is not known.

*Degenerative changes following rupture of the cyst.*—Once the cyst has ruptured, irritative pigmentary changes occur at the posterior pole. In elderly patients, the lesion may be quite extensive and may be misdiagnosed as "senile" macular degeneration (Fig. 125 *e*).

*Subjective symptoms*

Typically a macular cyst is an incidental finding, for the affection is silent except during the "acute attacks" and ultimately in the degenerative phases. During the symptomless stages there is no, or but slight, diminution of central vision, and no anomalies in dark adaptation or colour vision.

*Transient "acute attacks".*—During the "acute attacks" only one eye is generally affected; there is blurring of vision with recovery within weeks. The attacks may recur in the same eye or develop in the other eye. The frequency of these "acute attacks" is not known. It is likely that most patients do not experience them until vision begins to decline following rupture of the cyst, generally in middle life.

*Declining central vision.*—This is the beginning of the end stage in all patients and is the consequence of degenerative changes following rupture of the cyst. The onset is sometimes signalled by an "acute attack" from which there is no recovery. Vision steadily declines to around 6/60. At this stage, a persistent positive central scotoma is present. Similar symptoms may not develop in the other eye for several years. The peripheral field is not involved.

*Heredity*

Only dominant inheritance has been recorded so far (Fig. 127). Irregular dominance was present in the family studied by Best and his successors, in two of the five families recorded by Sorsby and colleagues (1956), and possibly also in that reported by Falls (1952). All other pedigrees have shown regular dominance.

The irregular dominance in Best's family and in one of the families investigated by Sorsby and colleagues could be more strictly regarded as intermediate

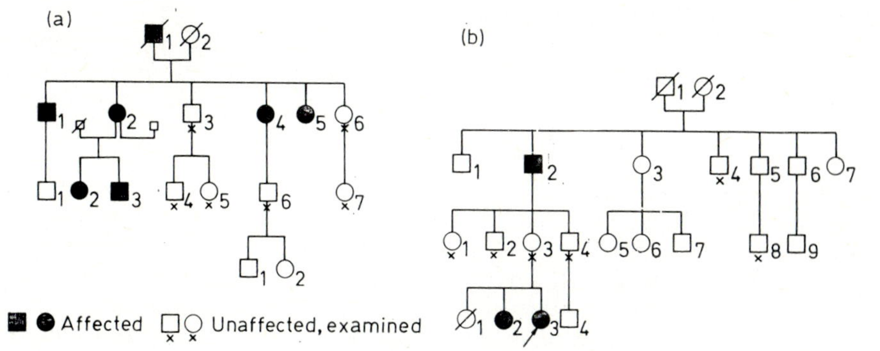


FIG. 127.—Macular cysts. (*a*) Pedigree showing dominant inheritance. (*b*) Pedigree showing irregular dominance. (*After Sorsby, Savory, Davey and Fraser*, 1956.)

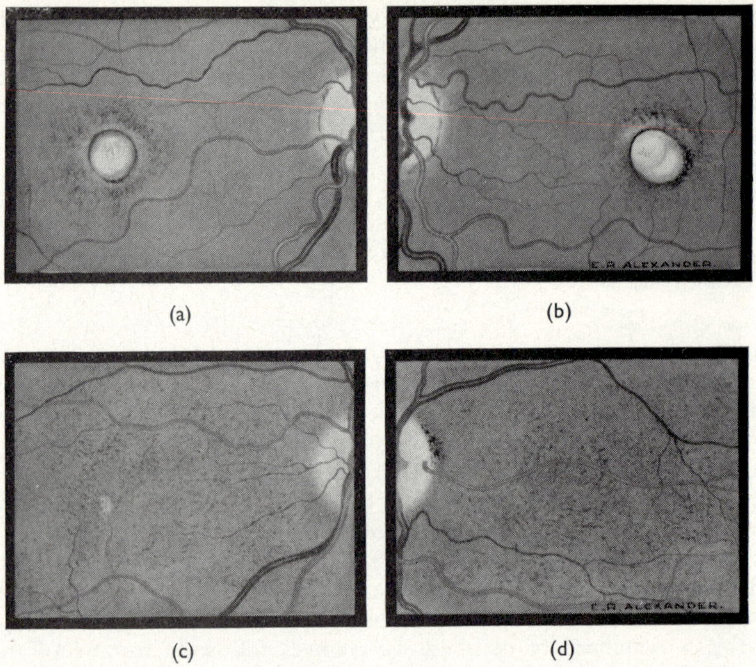


FIG. 128.—Dominant congenital cyst at macula. Typical lesion in a girl aged 14 and abortive appearances in her mother. (*a*) and (*b*) Right and left fundi of a girl at the age of 14. Visual acuity: right 6/9 partly, left 6/12 partly. This girl at 17 had been under observation for some 10 years and had shown no substantial changes. (*c*) and (*d*) Right and left fundi of her mother, aged 42. Vision full; diffuse mottling throughout posterior pole. (*After Sorsby, Savory, Davey and Fraser*, 1956.)

inheritance, for Best recorded two cases as mild and these were regarded by Jung on re-examination some 30 years later as showing "physiological variations" only. In the second family, a woman—the mother of an affected girl and sister of an affected man—showed diffuse mottling throughout the posterior pole without any visual disturbances (Fig. 128).

**Congenital sex-linked "pseudoglioma"**

In 1920 Ash and Fraser Roberts recorded a family with hereditary microphthalmia. A further study of this family was made by Roberts in 1937 and was recorded as showing blindness from microphthalmia with mental deficiency, the inheritance being in a recessive sex-linked manner. The hereditary aspect in this family was also discussed by Iles two years later. A pathological study of the eyes and brain in one of these cases was recorded by Whitnall and Norman in 1940, and it is now clear that the microphthalmia was merely an aspect of congenital pseudoglioma. Recognition of "familial congenital pseudoglioma" came from Heine in 1925 who recorded two affected brothers, but ascribed the familial incidence to "intrauterine infection" possibly tuberculous in origin. The first clear recognition of sex-linkage in congenital pseudoglioma came from the study by Wilson in 1949. Fig. 129 shows his striking pedigree in which a carrier woman had six affected sons by three men. In the same year sex-linkage was also stressed by Sjögren and

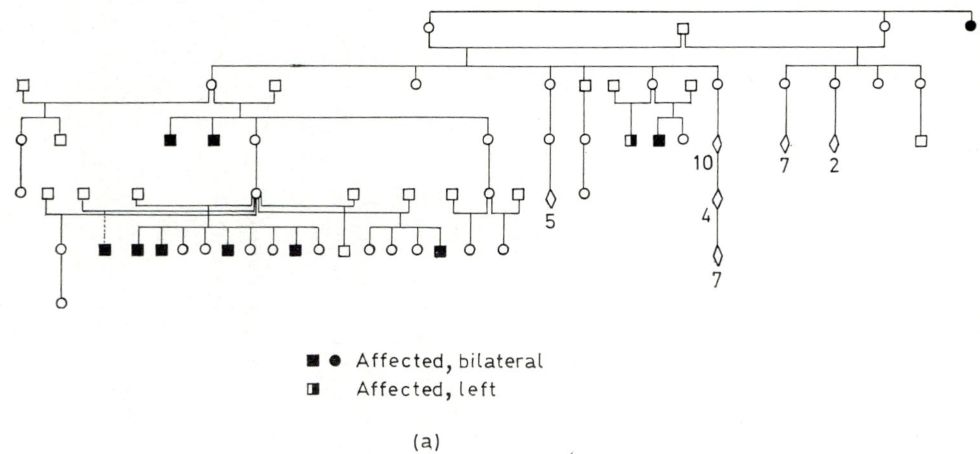


FIG. 129.—Congenital total detachment (pseudoglioma). Pedigrees suggestive of sex-linkage. *(a)* (*After Wilson*, 1949.) *(b)* (*After Clarke*, 1898.)

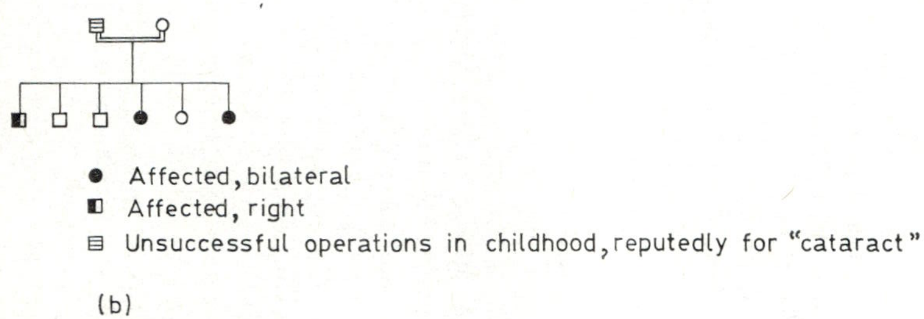

Larsson in their extensive study on "microphthalmos and anophthalmos with or without coincident oligophrenia"—a study which included several families with this affection.

Mette Warburg has drawn attention to the brief notes by Norrie in 1927 and 1933 of congenital blindness in boys in two families in Denmark. It is clear from Norrie's accounts and Warburg's subsequent studies that inheritance was in a recessive sex-linked manner, and that at least one of these families was suffering from congenital pseudoglioma.

A number of families of this disorder are now on record. The family originally studied by Ash and Roberts showed not only mental deficiency, but also epilepsy. Warburg has stressed mental deficiency and deafness in the Danish material. As in the early literature, some of the newer families have been reported under confusing appellations—such as Reese's retinal dysplasia by Winning, Coats' disease by Pajtas and Episcopi blindness by Taylor and his colleagues. The family reported by Lenz in 1955 may also have been an instance of this affection with additional defects of the heart, kidney and skeleton. It is clear that the affection is congenital and runs a progressive course during life, corneal opacities, band shaped keratopathy and cataract being common in addition to iritis. Histologically the retina is undifferentiated with proliferation of the pigment epithelium. The vitreous is hyperplastic and the optic nerves and possibly the whole optic tract are poorly developed. Warburg has found that there is nothing to suggest close linkage between the gene and the Xg locus. Eponymous designations such as Norrie's disease or Heine-Norrie disease do not appear to be either warranted or helpful.

**Congenital sex-linked polycystic detachment (retinoschisis)**

In 1935 Weve described falciform detachment of the retina, and Ida Mann vascular veils in the vitreous. It was thought at the time that these were different names for one and the same affection. Weve regarded falciform fold as a genetic anomaly as he had seen it in both members of a uniovular twin and had observed falciform fold and pseudoglioma in two brothers, a male cousin of whom also had pseudoglioma. In 1951 Sorsby and his associates showed that vascular veils in the vitreous were an aspect of a hereditary affection—congenital cystic detachment of the retina—which was sex-linked in its mode of inheritance, congenital in origin and progressive in character; they held that vascular veil in the vitreous was the anterior face of a ruptured cystic detachment. They also drew attention to sex-linked pseudoglioma or total detachment of the retina as described by Wilson in 1949 and suggested that falciform fold, congenital cystic detachment and congenital total detachment (pseudoglioma) are all different aspects of the same affection with some intra-familial stability. The report by Condon and Somerville-Large (1955) of a family with congenital cystic detachment, in which one member showed pseudoglioma, fits well with such an assumption. The occasional case of falciform fold in girls is readily explained by the fact that such lesions are now known to occur with retrolental fibroplasia and even toxoplasmosis.

Congenital cystic detachment does not always present as a cyst; more commonly there are characteristic sharp edges of what look like multiple disinsertions, and it is likely that at an earlier stage there were multiple cysts which have ruptures, and that the sharp edge is merely part of the torn anterior surface. In a ruptured cyst it occasionally happens that the anterior surface with its retinal vessels floats forward giving the appearance of vascular veils in the vitreous. Apart from

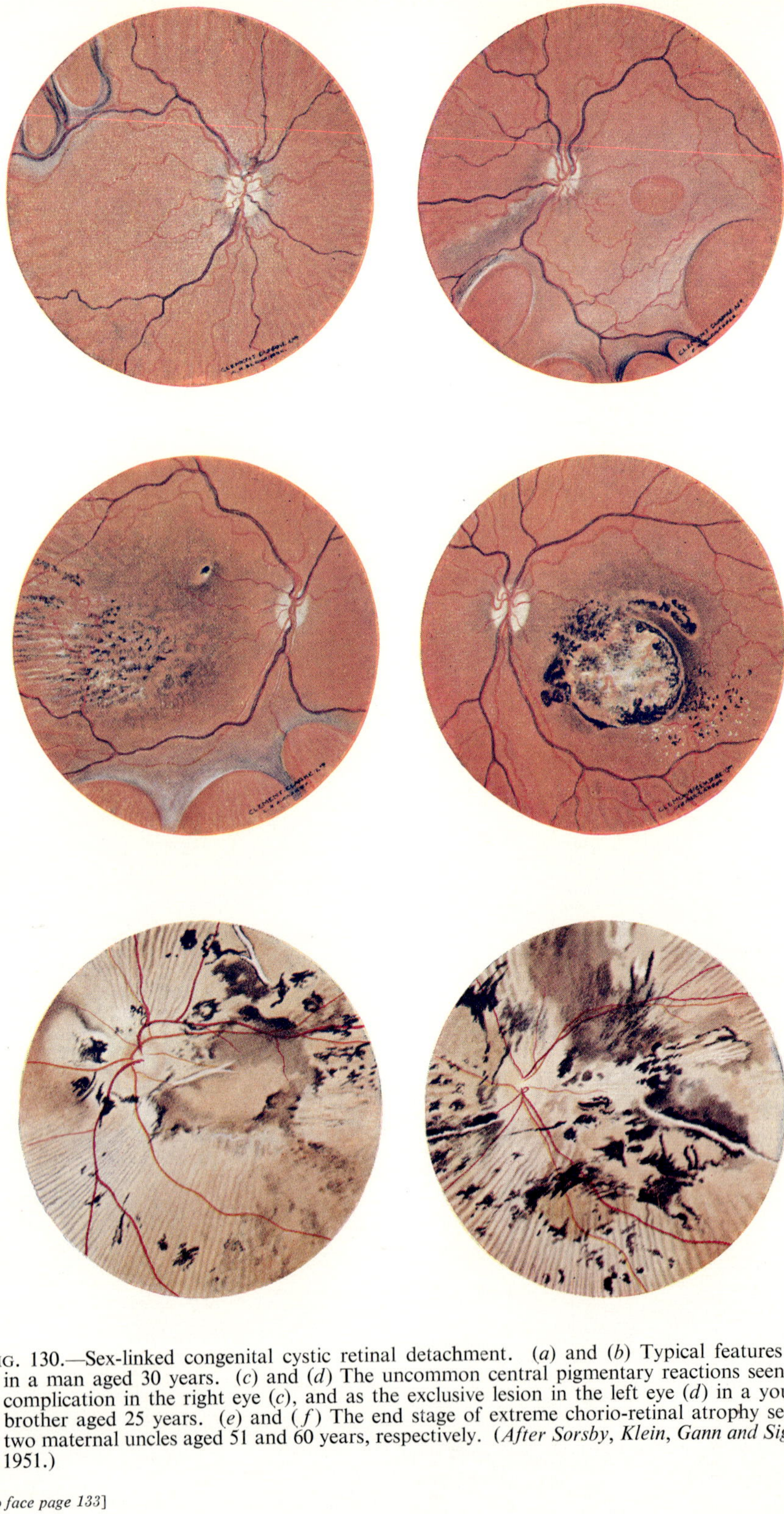


FIG. 130.—Sex-linked congenital cystic retinal detachment. (*a*) and (*b*) Typical features seen in a man aged 30 years. (*c*) and (*d*) The uncommon central pigmentary reactions seen as a complication in the right eye (*c*), and as the exclusive lesion in the left eye (*d*) in a younger brother aged 25 years. (*e*) and (*f*) The end stage of extreme chorio-retinal atrophy seen in two maternal uncles aged 51 and 60 years, respectively. (*After Sorsby, Klein, Gann and Siggins*, 1951.)

*To face page 133*]

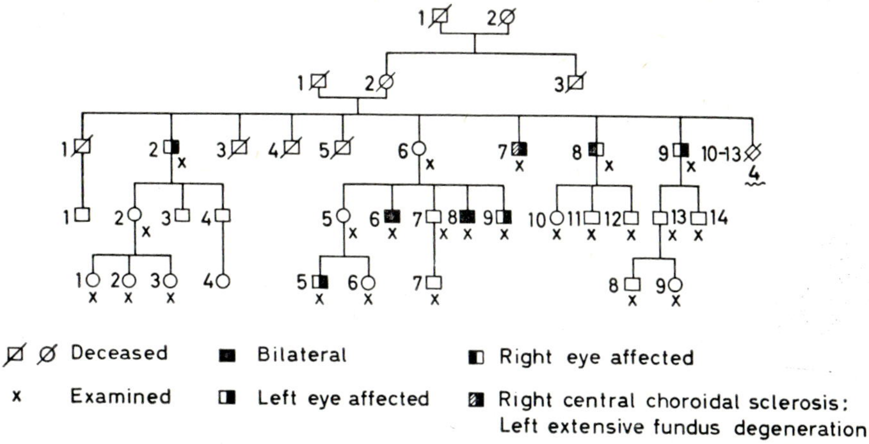


FIG. 131.—Congenital cystic retinal detachment. Pedigree of family illustrated in Fig. 130, showing sex-linkage and variable expression of the affection. (*After Sorsby, Klein, Gann and Siggins*, 1951.)

bursting and producing vascular veils, haemorrhage may occur into the cyst leading to the appearance of a tumour. The end stage shows a fundus lesion indistinguishable from a diffuse chorioretinal inflammation. The wide range of appearances in one family is shown in Fig. 130.

Sex-linkage (Fig. 131) helps in establishing the diagnosis: the female carriers do not apparently show any diagnostic features.

## ABIOTROPHIC DISORDERS

The classical forms of abiotrophic affections of the fundus are retinitis pigmentosa and macular dystrophy. Less common abiotrophic affections are gyrate atrophy of the retina and choroid, choroideremia, and the affection known as Doyne's choroiditis. Retinitis pigmentosa has a characteristic pigment reaction, and while the lesion in macular dystrophy is also pigmentary, there is mottling and atrophy instead of bone corpuscle reaction. In gyrate atrophy the reaction is almost entirely one of atrophy with exposure of white sclera. In choroideremia, fundamentally the same reaction is present, but on a more extensive scale with occasional bone corpuscle pigment. In Doyne's choroiditis, pigment proliferation is present, but in addition there are whitish "exudates", or possibly large colloid bodies. In all these affections the reaction is therefore essentially one of atrophy and relatively fine pigmentary disturbances, except that in Doyne's choroiditis an approach to an exudative reaction is observed.

In recent years a considerably wider range of reactions has come to be recognized in the abiotrophic lesions. Angioid streaks with the not infrequently associated haemorrhages and exudates bear no similarity to the classical reactions. In choroidal sclerosis the conversion of the choroidal vessels into white streaks is yet another unusual abiotrophic reaction. Still more striking are the exudative reactions recorded in macular dystrophy, whilst in generalized fundus dystrophy oedema, haemorrhages and exudates can be observed in the early stages and massive pigmentary proliferation in the late stages.

The variety of abiotrophic reactions is therefore so wide as to simulate almost any type of fundus reaction traditionally associated with affections of environmental origin. These developments have extended the range of abiotrophic lesions to considerably beyond the limited range of affections recognized in the past.

In retinitis pigmentosa it has been known for many years that the age of onset of the affection varies considerably in different families and that there are several modes of inheritance. In macular dystrophy the tendency has been to regard the classical form described by Stargardt which occurs in late childhood or at puberty, as an exclusive chronological and genetic type. That this view as to the age of onset is untenable was shown by Behr, who stressed the occurrence of macular dystrophy later in life. He held that macular dystrophy occurs at the critical periods of development: the first dentition, adolescence, early adult life, the climacteric, and possibly also in old age. Though somewhat schematic, Behr's teaching has the merit of emphasizing that in the macular dystrophies, perhaps even more than in retinitis pigmentosa, there is no one age at which the lesion may occur, and that the classical Stargardt form is merely one of many possible varieties. Likewise, though the recessive type is much the commonest, other forms of inheritance do occur—both regular and irregular dominance and sex-linkage. Furthermore the mottled or pigmentary reaction in the typical macular dystrophies are not the only reactions possible, any more than bone corpuscle pigment reaction is the only possible reaction in the retinal abiotrophies. In the macular dystrophies exudative reactions and gross pigmentary changes may replace the more commonly seen lesions.

## Retina

### The retinitis pigmentosa group

In view of the great diversity in clinical course and of the modes of inheritance seen with what passes ophthalmoscopically as retinitis pigmentosa, it is necessary to differentiate clear-cut clinical entities.

Four, and possibly six, modes of inheritance of retinitis pigmentosa without generalized associations are recognized. The relative frequency of these different types and the clinical differences between them are known only in broad outline.

#### *Genetic varieties*

*Recessive.*—Published pedigrees of retinitis pigmentosa tend to emphasize the exceptional families in which large numbers are affected and the affection is transmitted over several generations. There is no doubt, however, that the relatively infrequently recorded pedigrees of recessive inheritance stand for the bulk of the cases. In a consecutive series of 41 pedigrees of retinitis pigmentosa, Usher found that all but one were recessive. Fig. 132 *a* illustrates a typical pedigree.

*Dominant.*—The very large number of pedigrees published tends to give an exaggerated importance to the frequency of this mode of inheritance. In all the published pedigrees a striking feature has been the regular mode of inheritance without any skipping of a generation (Fig. 132 *b*).

*Sex-linked recessive.*—Relatively few pedigrees are available. Fig. 132 *c* illustrates the typical mode of inheritance. Available evidence would seem to suggest that retinitis pigmentosa with this mode of inheritance is a particularly severe affection. It would also seem that in some families the female heterozygotes are occasionally affected.

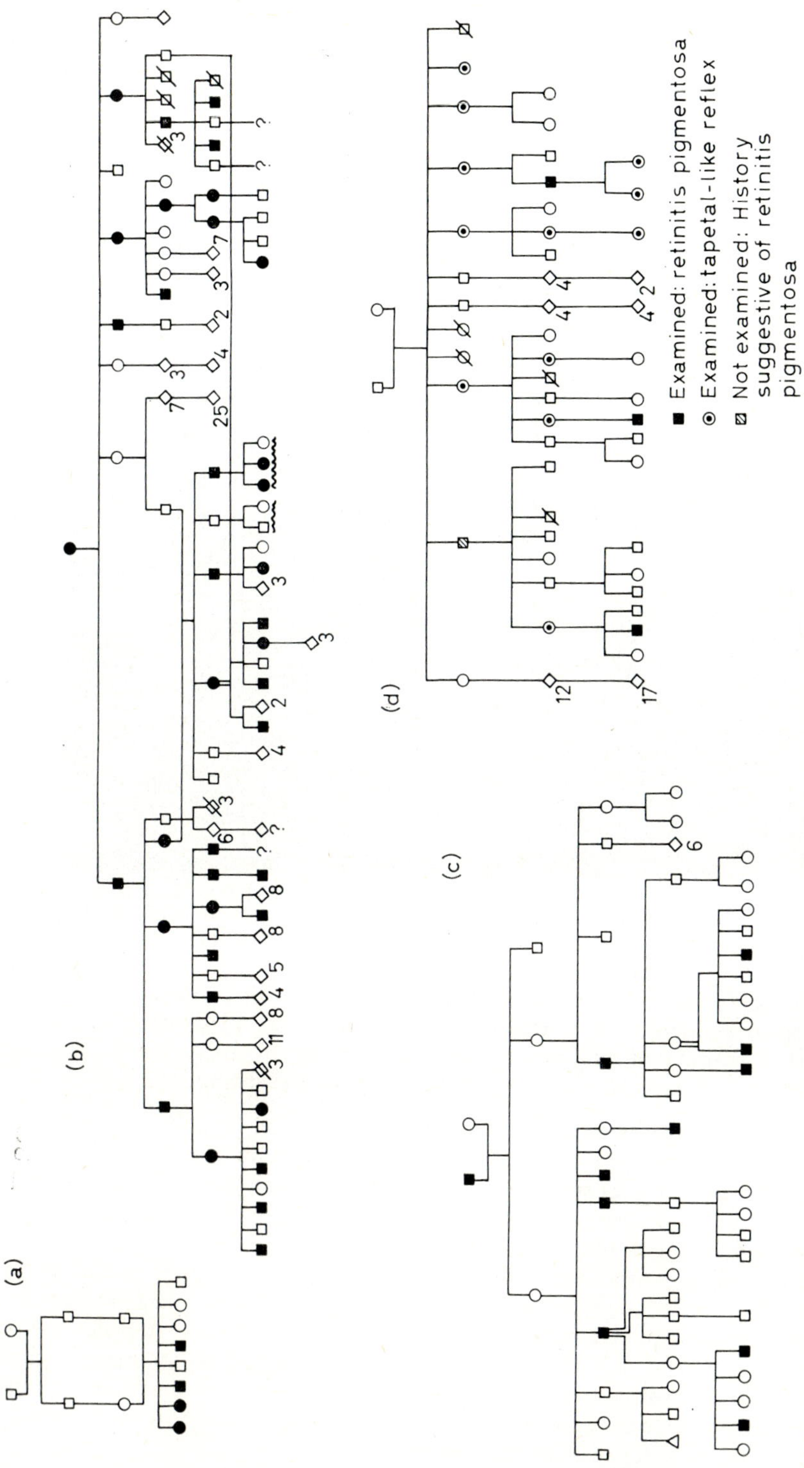


FIG. 132.—Retinitis pigmentosa. (*a*) Recessive inheritance. (*After Nettleship*, 1908.) (*b*) Dominant inheritance. (*After Nettleship*, 1908.) (*c*) Recessive sex-linked inheritance. (*After Usher*, 1935.) (*d*) Intermediate sex-linked inheritance. (*After Falls and Cotterman*, 1948.)

*Intermediate sex-linked.*—Falls and Cotterman (1948) drew attention to this variety of retinitis pigmentosa (Fig. 132 *d*). As in choroideremia, female heterozygotes can be recognized by ophthalmoscopic changes of no pathological importance. There is a characteristic highly glistening retinal reflex, somewhat reminiscent of the tapetal reflex of animals (Fig. 133). The exact significance of this heterozygous manifestation has still to be assessed. A marked tapetal reflex has been observed in a girl who subsequently showed typical retinitis pigmentosa.

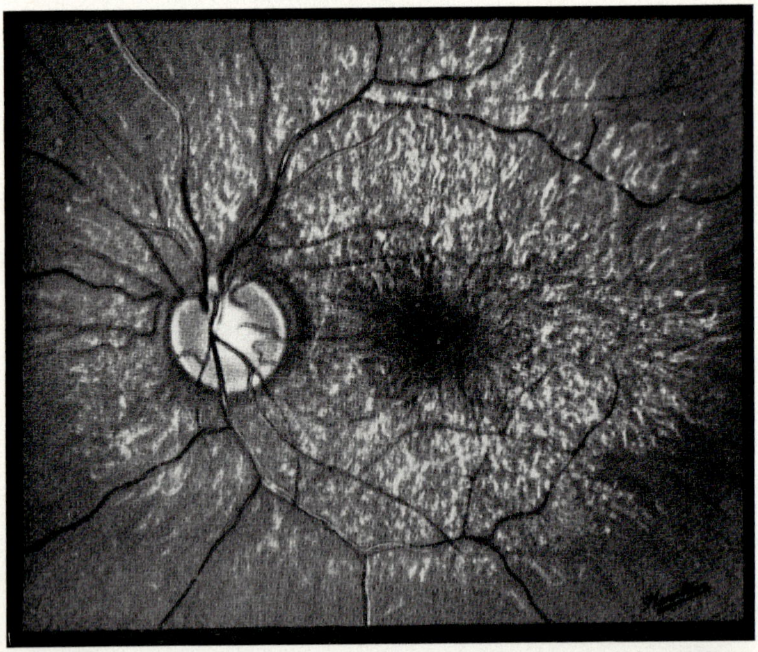

FIG. 133.—Intermediate sex-linked inheritance. "Tapetal reflex" in a woman aged 24 years with normal visual functions. She is a member of the family whose pedigree is shown in Fig. 132 (*d*). (*After Roberts and Sorsby*, 1951.)

Apart from these four modes of inheritance there are two further possibilities suggested by Haldane (1941): recessive and dominant partial sex-linkage. Fig. 134 supports a reading of dominant partial sex-linkage if cross-over is assumed; the evidence for recessive partial sex-linkage is even less definite.

*Ocular associations of retinitis pigmentosa*

*Glaucoma.*—The frequency of glaucoma as an association of retinitis pigmentosa has probably been overrated. There is evidence that such glaucoma is genetically determined and not merely incidental (Fig. 135 *a*). As noted earlier (p. 21), microphthalmos is a further association in some cases.

*Cataract.*—The general assumption that cataract is a secondary manifestation in retinitis pigmentosa is probably not valid. It is possible that cataract is a frequent and perhaps a constant association of dominant retinitis pigmentosa. Fig. 135 *b* shows a pedigree of fully developed cataract in dominant retinitis pigmentosa over three generations. In most individuals with dominant retinitis pigmentosa lens changes appear to develop early and to progress fairly rapidly, irrespective of the severity of the fundus lesion.

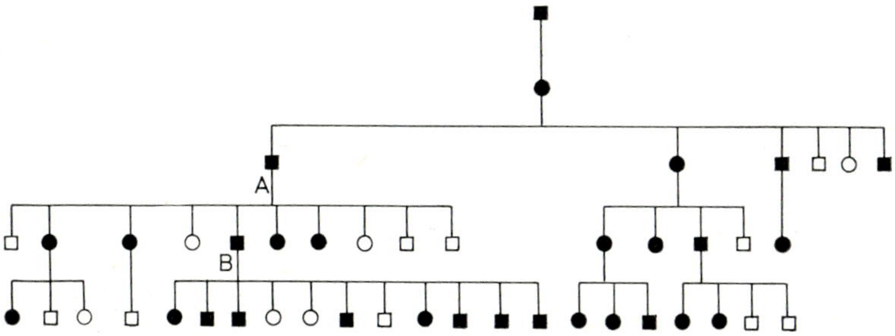


FIG. 134.—Presumed dominant partial sex-linkage: A pedigree of retinitis pigmentosa (as interpreted by Haldane, 1941).

On the assumption of dominant partial sex-linkage the affected man in the first generation carried the dominant gene on his X chromosome and can have only affected daughters. Such daughters in turn can contribute their abnormal X chromosomes to either sons or daughters. The man marked A in the third generation would again transmit it to all his daughters and to none of his sons. Actually two of his daughters are unaffected, and one son is affected. This can be explained by three cross-overs occurring in this generation. The affected son B in the fourth generation now carries the pathogenic gene on his Y chromosome and would therefore transmit the affection to his sons only. Actually one of his sons is normal and two of his daughters are affected. This, too, could have occurred as the result of a cross-over. (*After Snell*, 1903.)

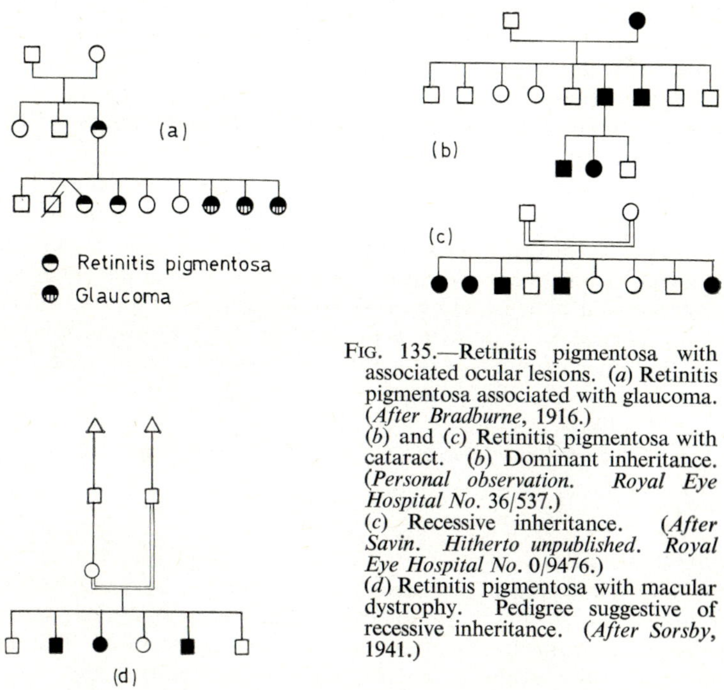


FIG. 135.—Retinitis pigmentosa with associated ocular lesions. (*a*) Retinitis pigmentosa associated with glaucoma. (*After Bradburne*, 1916.)
(*b*) and (*c*) Retinitis pigmentosa with cataract. (*b*) Dominant inheritance. (*Personal observation. Royal Eye Hospital No.* 36/537.)
(*c*) Recessive inheritance. (*After Savin. Hitherto unpublished. Royal Eye Hospital No.* 0/9476.)
(*d*) Retinitis pigmentosa with macular dystrophy. Pedigree suggestive of recessive inheritance. (*After Sorsby*, 1941.)

Cataract would appear to be less common in recessive retinitis pigmentosa. It is, however, possible that there is a variety of recessive retinitis pigmentosa in which cataract is a constant association. Fig. 135 *c* illustrates such a pedigree.

It would therefore appear that whilst at least four different genes are responsible for the modes of inheritance of retinitis pigmentosa in different families, the clinical varieties of the affection are even more complex. Intensive combined clinical and genetic studies are necessary for the elucidation of these problems. It is not unlikely that such ill-defined entities as "atypical retinitis pigmentosa" and "retinitis punctata albescens" will become more intelligible in the light of such studies.

*Ophthalmoplegia.*—There are case records of external ophthalmoplegia with or without ptosis associated with "atypical retinitis pigmentosa". Occasionally present at birth, the onset is most frequent at about puberty and the fundus lesion may be a macular dystrophy or "atypical retinitis pigmentosa" or both in combination. Nystagmus is present in the congenital cases. The affection has been seen in sibs, but the exact genetic status is uncertain. The association of elements of bulbar palsy with retinal changes recalls the retinal changes seen in the hereditary spino-cerebellar ataxias.

*Unusual forms of retinitis pigmentosa*

*Retinitis pigmentosa with macular dystrophy.*—The mode of inheritance of this affection is not known. Clinically it is sharply delineated from uncomplicated retinitis pigmentosa by the fact that central vision suffers early, with a consequent early total blindness. Fig. 135 *d* shows a pedigree that suggests recessive inheritance.

*Unilateral retinitis pigmentosa.*—There is nothing to suggest that the rare cases of unilateral retinitis pigmentosa represent a partial manifestation of the hereditary forms of retinitis pigmentosa. The available literature reveals neither an excessive incidence of consanguinity amongst the parents of such individuals, nor any definite family history of the affection. Some of the cases are probably of environmental origin—the consequence of mechanical or chemical injury. Others may represent a somatic mutation (Joseph, 1951).

*Quadrantic and sectorial retinitis pigmentosa.*—In contrast to unilateral retinitis pigmentosa, the rare cases of quadrantic or sectorial degeneration of the retinitis pigmentosa type are probably genetically determined. This is suggested by the symmetry of the lesion—generally in the inferior nasal quadrant, and by the not infrequent depression of the ERG and dark adaptation. In at least four families dominant inheritance was present and, judging by the spread of the lesion observed in the older members of some of these families, it would be reasonable to assume that these cases are examples of dominant retinitis pigmentosa with a mild course. It is likely that there is also a recessive variety, for in an isolated case on record deaf-mutism was present in the patients and there was also parental consanguinity.

**The macular dystrophies**

The classical form of macular dystrophy was described by Stargardt in a series of papers in 1909–17. It was Stargardt's merit that he isolated these purely retinal lesions from the juvenile forms of cerebro-macular degeneration that had been recognized previously. Formerly regarded as *formes frustes* of the more serious neurological disorders (the Batten–Mayou or the Vogt–Spielmeyer disease), it became clear that this was an independent disorder with clear-cut features.

As already noted following the isolation of macular dystrophy as a distinct entity, attempts were made to establish different types on the basis of age at onset, and by distinguishing exudative reactions from pigmentary changes. Whilst helpful, these classifications have proved of less value than differentiation by genetic behaviour. At least two and possibly three genetic forms have to be considered.

*Recessive macular dystrophy* (*Stargardt's disease*)

The original studies by Stargardt contain family records that would not now be admitted, either because the lesions extended beyond the macula, or showed symptoms different from those he recorded in his major cases. It is best to confine the name of Stargardt's disease to the recessive type (Fig. 136 *a* and *b*) occurring in late childhood at puberty.

*Clinical features.*—This affection is characterized by a sudden disturbance in central visual acuity, often declining to 6/36 or 6/60 within a few weeks, and either remaining at this level or possibly showing a slight improvement. Ophthalmoscopically there may be no lesion when vision has already declined, so that retrobulbar neuritis may be mistakenly diagnosed, but before long loss of foveal reflex and fine pigmentary changes become established at the macula (Fig. 137). There is little or no extension away from the central area. In longstanding cases temporal pallor of the optic disc may become a feature. There are no substantial anomalies in colour vision.

*Dominant macular dystrophy*

In the literature on macular dystrophy a number of records of dominant inheritance are available. Sorsby and Davey (1955) have shown that these dominant cases, though ophthalmoscopically similar to Stargardt's disease, constitute a distinct entity with characteristic features of their own (Fig. 136 *c*).

*Clinical features.*—The macular lesion is often present for years without any visual symptoms, except for crude anomalies of colour vision, markedly different from the usual red–green defect. Though visual acuity may occasionally decline in childhood, it is often not till adult life or early middle age that symptoms become troublesome. The affection does not set in acutely but takes a slowly progressive course; the end result over years is vision of the order of 6/60. In the elderly, the lesion has sometimes progressed to such an extent that it becomes indistinguishable from "senile macular degeneration" (Fig. 138).

*Sex-linked macular dystrophy*

The possibility of a sex-linked form of macular dystrophy is suggested by Fig. 136 *d* which records a family with typical macular lesions possibly associated with colour anomalies.

These macular lesions are all pigmentary in type. Exudative reactions do, however, occur, but are rare; of the two families reported one showed dominant and the other recessive inheritance (Sorsby, 1940). Classification by age is of significance in that in some families recessive macular lesions set in in adult life and do not always run a severe course. Many and perhaps most of the macular dystrophies

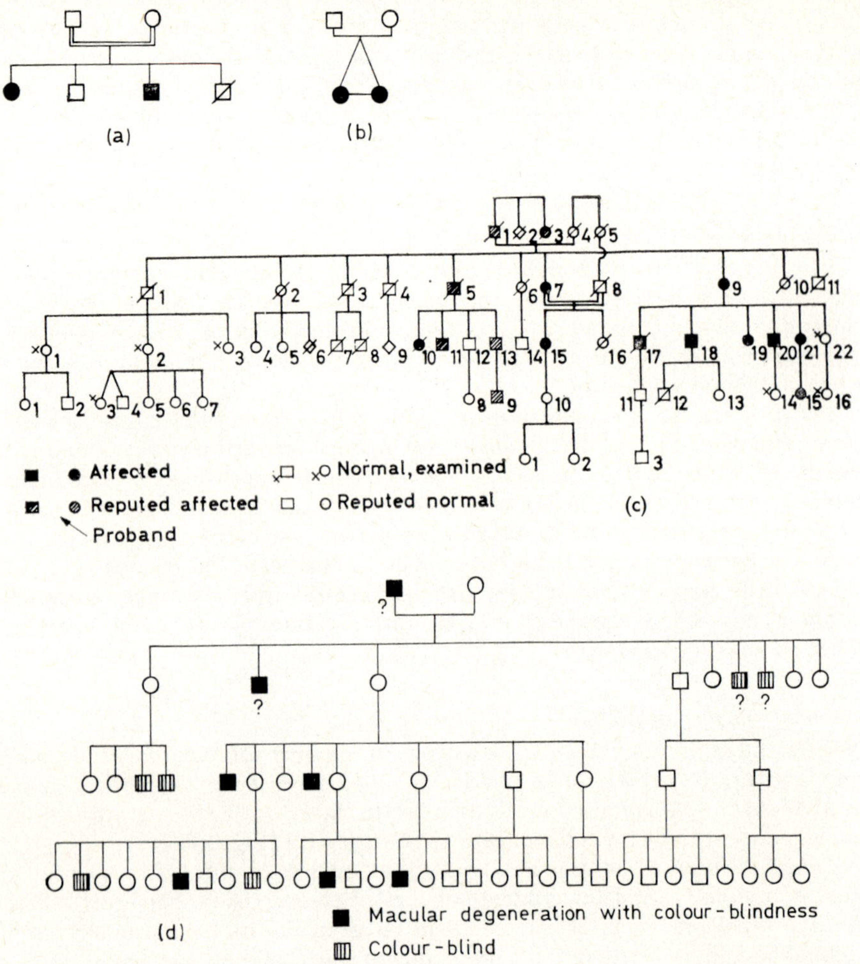


FIG. 136.—Macular dystrophies with atrophic reactions. Juvenile forms. Pedigrees. (*a*) Pedigree showing recessive inheritance. (Stargardt's disease). (*After Neame*, 1935.) (*b*) Pedigree chart showing the occurrence of the affection in a uniovular twin. (*Personal observation*. Fig. 137 illustrates the appearances observed in this twin.) (*c*) Pedigree of a family with dominant macular dystrophy. (*After Sorsby and Davey*, 1955.) (*d*) Pedigree chart showing recessive sex-linkage. (*After Halbertsma*, 1928.)

in middle-age are probably dominant, and often clinically silent for years. There is room for a clearer appreciation of these unusual morphological and chronological forms of macular dystrophy.

**"Idiopathic" retinal detachment**

There are many case reports of retinal detachment in sibs and over two generations, generally developing in middle-life but occasionally earlier on. Myopia—usually of the high type—is commonly present, but in many instances myopia was either slight or altogether lacking. Fig. 139 shows two representative pedigrees: in one family high myopia was present, and this was lacking in the second.

(a) (b)

(c) (d)

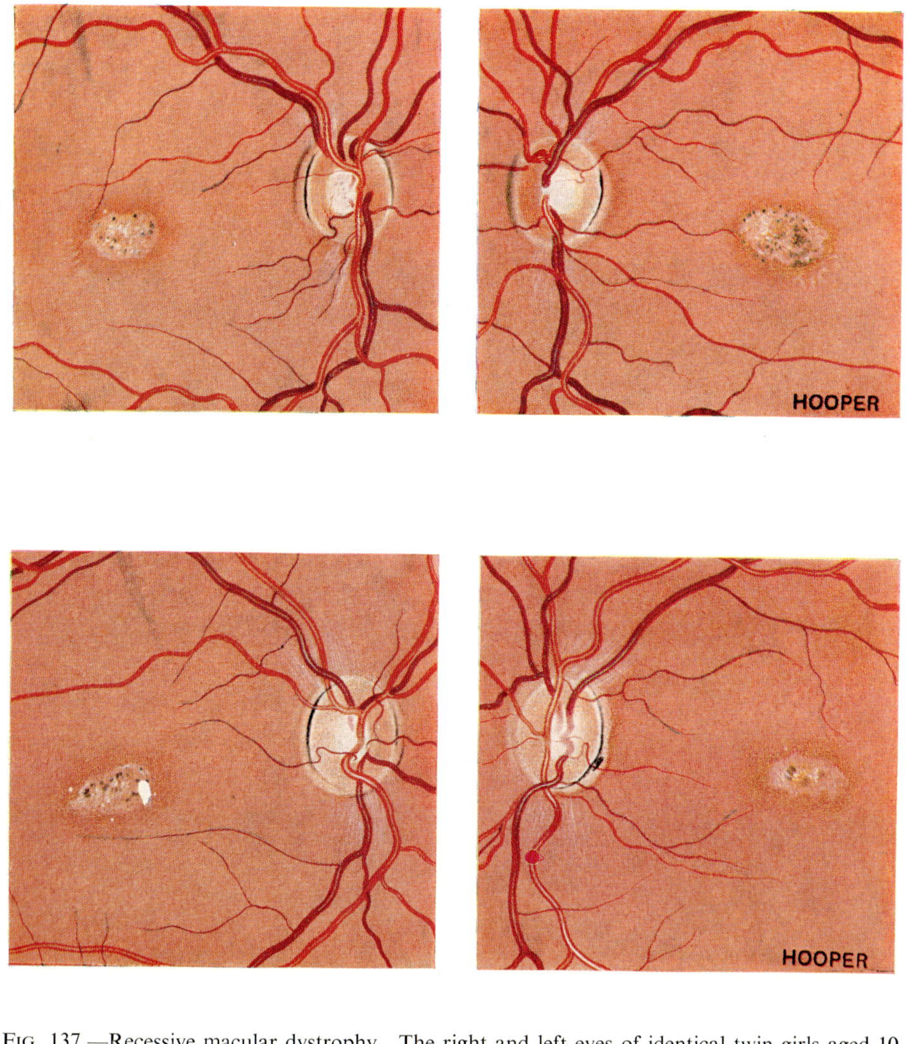


FIG. 137.—Recessive macular dystrophy. The right and left eyes of identical twin girls aged 10 years. Both showed exactly similar lesions.

[*To face page 140*

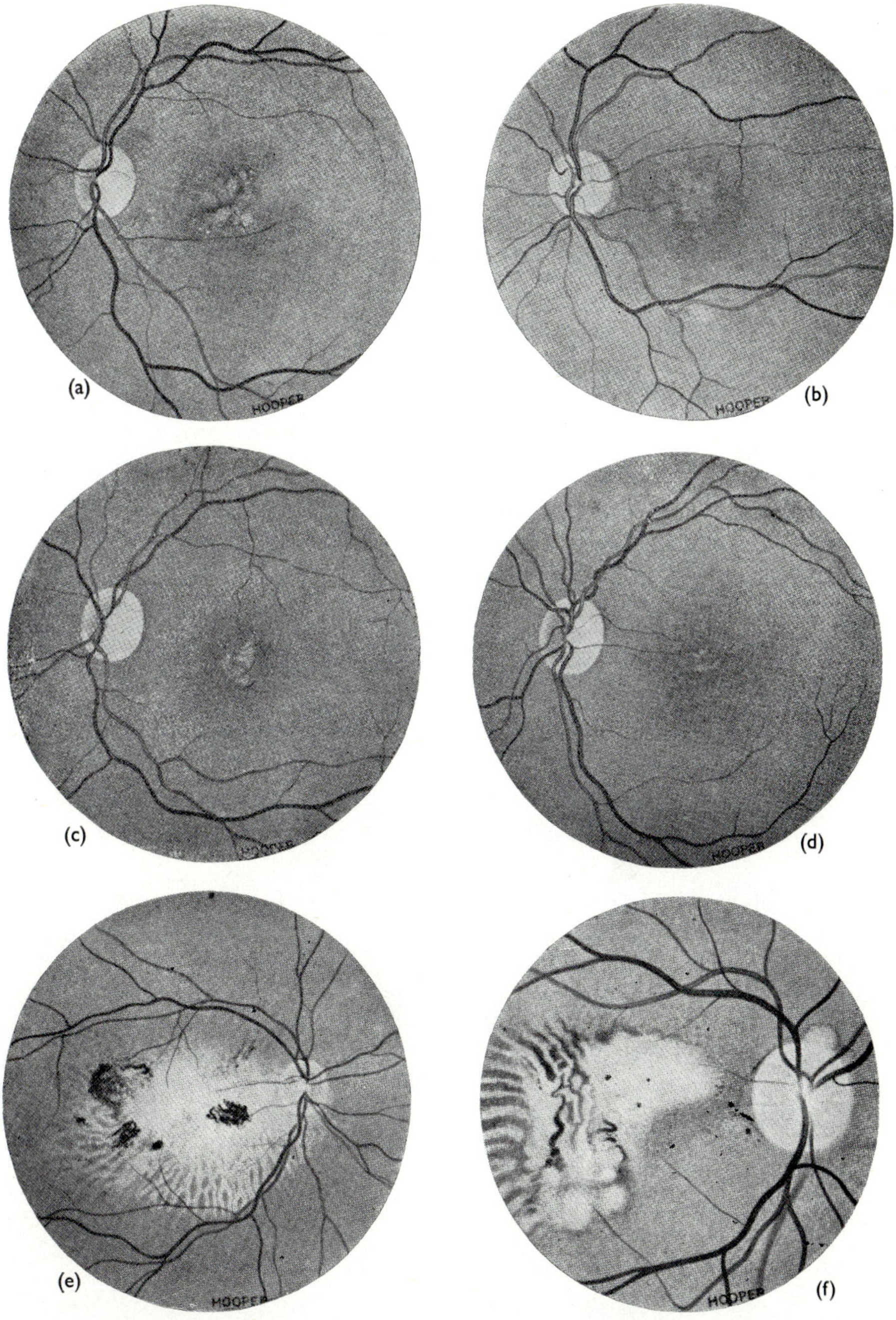


FIG. 138.—Macular dystrophy. The dominant type. Appearances in a family over three generations. (*a*) A man aged 51 years. (*b*) His mother aged 83 years. (*c*) His sister aged 49 years. (*d*) Her daughter aged 24 years. (*e*) A sister of the woman shown in (*b*), aged 86 years. (*f*) Her daughter aged 61 years. In all but the patient shown in (*d*) vision was grossly affected; gross colour defects were present in all patients. (*After Sorsby and Davey*, 1955.)

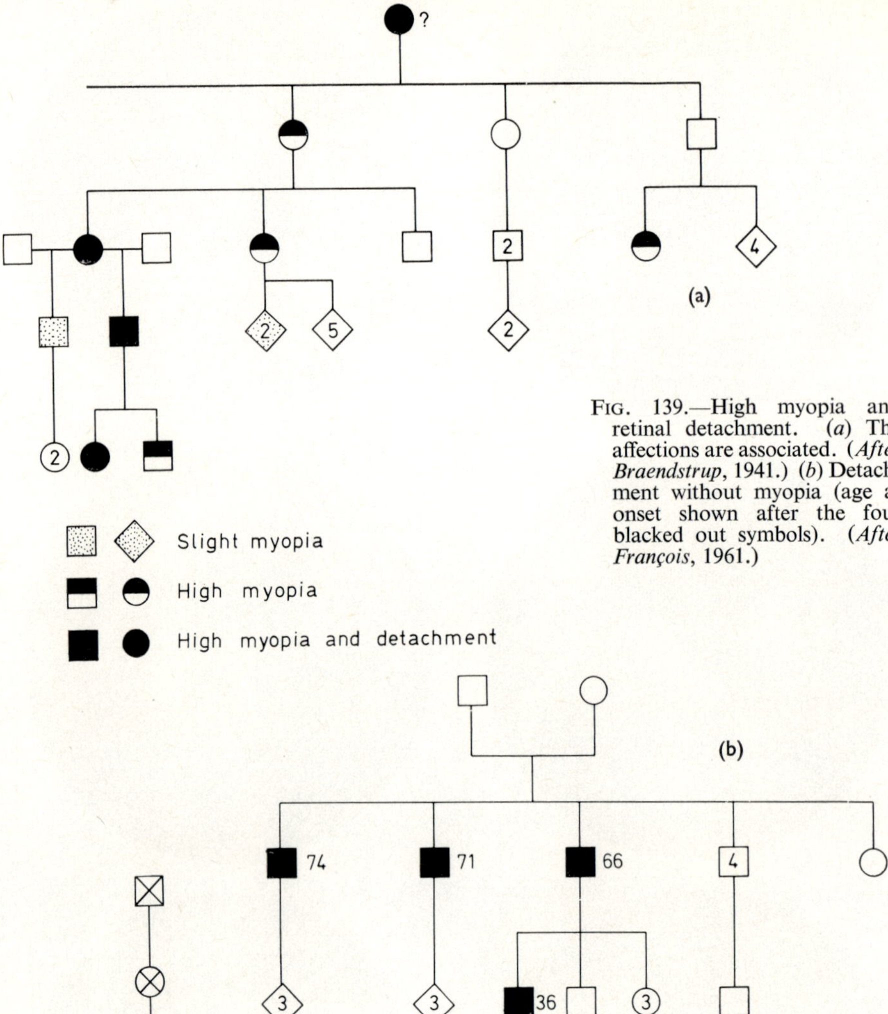


FIG. 139.—High myopia and retinal detachment. (*a*) The affections are associated. (*After Braendstrup*, 1941.) (*b*) Detachment without myopia (age at onset shown after the four blacked out symbols). (*After François*, 1961.)

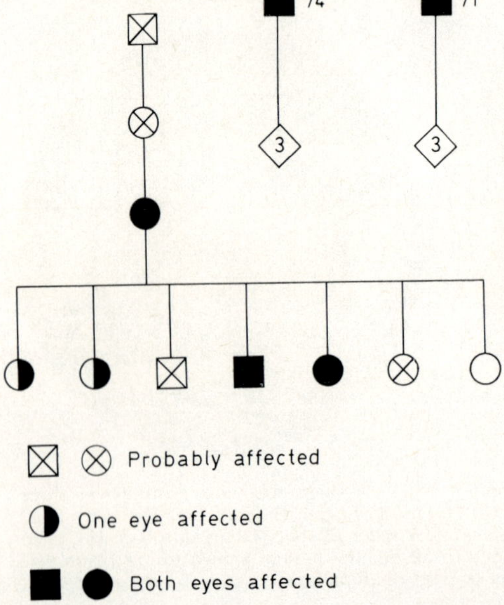


FIG. 140 (*left*).—Retinal detachment in eyes with dystrophic areas at the periphery of the retina. (*After Friedman*, 1-39.)

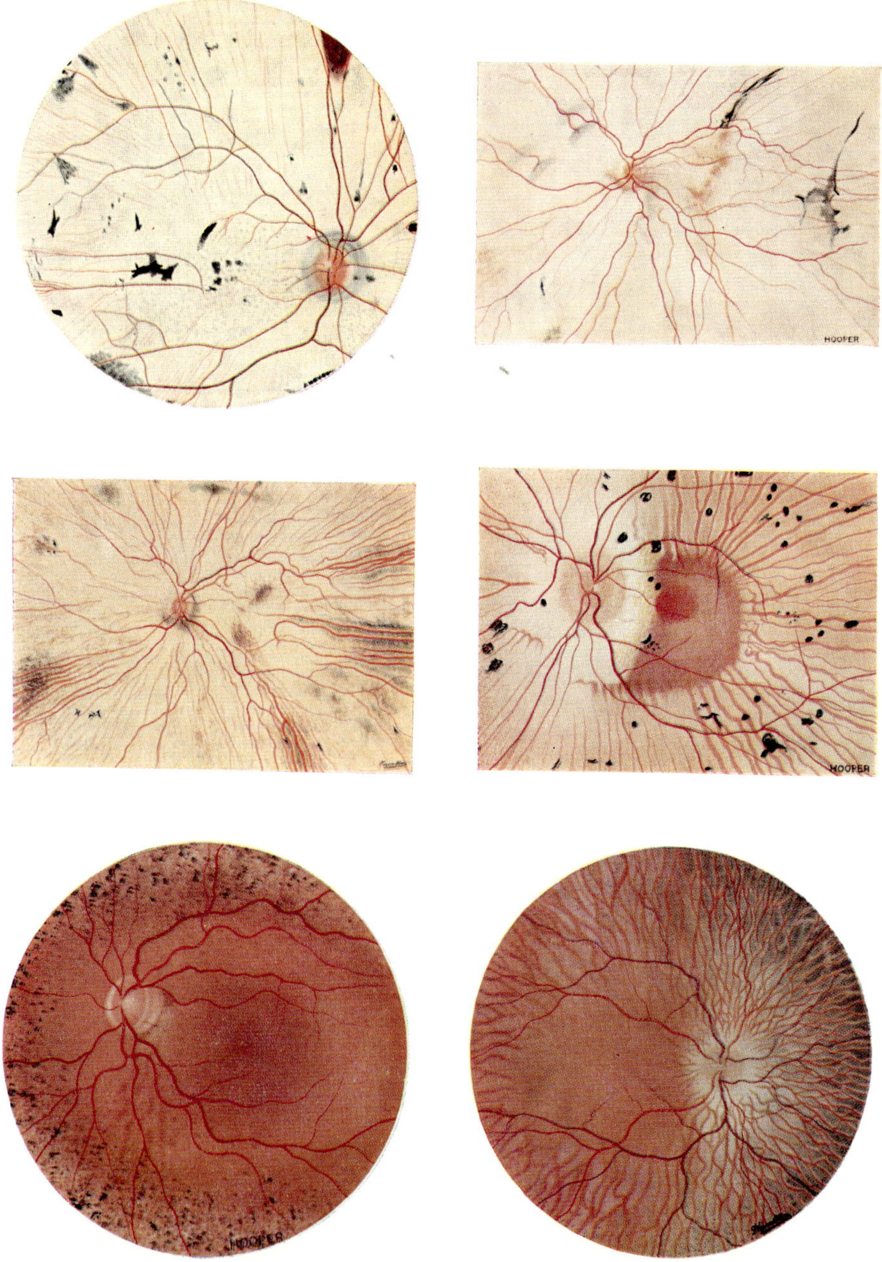


(a) (b) (c) (d) (e) (f)

FIG. 141.—Progressive choroidal atrophy ("choroideremia"). Range of appearances in males. (*a*) Appearances in a man aged 57 years. (*b*) Appearances in a cousin aged 41 years. (*c*) Appearances in the man shown in (*b*) 13 years previously. (*d*) Appearances in a man (in an unrelated family) aged 35 years. (*e*) Appearances in a youth (in another unrelated family) aged 18 years. (*f*) Appearances in a boy aged 4 years, a member of a collateral branch of the family illustrated in (*a*), (*b*) and (*c*). (*After Sorsby, Franceschetti, Joseph and Davey*, 1952.)

[*To face page 142*

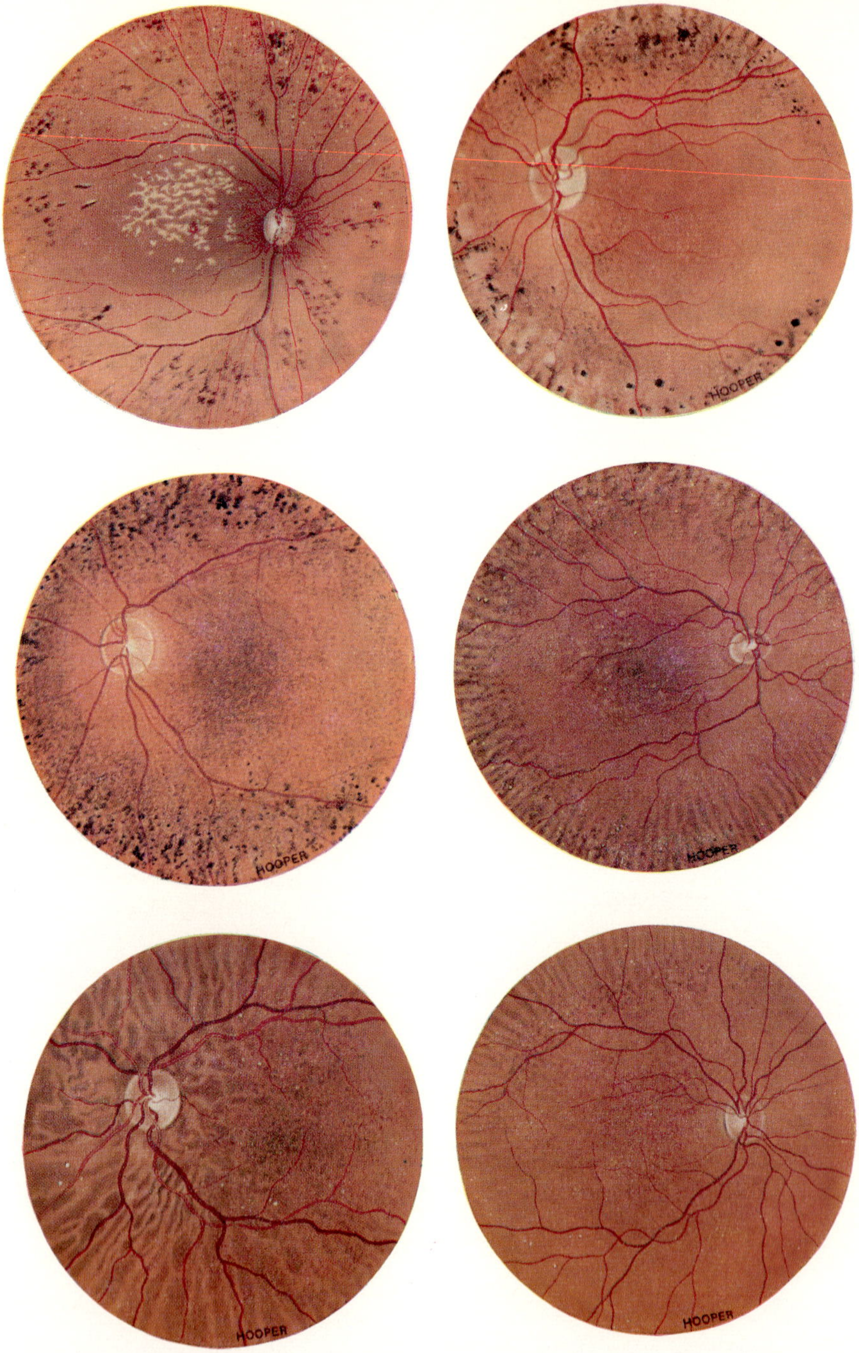

(a) (b) (c) (d) (e) (f)

FIG. 142.—Progressive choroidal atrophy ("choroideremia"). Range of appearances in female carriers. (*a*) Appearances in a woman aged 23 years—a member of the family depicted in Fig. 141 *a*. (*b*), (*c*) and (*f*) Vision was unaffected in spite of the central lesion. (*b*) Appearances in a woman aged 45 years, the mother of the youth shown in Fig. 141 *e*. (*c*) Appearances in a girl aged 3 years, the daughter of the man shown in Fig. 141 *d*. (*d*) Appearances in a girl aged 14 years, daughter of the woman shown in (*f*) and a cousin of the youth shown in Fig. 141 *e*. (*e*) Appearances in a woman aged 65 years, mother of the man shown in Fig. 141 *b* and *c*. (*f*) Appearances in a woman aged 39 years, mother of the girl shown in (*d*) and sister of the woman shown in (*b*). (*After Sorsby, Franceschetti, Joseph and Davey*, 1952.)

*To face page 143*]

No adequate studies on unselected families or twin series are available. Fig. 140 is of interest in bringing out the presence of peripheral retinal lesions in some of the apparently normal members of an affected sibship. It is possible that this—rather than the actual detachment, which may well be precipitated by environmental factors—is the lesion which is inherited, presumably as an abiotrophic defect. A contrary reading is suggested by other families with such retinal lesions but no detachment (Everett, 1968).

## CHOROID

### Choroideremia (progressive choroidal atrophy of the choroid)

As the name implies, the affection when it was first recognized was regarded as a congenital anomaly due to absence of the choroidal vessels—somewhat parallel to the non-pigmented coloboma of the macula. That the affection was, however, progressive in character, became evident as cases accumulated and less extreme aspects of the disorder were recognized as part of an evolutionary course. The presence of night-blindness as a cardinal sign of the affection and the pigmentary disturbance seen during the course of development, before the ultimate stage of atrophy of the choroidal vessels, led to the assumption that choroideremia was related to retinitis pigmentosa—a reading supported by the fact that at the end stage there was narrowing of the retinal arteries. Further confusion between choroideremia and retinitis pigmentosa came from descriptions of "atypical retinitis pigmentosa" in some members of families with choroideremia.

These difficulties have now been resolved, and the status of choroideremia as an independent affection, abiotrophic in type, is now unquestioned. Choroideremia shares with retinitis pigmentosa the symptom of night-blindness and retention of central vision until towards the end; otherwise the two affections differ considerably. The mode of inheritance of choroideremia has been shown to be sex-linked, and the "atypical retinitis pigmentosa" observed in families with choroideremia has been recognized as instances of the carrier state in women (McCulloch and McCulloch, 1948).

The mildest changes of choroideremia have been observed in boys in the first years of life when the fundus shows fine granular changes, indistinguishable from the changes seen in carrier women. The progressive nature of these changes is illustrated in Fig. 141, whilst the essentially stationary character of the carrier state is shown in Fig. 142. Although the affection in males is relentlessly progressive, the severity is not directly related to age: blindness may supervene as early as the twenties, or not until as late as the sixties. There is nothing to suggest that the changes seen in the carrier state are progressive: the mild carrier state has been observed in elderly women, whilst young girls have shown marked changes. That choroideremia should give the symptoms of retinitis pigmentosa and ultimately the narrowing of arteries and the optic atrophy reminiscent of retinitis pigmentosa is not unexpected in view of the fact that there is a slow cutting off of the blood supply to the retina, so that inevitably there is a slowly developing death of the retina with attendant progressive loss of function and structure.

At the end stage the picture of choroideremia is unmistakable: the white glistening sclerotic dominates the fundus background, broken only here and there by tufts of choroidal vessels and mild pigment changes, whilst the disc is atrophic and the retinal vessels narrow. Choroidal vessels persist longest at the central area. Before the end stages, the diagnosis presents considerable difficulty, as narrowed or obliterated choroidal vessels are seen against the fundus background and the diagnosis of choroidal sclerosis is feasible. At an earlier stage still the mottled reaction of the fundus, particularly towards the periphery, is, as already mentioned, indistinguishable from the marked carrier state and in mild cases may well be regarded as a physiological variation, and in more severe cases as a variant of "pepper and salt" fundus.

In the carrier state the peripheral pigmentary mottling is highly suggestive and may be mistaken for a physiological variation. It is readily distinguished from the characteristic tapetal reflex seen in the carrier state of retinitis pigmentosa.

As choroideremia is inherited in an intermediate sex-linked manner (Fig. 143), it is possible to recognize the carrier women readily by the characteristic fundus appearances. It should be noted, however, that these appearances may be minimal and easily missed. Occasionally carriers show the full affection (Kurstjens, 1965; Fraser and Friedmann, 1968).

The gene for the affection is far apart from the Xg locus on the X chromosome (Øther, 1968).

**Choroidal sclerosis**

Sclerosis of the choroidal vessels is an aspect of many fundus disturbances. Involutionary changes of the atherosclerosis type in the choroidal vessels are histologically a normal feature of senescence, and are apparently present as early as the age of 40. Pathological obliteration of the choroidal vessels is suggested when the choroidal vessels stand out ophthalmoscopically as white streaks against the fundus background, but histologically in some such cases the choroidal vessels have been found patent and the sheathing along the vessels the result of connective tissue proliferation in between the vessels. Appearances suggestive of choroidal sclerosis are also seen in generalized fundus dystrophy and, as already noted, during the evolution of choroideremia. In the literature on retinitis pigmentosa there is the repeated suggestion that there are two types of this affection, a choroidal or mesodermal type and a retinal or ectodermal type—the choroidal type being characterized by obvious choroidal sclerosis not generally seen in the retinal type. Likewise, in the normal fundus it is not easy to distinguish *fundus tigré* with its normal choroidal circulation from early choroidal sclerosis producing an ophthalmoscopically similar patterning. Nonetheless there is apparently a genuine counterpart to choroideremia in so far that there is a primary choroidal disturbance shown not by the disappearance of the choroidal vessels as in choroideremia, but by their conversion into obliterated white cords. Choroidal sclerosis as a clinical entity has been well established for years, but its genetic character has been recognized only fairly recently.

Three hereditary forms of choroidal sclerosis can be distinguished.

*Central choroidal sclerosis*

The characteristic appearances of a sharply delineated circular or transversely oval patch of choroidal sclerosis was known to Liebreich as early as 1862, and was described by Nettleship in 1884 under the designation of central senile areolar choroidal atrophy. It is clear that the designation "senile" is inapplicable, and that the earliest changes may occur by the age of 20 or before, and take the form of white dots over the central area. A number of families studied are now available and whilst recessive inheritance appears to be the rule (Fig. 144 *a*), families are known in which it occurred as a dominant disorder (Fig. 144 *b*).

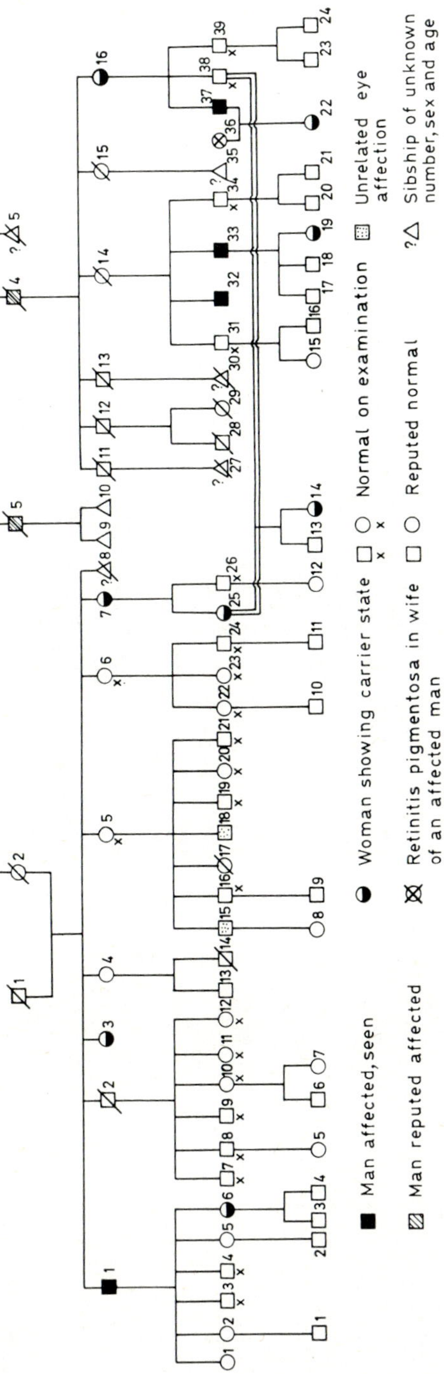


FIG. 143.—Choroideremia. Pedigree showing intermediate sex-linked inheritance. (*After Sorsby, Franceschetti, Joseph and Davey*, 1952.)

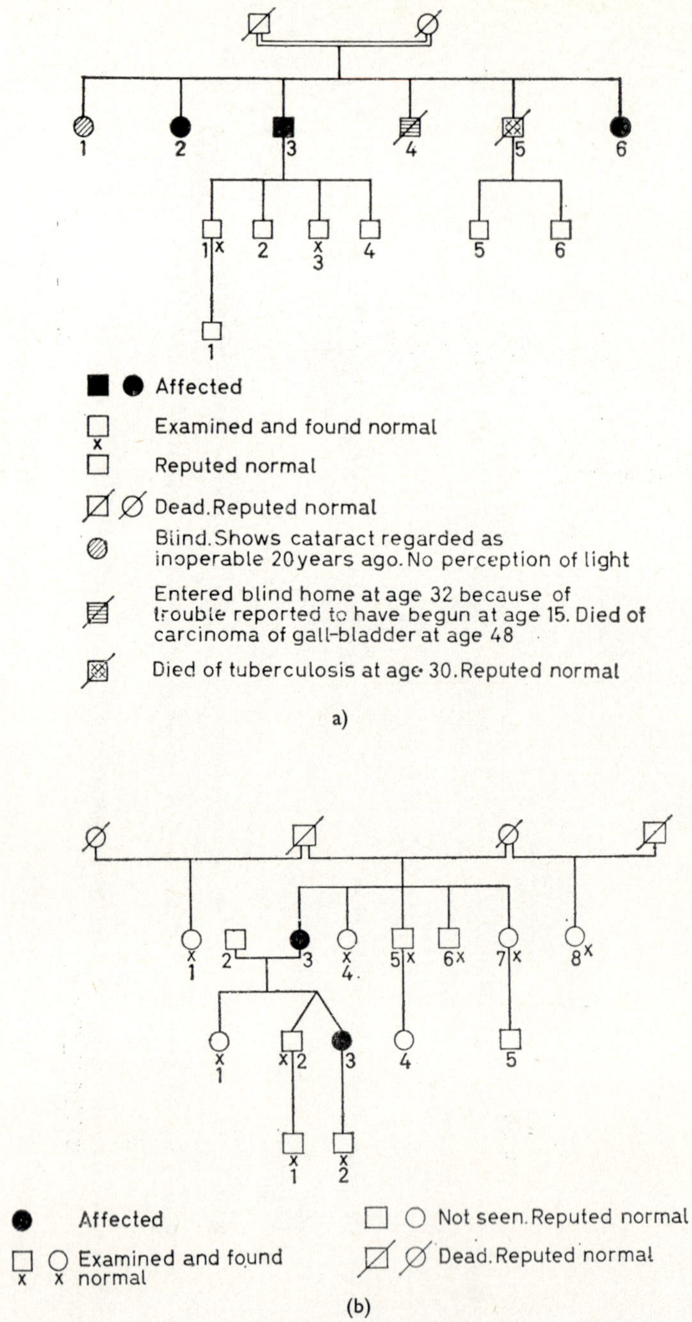


FIG. 144.—Central choroidal sclerosis. (*a*) Recessive inheritance. (*b*) Dominant inheritance. (*After Sorsby and Crick*, 1953.)

Whilst the affected area is generally sharply delineated from the rest of the fundus, individual cases do show some ill-defined choroidal sclerosis extending beyond the central area; this, however, is exceptional.

*Subjective symptoms.*—There is no night-blindness and the visual symptoms follow on the slow shutting off of the blood supply to the central area, so that central vision declines and at the height of the affection is reduced to counting fingers; the peripheral vision remains intact.

*Morbid histology.*—The one study available suggested that the choroidal vessels were not grossly affected but patterned by exudation. It is difficult to fit this with the ophthalmoscopic appearances and clinical course.

*Generalized choroidal sclerosis*

This group is not so well defined as central choroidal sclerosis. The ophthalmoscopic appearances of the choroidal vessels as white streaks is indeed unmistakable, and the distribution of these white streaks all over the fundus justifies the designation of generalized choroidal sclerosis. The earliest stages of this affection—as the earlier stages of central choroidal sclerosis—are represented by white dots over the fundus, with possibly mild pigmentary disturbances; these are indicative of the slow dying of the overlying retina. The difficulty is to know whether these appearances will ultimately lead to the fairly clear-cut picture of conversion of the whole of the choroidal pattern into white streaks, or whether the intermediate stages ultimately finish in either the picture of choroideremia or generalized fundus dystrophy—or even retinitis pigmentosa. Family studies are therefore particularly important in the diagnosis of choroidal sclerosis, and further studies are needed on the subjective symptoms, particularly on night-blindness.

*Heredity.*—It is likely that generalized choroidal sclerosis is dominant (Fig. 145), a point that helps to distinguish it from retinitis pigmentosa (with its usual recessive course) and from choroideremia with its sex-linkage.

*Peripapillary choroidal sclerosis*

In one sibship, two sisters were affected with a marked peripapillary choroidal sclerosis reminiscent of *Caput Medusae* of the early ophthalmological literature. Further studies are needed.

**Myopic chorio-retinal atrophy**

Myopic chorio-retinal atrophy sets in in middle-life, many years after the actual progression in myopia has occurred in childhood, adolescence and early adult life. Seeing that myopia itself—including moderate and high myopia in which this chorio-retinal atrophy is seen—is hereditary in character it is likely that the atrophy is one of the late abiotrophies. Adequate family studies, however, are not available.

## Abiotrophies of Uncertain Origin

The five affections described in this section are of uncertain anatomical origin. Such histological evidence as is available suggests that generalized fundus dystrophy may follow on changes in the membrane of Bruch, linking it histologically but not clinically nor genetically with disciform degeneration of the macula. The nature of Doyne's choroiditis is also unknown. The one study available suggests that it is due to massive colloid formation, again at the membrane of Bruch. The

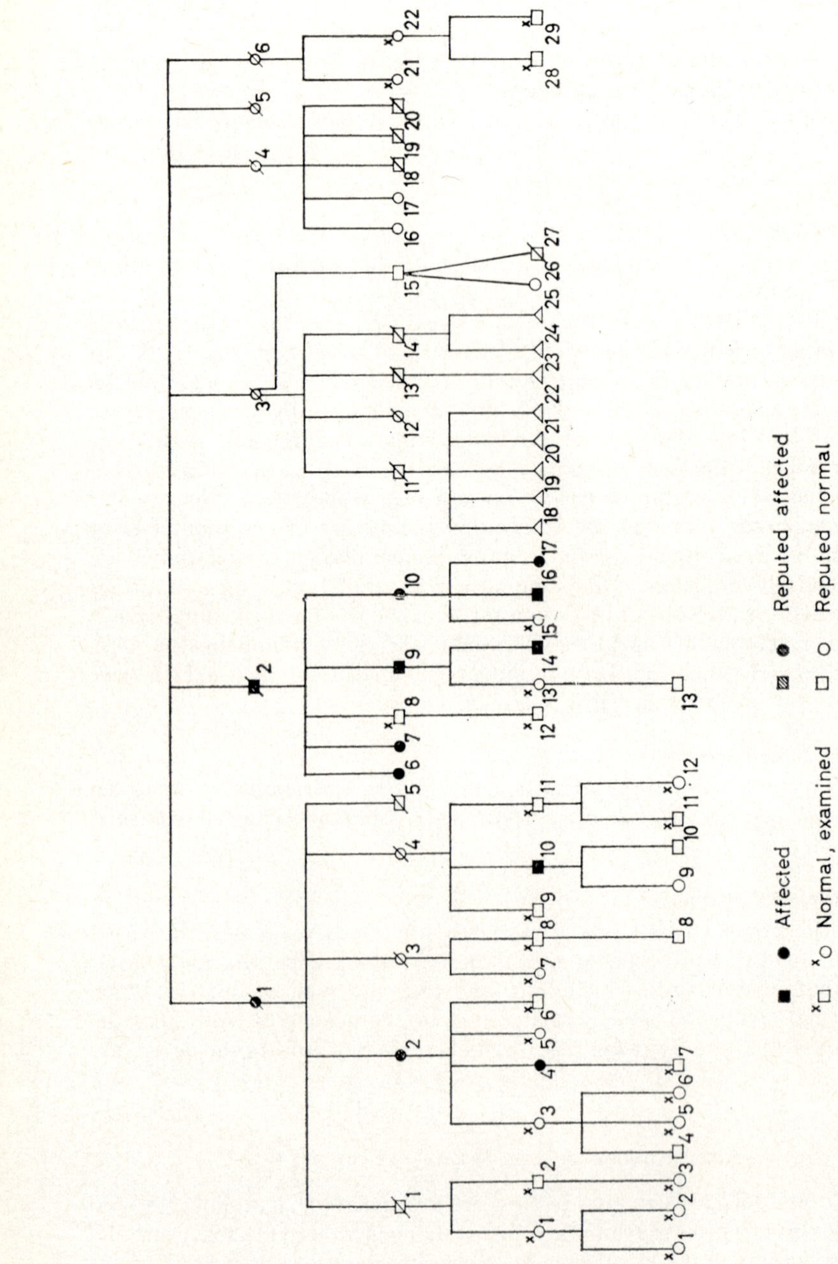


FIG. 145.—Generalized choroidal sclerosis. Dominant inheritance. (*After Sorsby and Davey*, 1955.)

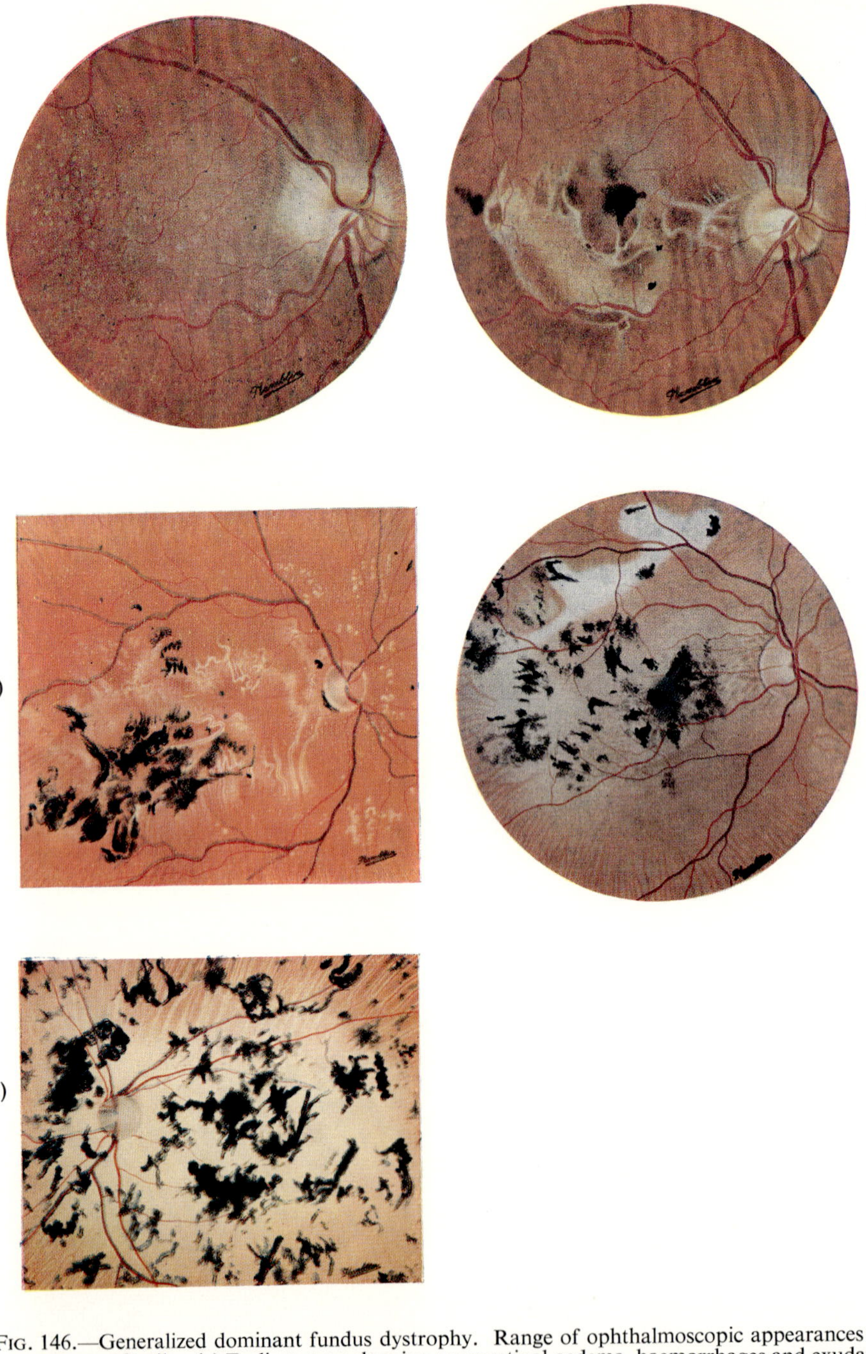

(a) (b) (c) (d) (e)

FIG. 146.—Generalized dominant fundus dystrophy. Range of ophthalmoscopic appearances as seen in one family. (*a*) Earliest stage showing neuroretinal oedema, haemorrhages and exudates in a patient aged 41 years. (*b*) The same eye 22 months later, showing scar formation. (*c*) Appearances in a cousin of the patient at the age of 68 years; patterned exudates, pigmentary reaction, and early choroidal sclerosis are all evident. (*d*) Appearances in an uncle at the age of 57 years. There is considerable atrophy. (*e*) Appearances in an aunt at the age of 77 years. There is extensive atrophy and considerable choroidal sclerosis, and some pigmentary disturbance. There is also coincidental glaucomatous optic atrophy. (*After Sorsby and Joll Mason*, 1949.)

*To face page 149*]

pathological basis of the so-called senile macular lesions is obscure, though some at least are the result of primary retinal lesions, as are the macular lesions seen in the elderly members of families with dominant macular dystrophy. As for gyrate atrophy, its very existence as a separate entity is in question, and in Wagner's disease the vitreous as well as the retina appears to be implicated.

**Dominant generalized fundus dystrophy**

The affection was described by Sorsby and Mason in 1949. Few case reports have as yet appeared, but the condition is not uncommon. The intermediate stages show an extremely wide range of appearances, presenting considerable difficulties in the diagnosis of individual cases.

*Clinical features.*—The affection commonly begins at about the age of 40 years. The first subjective symptoms are blurring of central vision in one eye followed by the same symptoms in the other eye within a matter of months, or perhaps within a few years. It is not known whether the two eyes may be affected simultaneously. Central vision rapidly declines, but there is no involvement of peripheral vision or colour vision at this stage. There are no symptoms of night-blindness early on or during the course of the affection.

Objectively the first signs are oedema, haemorrhages, and exudates in the central area (Fig. 146). This progresses to scar formation with a varying amount of pigment proliferation, which may be exceedingly massive. The choroidal vessels become exposed and show some sclerosis. Over the course of years the process extends peripherally, choroidal sclerosis generally becomes more manifest and sometimes dominates the picture. During its spread peripherally, exudates—sometimes patterned—may appear. Occasionally, widespread glistening "colloid" bodies may be a pointing sign. The end-stage is extensive disappearance of the choroidal vessels exposing the sclerotic covered irregularly by proliferating pigment. The terminal stage produces practically total blindness. The full course of the affection spreads normally over about 35 years. The process may, however, be milder or more severe in individual cases.

The polymorphism of the fundus reactions is such that any stage of oedematous and inflammatory fundus lesions as well as diffuse choroidal sclerosis can be simulated.

*Histology.*—Ruptures in the membrane of Bruch were the outstanding features in two sisters with this affection (Ashton and Sorsby, 1951). Clinically these cases were not quite conclusive examples of the affection; further studies are needed.

*Heredity.*—Genetically the condition is a simple autosomal dominant (Fig. 147).

**Doyne's "choroiditis"**

This patterned form of central retinal dystrophy (Fig. 148) has these unusual features:

(1) The lesion is much more extensive than Stargardt's disease or dominant macular dystrophy, though it never becomes a generalized disorder extending over the whole of the fundus.

(2) Instead of pigmentary reaction there are white reactions of the colloid body type, occasionally becoming patterned into the "honeycomb" described by Doyne. The "honeycomb" itself is exceptional, but the white patterned lesion is characteristic.

(3) At the later stages fine lines of pigment proliferation appear.

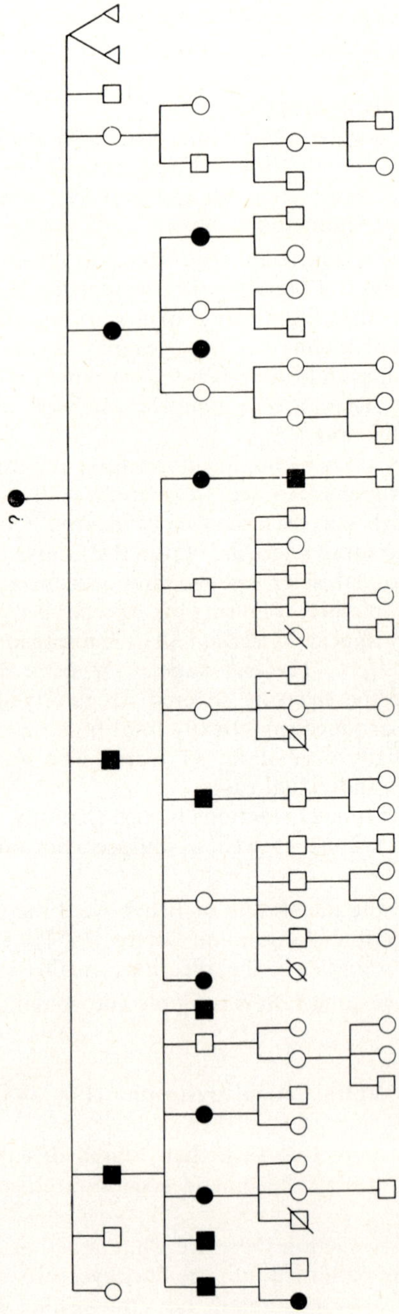


FIG. 147.—Generalized fundus dystrophy. Pedigree showing dominant inheritance (most of the members of the fourth and fifth generations have not yet reached the age of manifestation of the affection). (*After Sorsby and Mason*, 1949.)

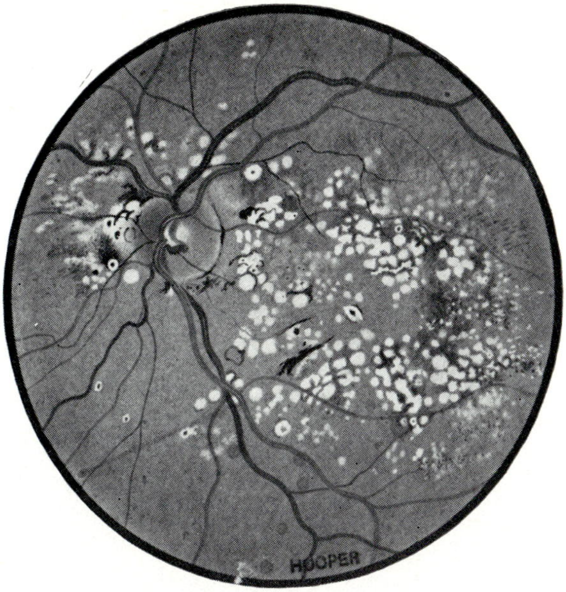


FIG. 148.—Doyne's choroiditis. Fundus in IV, 1, in Fig. 149.

The affection is dominant (Fig. 149) and has been recorded in Switzerland under the name *Maladie Leventinese*. It is apparently not common, though its frequency may be under-estimated owing to the fact that most cases run a mild course and many sufferers are unaware of the existence of their trouble. In only a minority of patients is central vision affected. Commonly, in addition to the macular and paramacular lesion, colloid bodies are also to be observed on the nasal edge of the disc. When present they are of considerable diagnostic significance.

Doyne's choroiditis, when it does give trouble, is unlikely to do so before middle-life, though ophthalmoscopic evidence of the affection may be present very much earlier—as early as twenty or before.

**"Senile macular degeneration"**

It has already been observed that the end-stage of dominant macular dystrophy may simulate so-called senile macular degeneration. It is possible that some cases of macular lesions in the elderly are genetically determined; the evidence is as yet indefinite.

**Gyrate atrophy**

It is unlikely that gyrate atrophy is a stage in the development of choroideremia, as has been repeatedly suggested. Although many cases of gyrate atrophy have been followed up, in no cases is there a record of choroideremia as the end-result. Ophthalmoscopically, a plexus of blood vessels at the macula is common in choroideremia, but is not seen in gyrate atrophy. Moreover, the two affections have a different mode of inheritance: gyrate atrophy is said to be recessive, choroideremia is clearly sex-linked. High myopia is said to be common in gyrate atrophy.

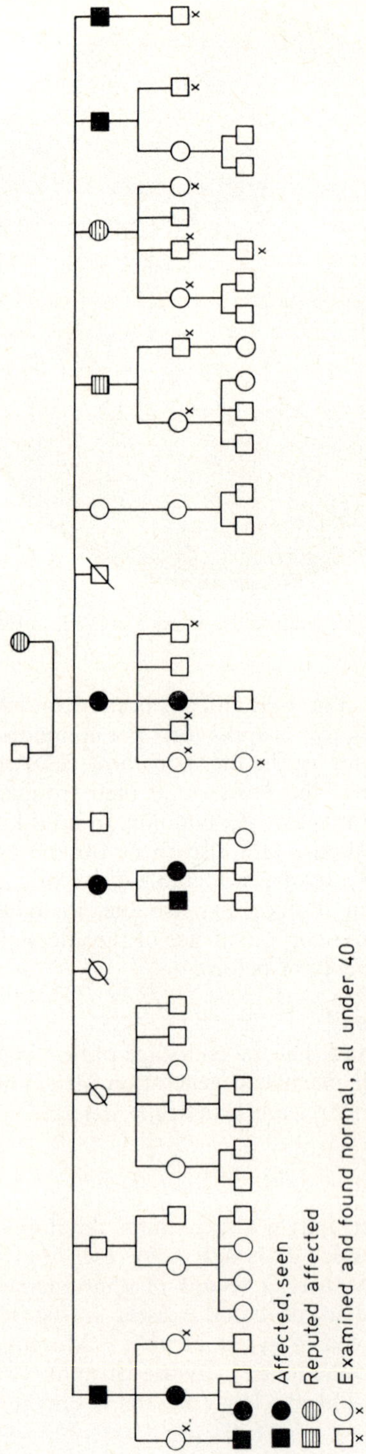


FIG. 149.—Doyne's "choroiditis". Dominant inheritance. (*Personal observation, unpublished.*)

**Wagner's disease**

In 1938 Wagner reported on a Swiss family in which 13 members were affected with unusual vitreous and retinal lesions. The vitreous was liquefied and optically almost empty, containing only a few punctiform fibrils. Adhesions to the internal limiting membrane were, however, present and are illustrated in Fig. 150, which also shows the reticulated nature of some of the adhesions. The retina itself showed peripheral pigmentation, whilst some of the retinal vessels carried white

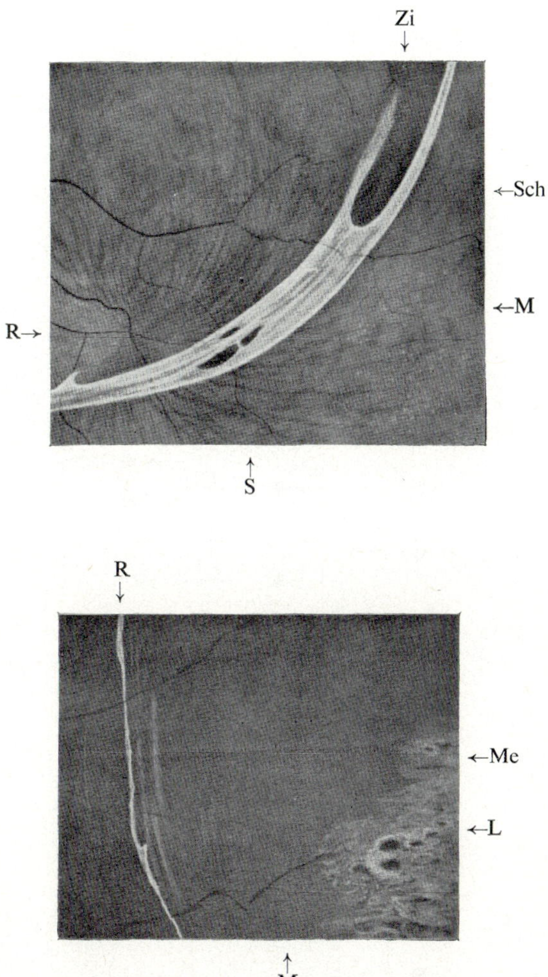


FIG. 150.—Degeneratio hyaloideo-retinalis. Zi = rag-like adhesions of the vitreous "membrane" (M, Me and R) to the membrana limitans interna, showing some holes (S, Sch). L = holes and condensation of the vitreous "membrane". (*After Wagner*, 1938.)

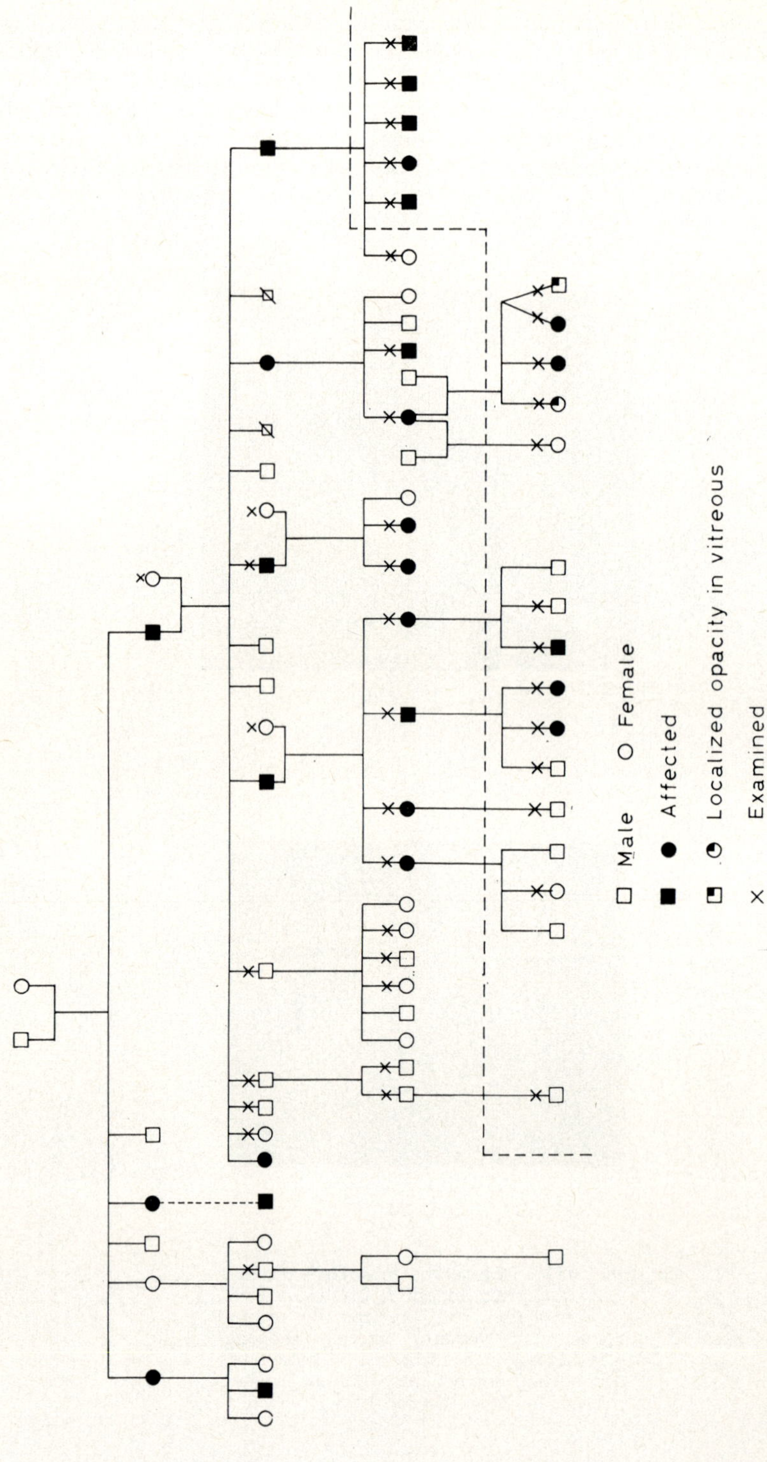


FIG. 151.—Pedigree showing dominant inheritance of Wagner's disease. The pedigree above the broken line was recorded by Wagner (1938) and below it by Boehringer, Dieterle and Landolt (1960). (*After Ricci*, 1961.)

streaks. Some of the patients showed further degenerative changes, such as atrophic choroidal areas with sclerosed vessels, and even optic atrophy. All patients but the youngest showed posterior cortical lens changes, progressing to complicated cataract later in life. Vision was generally good until the late degenerative changes set in, though scotomata were present in some cases earlier on. All patients showed low myopia (about 3 to 4 D). The affection was clearly dominant and was designated by Wagner as *Degeneratio hyaloidio-retinalis heredetaria.*

The family recorded by Wagner has been studied subsequently by Boehringer, Dieterle and Landolt in 1960 and by Ricci in 1961. The completed pedigree is shown in Fig. 151. The dominant autosomal inheritance is beyond question.

As yet other studies are few. Holste, in 1939, briefly recorded two cases, and a family was studied by Jansen in Holland (Waardenburg, Franceschetti and Klein, 1963). Little has been added to the clinical picture as given by Wagner. It would appear that an almost pathognomonic feature is the presence of condensed streaks in the posterior limiting membrane of the vitreous, giving rise to pre-retinal concentric peripheral striae (Fig. 152). Arcuate scotomata are not uncommon, but

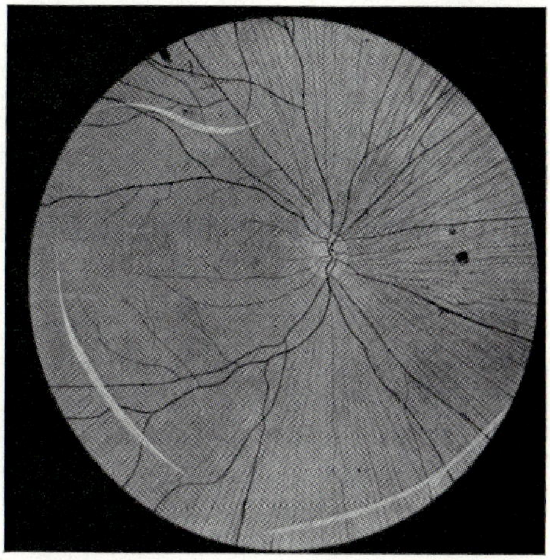

FIG. 152.—Vitreous streaks and polymorphous pigmentation in a case of Wagner's disease. (*After Boehringer, Dieterle and Landolt*, 1960.)

dark adaptation and the ERG are normal, or but slightly reduced. Both a high myope and a high hypermetrope were observed in these subsequent studies, and vitreous opacities were noted by Boehringer, Dieterle and Landolt as the only lesions in two sibs of an affected family group.

A histological study made by Babel is recorded by Ricci and by Franceschetti, François and Babel (1963). It concerns one of the cases described by Wagner and followed up by Boehringer. The lesion was most marked at the equator where a fine glial membrane covered the internal limiting membrane; it split into two leaves, one extending towards the retina and the other towards the vitreous, leaving empty spaces in between. There was cellular infiltration into the layers of the retina which itself was not greatly disturbed; the neuro-epithelium in itself appeared normal, but there were some changes in the pigment epithelium and choroid. These findings are not dissimilar to those recorded by Wagner in 1941.

## TUMOURS

### "Sarcoma" of the choroid

This has been observed in sibs and over two and even three generations. It is said that these rare genetically determined cases occur earlier than the sporadic cases (Lynch and colleagues, 1968) (Fig. 153).

### Retinoblastoma

Towards the end of the last century familial occurrence of retinoblastoma began to be reported with increasing frequency, and de Gouvea in 1896 recorded the occurrence of the affection in both eyes in three out of seven children born to a man who had lost an eye in infancy from retinoblastoma. A substantial number of pedigrees, mostly showing affected sibships, are now available. From the accumulated literature it appears that there is no high rate of parental consanguinity in affected sibships, that some of the affected sibs are now known to have themselves transmitted the disease, and that there are now many pedigrees with transmission over two or three generations. The available material gives little support for recessive inheritance and suggests dominance with incomplete expressivity and penetrance (Fig. 154). Whilst the occurrence of both unilateral and bilateral cases and the occasional occurrence of spontaneous cure add to the difficulties of analysis, it is, however, clear that frankly hereditary cases are exceptional, the sporadic case being the rule.

The highly lethal character of untreated retinoblastoma, and the high mortality of treated cases, raised the possibility that every fresh case of this infantile disease represented a germinal mutation. Vogel in 1954 and 1957 questioned the validity

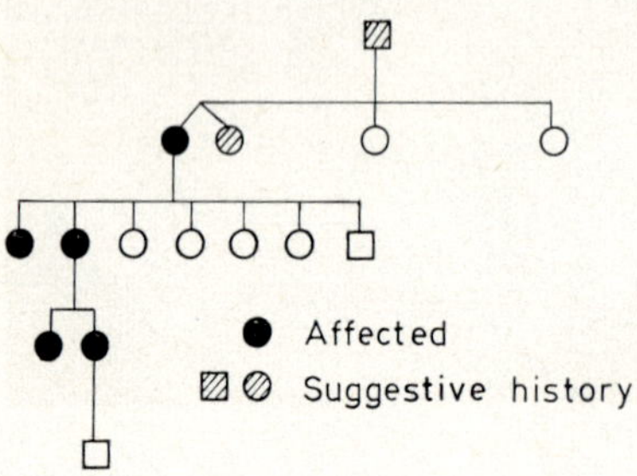


FIG. 153.—Sarcoma of choroid. Pedigree showing dominant inheritance. (*After Davenport*, 1927.)

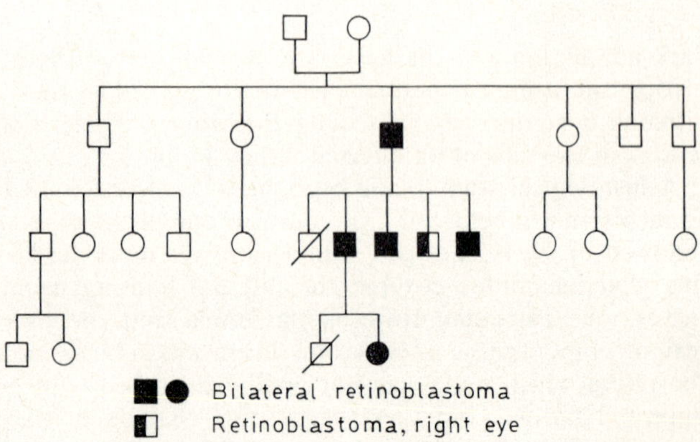


FIG. 154. — Retinoblastoma: mutation. In the second generation there is an isolated occurrence of retinoblastoma, presumably due to a fresh mutation. Dominant inheritance is seen fom the subsequent course. (*After Griffith and Sorsby*, 1944.)

of this assumption and holds that germinal mutations account for only a minority of the cases of retinoblastoma, most cases being genuinely sporadic.

Most cases of retinoblastoma are unilateral and it is likely that these cases are determined genetically only exceptionally. It is assumed that they represent a somatic mutation (Vogel). This view is based on the fact that a high proportion of family groups with retinoblastoma show the disease in the bilateral form, whilst the starting point of new lines of retinoblastoma have almost invariably been in survivors who have lost both eyes from the affection. It has been computed that the risk of transmission with an apparently sporadic case of unilateral retinoblastoma is of the order of 4 per cent; the risk of transmission is considerably higher in apparently sporadic cases with both eyes affected. The risk of transmission by a member of a known retinoblastoma family, whether affected in one eye or both, is rather less than the 50 per cent characteristic of dominance, owing to incomplete penetrance and expression of the gene.

The wide range of ophthalmoscopic appearances in the hereditary affections of the retina and choroid—as isolated disorders or in association with general disturbances—is shown in summary form in Table X. It is clear that no single criterion—clinical, pathological or genetic—is definitive.

## ANOMALIES OF COLOUR VISION

In trichromatic vision any colour (or spectral light) can be matched by a mixture of three primary colours (or spectral lights). Dichromats can match any light with a mixture of two primary lights. In monochromatic vision any light can be matched by any other light, merely by adjusting intensities.

Normal trichromatic vision is present in about 92 per cent of men and about 99·5 per cent or more of women. Of the 8 per cent or so defectives amongst men, most have trichromatic vision: they match a light with a mixture of three primary lights, but their trichromatic coefficient curves are of a different shape and their colour vision differs in some details from the normal trichomats (anomalous trichromatism). Only 2·6 per cent of men are dichromats. Monochromats are rare, and there does not appear to be any definite excess of men over women.

**Monochromatism** (total colour-blindness; day-blindness)

The classical form of total colour-blindness is an aspect of a severe symptom-complex, which includes photophobia, low visual acuity, and nystagmus. Luminosity curves and such sparse or ill-formed histological evidence as is available suggest that cones are lacking. It is now clear that the severity of the affection —designated rod monochromatism—may vary considerably, giving the so-called "incomplete form" of the disorder. Vision may be as high as 0·4, possibly because of a milder degree of nystagmus.

The familial occurrence of the affection was noted by Nettleship as early as 1880, when he also stressed the frequences of consanguinity in the parents. The available pedigrees show it as essentially a familial affection, and there are a not inconsiderable number of isolated cases. A high degree of consanguinity is recorded: around 30 per cent in most European series, and even more elsewhere.

## TABLE X

HEREDITARY AFFECTIONS OF THE RETINA AND OF THE CHOROID: CLINICAL CLASSIFICATION

| *Affection* | *Mode of inheritance* | *Remarks* |
|---|---|---|
| | 1. OPHTHALMOSCOPICALLY NEGATIVE | |
| Retinal aplasia—early stages | Recessive | "Cortical blindness" |
| | 2. INDEFINITE OEDEMA | |
| Infantile amaurotic idiocy—early stages | Recessive | A gross metabolic disorder—infiltration of ganglion cells with lipoids |
| | 3. PIGMENTARY DISTURBANCES | |
| | A. *The retinitis pigmentosa group* | |
| *Uncomplicated* | | |
| Classical retinitis pigmentosa | Recessive<br>Dominant<br>Sex-linked intermediate<br>Sex-linked recessive | |
| *With ocular associations* | | |
| with a macular lesion | Recessive | |
| with cataract | Recessive<br>Dominant | |
| with glaucoma | Recessive | |
| with diffuse ocular lesions (keratoconus, drusen, microphthalmos) | ? | Ill-defined affections |
| *With general associations* | | |
| with deaf-mutism | Recessive | |
| with mental deficiency | Dominant*<br>Recessive | |
| with lipoid metabolic disorders: Stock-Spielmeyer disease with various neurological disorders: | Recessive | |
| Mid-brain lesion: external ophthalmoplegia | ? | Requires elucidation |
| Spino-cerebellar lesions: | | |
| Friedreich's ataxia | Recessive | |
| Marie's ataxia | Dominant | |
| | B. *The macular dystrophies* | |
| (1) Stargardt's disease | Recessive | Onset in childhood |
| (2) Dominant macular dystrophy | Dominant | Onset of symptoms generally in adult life |
| (3) Sex-linked | ? | Requires elucidation |
| | C. *Combined peripheral and central* | |
| (1) Retinitis pigmentosa and macular dystrophy | Recessive | ? Associated with cystinuria |
| (2) Spreading macular dystrophies | ? | Requires elucidation |
| (3) Gyrate atrophy | ? Recessive | Requires elucidation |
| | D. *Retinal aplasia group* | |
| *Uncomplicated* | | |
| "Cortical blindness" progressing to "atypical retinitis pigmentosa" | Recessive<br>Dominant* | |
| Milder forms | Recessive<br>sex-linked | Intrafamilial variation. A clear-cut variant (Hoare, 1965) |

* Rare or uncommon.

TABLE X (*continued*)

HEREDITARY AFFECTIONS OF THE RETINA AND OF THE CHOROID: CLINICAL CLASSIFICATION

| *Affection* | *Mode of inheritance* | *Remarks* |
|---|---|---|
| *With ocular associations* | | |
| Cataract | Recessive | Require further elucidation |
| Keratoconus | Recessive | |
| ? Other | | |
| *With general associations* | | |
| Gross mental deficiency | Dominant | ? irregularly |
| Syndromes: | | |
| Laurence–Biedl | Recessive | |
| Alström | Recessive | |
| Hallgren | Recessive | |
| Refsum | Recessive | Tetramethyl hexadecanoic acid infiltration |
| Sjögren–Larsson | Recessive | |
| Cockayne | Recessive | |
| Bassen–Kornzweig | ? Intermediate | Congenital absence of beta-lipoprotein in serum |
| Senior–Friedmann–Braudo | ? Intermediate | |
| 4. HAEMORRHAGIC-EXUDATIVE REACTIONS | | |
| Angioid streaks | Recessive | Part of a syndrome (Grönblad's syndrome or elastosis dystrophica) |
| Generalized fundus dystrophy | Dominant | Onset in middle life |
| 5. PROGRESSIVE OBLITERATION OF CHOROIDAL VESSELS (Choroidal sclerosis) | | |
| Choroidal sclerosis: | | |
| Central areolar | Recessive | Not "senile" |
| | Dominant | a long asymptomatic course |
| Peripapillary ("Caput medusae") | Recessive | Massive choroidal haemorrhages |
| Generalized | Recessive | Varying rates of development. Asymptomatic white dots if slow |
| | Dominant | Retinitis pigmentosa appearances if moderate |
| | (?) Sex-linked | (?) "Choroideremia" if rapid and severe |
| 6. RETINOSCHISIS | | |
| Peripheral cyst formation | | |
| Multiple congenital cyst formation with rupture and haemorrhages | | A progressive affection. "Vitreous veils" a transient aspect |
| | | Macular lesions |
| | | End stage: gross retinal atrophy |
| (?) Symmetrical inferior temporal cysts | ? | Require elucidation |
| Central | | |
| (? Congenital) macular cysts | Dominant | (1) Episodes of inflammatory reaction |
| | Irregularly dominant | (2) Vitelliform disc or cyst |
| | | (3) Rupture at about 40 |
| Total retinal detachment | | |
| "Pseudoglioma" | Sex-linked | Mental deficiency probably not uncommon |

(*continued*)

TABLE X (*continued*)

HEREDITARY AFFECTIONS OF THE RETINA AND OF THE CHOROID: CLINICAL CLASSIFICATION

| *Affection* | *Mode of inheritance* | *Remarks* |
|---|---|---|
| | 7. WHITE DOTS | |
| Retinitis albi punctatus | Recessive | Probably an enzyme deficiency for vitamin A in the retinal pigment epithelium<br>To be distinguished from retinitis punctatus albescens and early choroidal sclerosis |
| Central | | |
| Doyne's choroiditis | Dominant | Severe form characterized by pigment reaction is exceptional |
| Urbach–Wiethe's hyalinosis | Recessive | Probably a systemic hyalinization<br>Lipoprotein disturbance |
| | 8. COLOBOMATA | |
| Typical choroidal coloboma | Dominant | Variable manifestation of a complex that extends from minimal iris notches to "anophthalmos" |
| Macular coloboma | Dominant | A choroidal defect |
| | 9. TUMOUR FORMATION | |
| Retinoblastoma, bilateral | Dominant | Most commonly a non-hereditary somatic mutation affecting one eye |
| Choroidal melanoma | | Rare hereditary cases |

A Japanese pedigree involving three collateral sibships is shown in Fig. 155 *a*. Isolated cases in collateral branches are shown in Fig. 155 *b*; in each case the parents were not consanguineous, but both the mothers had a common descent. In contrast, consanguinity of parents is shown in an isolated case in Fig. 155 *c*. The fullest pedigree has come from Holm and Lodberg. It shows pseudo-dominance, readily explained by the fact that the family derives from a closed community of some 1,600 on the Danish island of Fuur, where 1 in 5 of the inhabitants is probably a carrier of the affection.

The pedigree recorded in Fig. 156 shows the occurrence of the affection in all the four members of a sibship; two of the members also suffered from labyrinthine deafness, which appears to have been inherited independently in a dominant manner. The parents of the affected sibs were unrelated.

In this last pedigree, as in many others, mental defect and various physical deformities, such as syndactyly and club foot, were frequently observed.

In the more recently recognized cone type of monochromatic vision patients have good visual acuity at high illumination, but have only vestiges of colour sensation. It is considered that they see colour scenes in the way colour-normal people see black and white photographs. Genetically, these rare cases might be the result of the fortuitous inheritance of the three different forms of dichromatic vision.

**Dichromatism and anomalous trichromatism**

The hereditary nature of "colour-blindness" has been known since 1778. John Dalton and two of his brothers were affected, and Dalton reported "extraordinary

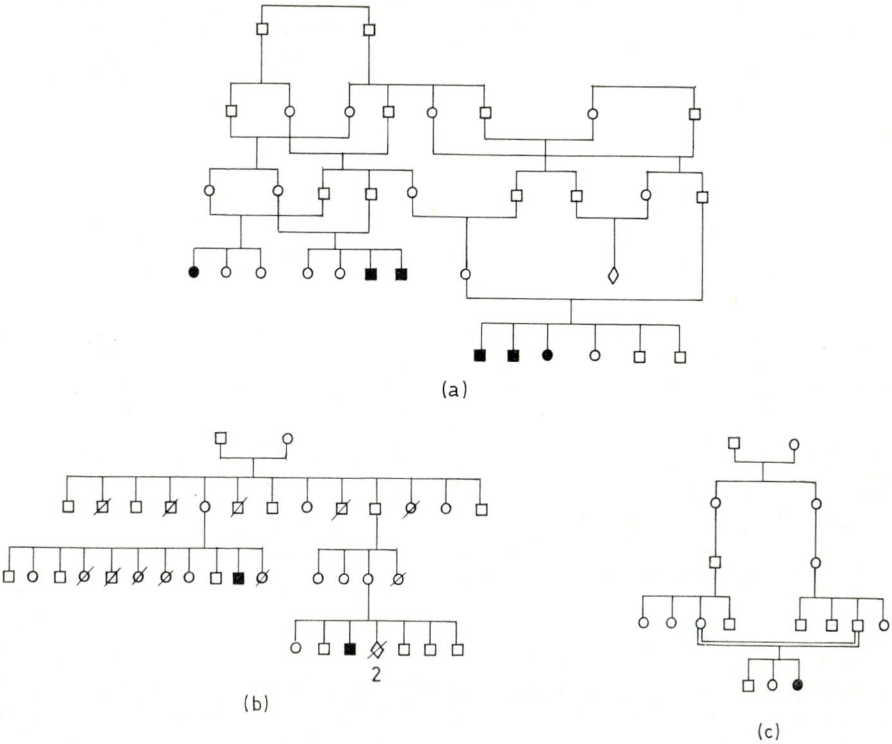


FIG. 155.—Total colour blindness. (*a*) Recessive inheritance in three collateral branches of a family heavily intermarried. (*After Maeda*, 1934.) (*b*) Inheritance in two isolated cases with a common ancestor. (*After Peter*, 1926.) (*c*) Isolated case in a sibship derived from a second-cousin marriage. (*After Vogt*, 1922.)

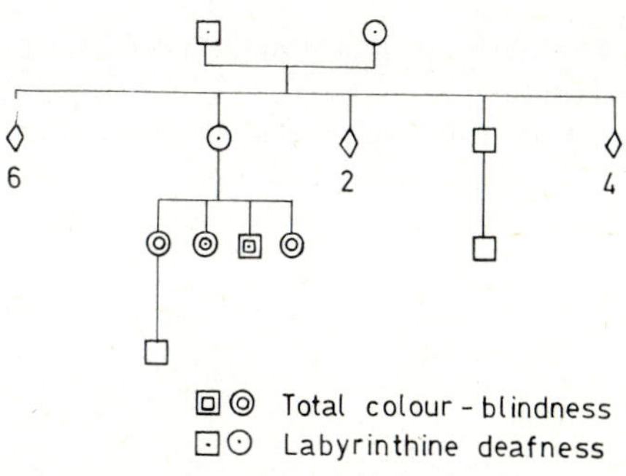


FIG. 156.—Total colour-blindness, inherited presumably in a recessive manner, with independent inheritance of dominant labyrinthine deafness. (*After Andersen*, 1946.)

facts relating to the vision of colours" in 1794. The early observers were well acquainted with the fact that the condition occurred largely in men, and Sedgwick in 1861 recognized the essentials of what is now called sex-linked inheritance in relation to this affection. Fig. 157 is from Horner, who in 1876 showed that colour-blindness is transmitted in the same way as Nasse had shown haemophilia to be inherited, and he also explained the apparent contradiction of direct transmission from father to son, for in his pedigree where this occurred the mother was a carrier.

The large number of pedigrees on colour-blindness show almost without exception regular recessive sex-linkage. Such pedigrees as appeared to depart from

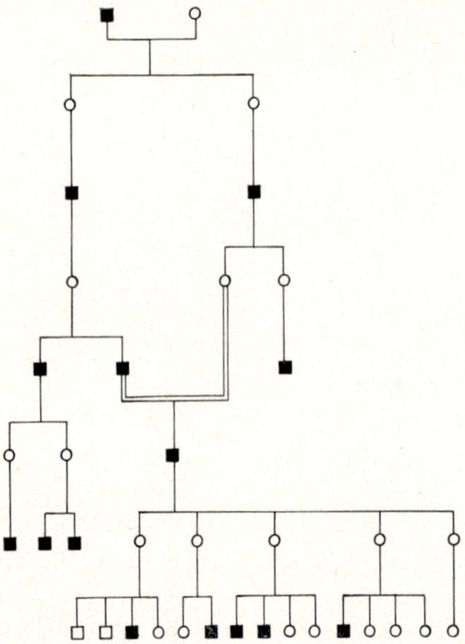

FIG. 157.—Dichromatism. Early pedigree showing recessive sex-linked mode of inheritance. (*After Horner*, 1876.)

this mode of linkage were shown by Döderlein and by Schiotz to be largely due to incomplete or mistaken statements. "Colour-blindness" is, in fact, one of the outstanding examples of sex-linkage. It has a special place in medical genetics as it was one of the conditions which appeared to invalidate the application of mendelian rules to Man, until the discovery of sex-linkage in Drosophila turned an apparently insuperable objection into a brilliant confirmation.

## Dichromatism

*Protanopia and deuteranopia*

The older literature made no distinction between protanopia and deuteranopia, or between dichromatism and anomalous trichromatism. Most recent observers agree on a distribution such as is shown in Table XI from Waaler, derived from an investigation on 9,049 boys and 9,072 girls.

That all these forms are sex-linked has to be accepted from the fact that the

TABLE XI

Incidence of Dichromatism.

| *Condition* | *Percentage distribution* | | | |
|---|---|---|---|---|
| | *Boys* | | *Girls* | |
| Protanopia – – – – – | 0·88 | 1·92 | — | 0·033 |
| Protanomaly – – – – | 1·04 | | 0·033 | |
| Deuteranopia – – – – | 1·03 | 6·09 | 0·011 | 0·401 |
| Deuteranomaly – – – – | 5·06 | | 0·39 | |
| "Colour-blind" – – – – | | 8·01 | | 0·434 |

After Waaler, 1927.

older literature does not record any inheritance but sex-linkage, and the more recent investigators conform to the older findings (Figs. 158 *a*, *b*, *c* and *d*).

Most of the exceptions to the usual transmission by an affected man through his carrier daughters to 50 per cent of his grandsons, find their explanation in the theoretical possibilities of transmission of recessive sex-linkage in unusual situations. In some cases the heterozygous (carrier) state of the clinically unaffected mother must be assumed; in others it can be reasonably deduced from a study of her pedigree.

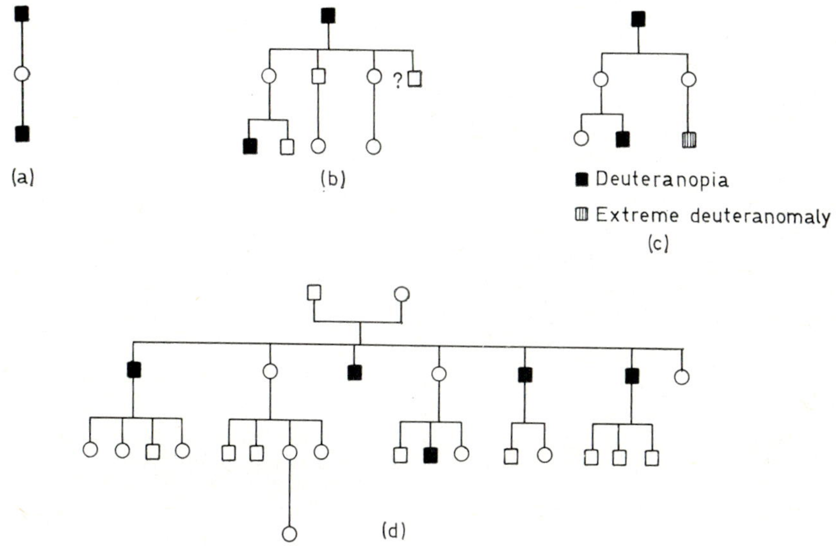


FIG. 158.—Deuteranopia and protanopia. Pedigrees showing recessive sex-linkage. (*a*) Protanopia. (*After Brunner*, 1930.) (*b*) Protanomaly. (*After Brunner*, 1930.) (*c*) Deuteranopia. (*After Brunner*, 1930.) (*d*) Deuteranomaly. (*After Wolfflin*, 1923.)

There are cases of colour-blind daughters of clinically unaffected parents. Theoretically this could not come about unless the father was affected and the mother a carrier. To explain these cases on the adage *pater semper incertus* is an easy—all too easy—way out of a difficulty. It is more likely that all such cases are to be explained by the occasional full expression of the heterozygous state. There is ample evidence that female heterozygotes are not always completely normal in their colour vision, and apparently they can be phenotypically fully affected. This is shown by such facts as the occurrence of a colour-blind daughter of a colour-blind father and a mother who is apparently not a carrier. Fig. 159 shows such a pedigree. On the one hand, the two affected grandsons of an affected man conform to rule in so far as their mothers are unaffected. On the other hand, the affected daughter should be homozygous, in which case her son ought to be affected—but he is not. It may be assumed that the daughter is indeed heterozygous and in spite of this manifests the affection. Presumably the total genetic environment comes into question in such cases.

It may therefore be taken that recessive sex-linkage with occasional expression in heterozygous women explains all aspects of inheritance in protanopia and deuteranopia.

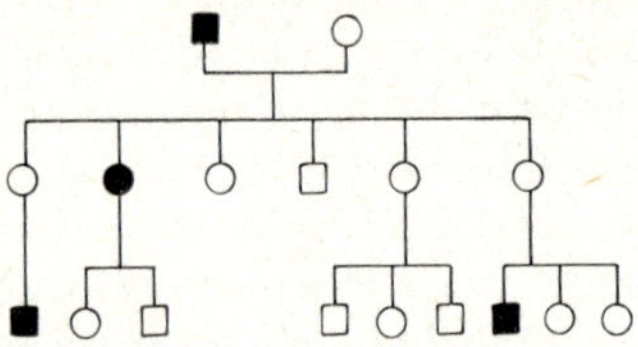

FIG. 159.—"Colour-blindness". Pedigree chart showing an affected heterozygous woman. (*After Siemens*, 1926.)

*Tritanopia*

Although known since 1897 when König first described this disorder, and also reported that the fovea itself is normally tritanopic, this colour defect has attracted little attention until recent years, mainly because neither the Ishihara tables nor the ordinary anomatoscope reveal it. The Farnsworth plates have made detailed studies feasible and, contrary to expectation, inheritance is in an autosomal dominant manner.

**Anomalous trichromatism**

*Deuteranomaly and protanomaly*

Sex-linked recessive inheritance applies to deuteranomaly and protanomaly as it does to deuteranopia and protanopia.

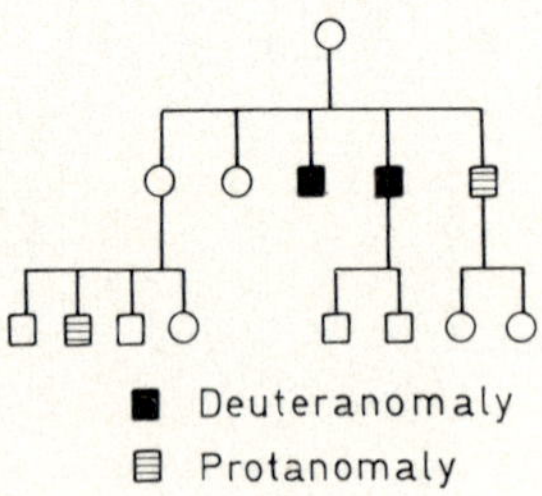


FIG. 160.—Deuteranomaly and protanomaly transmitted independently by a woman carrier of both genes. (*After Brunner*, 1930)

It is an old observation that within the same family, the same type of anomaly of colour vision occurs. There are, however, exceptions, and these have helped to elucidate the relationship of the different anomalies of colour vision to each other.

*Deuteranomaly and deuteranopia.*—In a pedigree of Wölfflin the daughter of a deuteranope married a deuteranomalous man. Their daughter showed deuteranomaly. Apparently she received from her father an X chromosome carrying deuteranomaly and from her mother an X chromosome carrying deuteranopia. On the assumption that the two genes are allelomorphs, deuteranomaly is dominant over deuteranopia.

*Protanomaly and protanopia.*—Similar relationships have been established between these two affections.

*Deuteranomaly and protanomaly.*—In a pedigree of Brunner (Fig. 160) a woman had 2 normal daughters and 3 sons, two of whom showed deuteranomaly and one protanomaly. It is assumed that the mother—who was clinically unaffected—carried both these genes but on different loci on her two X chromosomes. This supposition is strengthened by the fact that her daughter transmitted protanomaly to one of her sons. The two affections are therefore inherited independently.

The general conclusions that these and similar pedigrees allow are:

(1) Deuteranopia and protanopia are genetically distinct entities, the gene for each being carried by the non-homologous portions of the X chromosome.

(2) The gene determining deuteranopia is allelomorphic to that determining deuteranomaly. Likewise the gene for protanomaly is an allele of that for protanopia.

(3) The gene determining normalcy is dominant over the pathogenic alleles; and of these the allele which determines the less severe anomaly is dominant over that for the more severe anomaly.

FIG. 161.—Anomalous trichromatism. Sex-linked inheritance in tritanomaly. (*After Hartung*, 1926.)

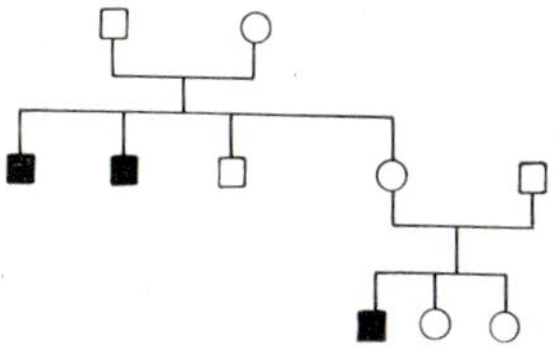

These relations are shown schematically as follows:

Normal > deuteranomaly > deuteranopia
Normal > protanomaly > protanopia

*Tritanomaly*

Unlike tritanopia, inheritance is sex-linked, as shown by the early pedigree recorded in Fig. 161 and by subsequent observers. It has not been studied deeply, possibly because of the difficulties in diagnosis and its relatively little practical importance.

**Extreme anomalous trichromatism**

It is uncertain whether extreme deuteranomaly and extreme protanomaly are distinct entities or merely anomalous states observed under conditions of fatigue. If they are genetically distinct, they are determined by alleles, and their position as regards dominance would presumably be between the anomalous state and the anopia state.

## STUDIES ON AFFECTIONS SIMULATING RETINITIS PIGMENTOSA

The lesions caused by therapeutic and experimental retinotoxic agents, like the lesion seen in hereditary retinal affections in animals, involve both the rod layer and the pigment epithelium. Anatomically they are therefore tapeto-retinal disorders, and thus bear on the problem of retinitis pigmentosa and allied affections.

### TAPETO-RETINAL DYSTROPHIES IN THE MOUSE, RAT AND DOG

The earliest recognition of a hereditary affection of the retinitis pigmentosa type in animals was that recorded in the dog by Magnusson in 1917. Observations on the mouse came from Keeler in 1928 and on the rat from Bourne, Campbell and Tansley in 1938. In the dog and the rat the affection was clearly recognized as simulating retinitis pigmentosa histologically, but in the mouse Keeler stressed the end-stage—"rodless retina"—which he regarded as a congenital anomaly, a mistaken view in the light of later observations. The appearances in the rat—a degenerative lesion following on an apparently normal development of the retina—

was considered by Bourne and her associates as evidence in support of the hypothesis of "abiotrophy", i.e. degeneration in fully developed tissue.

## Histological studies

*Retinitis pigmentosa-like affections as arrested development of the rods with consequent progressive degeneration of the retina*

In 1954 Sorsby and colleagues showed that the retina in the mouse with hereditary degeneration had not in fact developed normally: the different layers of the retina had become differentiated by the eleventh day after birth, but final development of the rods had not occurred before the degenerative process—complete by about 28 days after birth—had set in to lead to "rodless retina" (Fig. 162). They also reported similar findings for the dog (Irish setter) and the rat. Parallel and confirmatory studies by other observers were followed by electron microscopy investigation by Lasansky and de Robertis in 1960. These observers have shown that in the mouse the outer segment of the rod in the normal animal proceeds from a primitive cilium to the formation of membraneous material and then to remodelling and reorientation of the sacs that finally build up the definite regularly layered structure. In the dystrophic mouse only the first stage proceeds normally; anomalous changes occur in the second stage and the third stage is never reached—there is, instead, involution and cell death.

Further support has come from electroretinographic studies. In the Irish setter (in which maturation of the rod is not reached until 28 days after birth) a normal retinogram has been obtained in the normal animal at 21 days, but in the dystrophic animal there is no electroretinographic response, for the retina is already degenerate (Parry, Tansley and Thomson, 1955). In the normal rat Bonting, Caravaggio and Gouras (1961) found that the electroretinographic response is first obtained at 12 days after birth and the amplitude more than doubles between 12 and 22 days (when maturation of the rod is proceeding).

Whilst arrested development of the rods (or possibly the rods and pigment layer) without subsequent progressive degeneration throughout the retina is accepted as the basis of the retinal dystrophy in these different animals, there is still some uncertainty whether the lesion is identical in these strains. These histological studies have made possible extensive biochemical investigations on the developing retina in the normal rat as contrasted with the rat bred for the retinal dystrophy. Similar studies in the dog and mouse present considerable technical difficulties.

## Biochemical studies

*Carbohydrate metabolism*

The heavy dependence of the retina on carbohydrate for its energy supply suggested that its carbohydrate metabolism might profitably be investigated over the critical period of development when the rods grow to maturity. Several such studies on anaerobic glycolysis are available and they are rather inconclusive.

Using radioisotopic procedures involving radio-paper-chromatography Reading and Sorsby in 1962 and 1964 found that as regards glucose metabolism there was no significant quantitative or qualitative differences in the overall pattern in normal and dystrophic retinae—as judged by the processes of respiration, glucose utilization, glycolysis, citric acid cycle and the production of amino acids from glucose—during the period 10–21 days after birth, when degeneration is proceeding rapidly

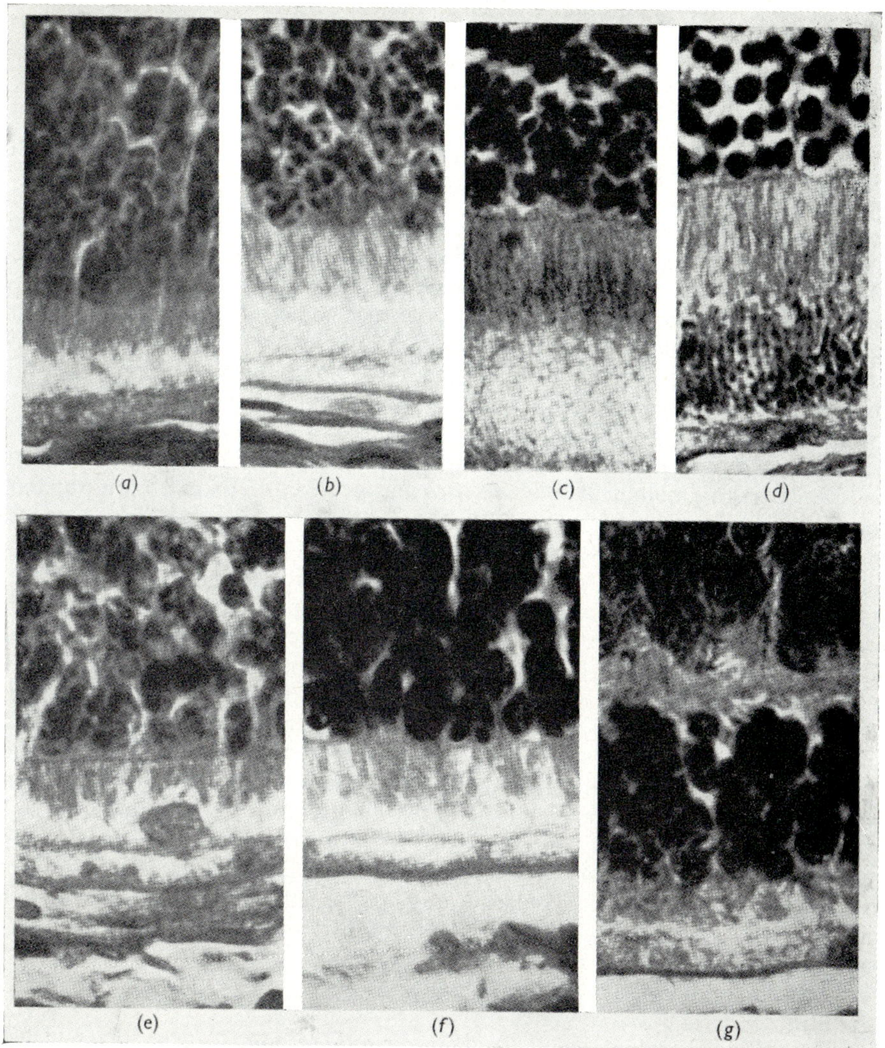


FIG. 162.—Abiotrophy as a minimal congenital defect with post-natal course. Recessive retinal dystrophy of the retinitis pigmentosa type in the mouse. Post-natal development of rod and outer nuclear layers of retina in normal and affected mouse. (*a*), (*b*), (*c*) and (*d*) Development in normal mouse at 12, 14, 21 and 28 days. Note that whilst rod and nuclear layers are already differentiated at 12 days after birth there is considerable post-natal development so that at 28 days the rods are clearly differentiated into two segments. (*e*) (*f*) and (*g*) Development in affected mouse at 11, 13 and 14 days. Note that in contrast to normal mouse post-natal development beyond the 11th or 12th day, there are rapidly developing regressive changes in the rods. At 28 days, when normal retina has reached full development, the rods and outer nuclear layers in affected mouse are completely degenerate. In retinal dystrophy in the mouse, which genetically and histologically simulates human retinitis pigmentosa, the evidence is, therefore, that whilst the retina becomes differentiated into its various layers, the rods do not develop fully. The tissue is "jerry" built and degenerative changes set up in tissue that has never been normal. (*After Sorsby, Koller, Attfield, Davey and Lucas*, 1954.)

in the dystrophic rat. Thereafter, up to 60 days, the activities of these processes reached a steady level in the dystrophic retina, whilst corresponding activities in the normal tissue increased: these differences in metabolic activity were regarded as secondary to the cell degeneration.

*Faulty protein synthesis*

There were, however, considerable differences in protein metabolism. In the normal retina, aspartic, glutamic and aminobutyric acids formed from glucose were progressively retained within the cells, whereas these acids, formed in the dystrophic retina, had diffused freely into the surrounding medium. Alanine and glutamine had diffused out into the medium in all cases. They held that failure of the dystrophic retina to retain intracellularly formed amino acids, together with a late decline in glutamine formation, was indicative of a breakdown in the mechanism for the proper utilization of energy—a mechanism which involves the participation of high-energy phosphate compounds in active transport and synthetic reactions.

Subsequently using $^{14}C$ labelled glycine, they studied the rate of protein synthesis and transport of amino acids both *in vitro* and *in vivo* in retinae from normal and from dystrophic rats and found that the dystrophic retina at six to eight days after birth—well before the onset of histological changes, or in fact before the full differentiation into layers—showed a marked diminution in the incorporation rate (protein synthesis) and in addition a slower rate of protein breakdown. Amino acid transport into the retina was equal in the normal and dystrophic animal. The work of Graymore in 1964 is relevant in this context. He found that one of the five isoenzymes (fraction 5) is lowered by about 40 per cent in retinal dystrophy, both in the immature and mature animals. This enzyme normally declines by about one third between six and twelve days, and the extra deficiency in the dystrophic animal occurred by the ninth day after birth. Reading's observation that protein binding of retinene in the developing retina reacts differently to light in the dystrophic retina as compared with the normal, is yet further evidence of anomalous protein synthesis in retinal dystrophy. The finding recorded below that retinotoxic agents act by denaturation of retinal protein (*see* p. 174) is of interest in this context.

## Drug-induced Retinopathy

Four agents, or groups of agents, come into consideration.

### Pregl's solution (Septojod)

This is now a matter of historical interest only. It was used to combat puerpural sepsis. Pigmentary degeneration of the retina followed occasionally on a single, relatively small intravenous dose. It was held that massive uterine haemorrhage was a predisposing cause. The composition of Pregl's solution appears to have been kept secret; it was believed to liberate nascent iodine.

### Diaminodiphenoxyalkanes

This group of agents has been explored extensively by pharmacologists as possible therapeutic agents in schistosomiasis. In unrecorded clinical trials with 1:7 di(*p*-dimethylaminophenoxy) heptane, retinal complications of the pigmentary type have been observed. These agents do not appear to have been released for general use.

Typically the diaminodiphenoxyalkanes have the structural formula:

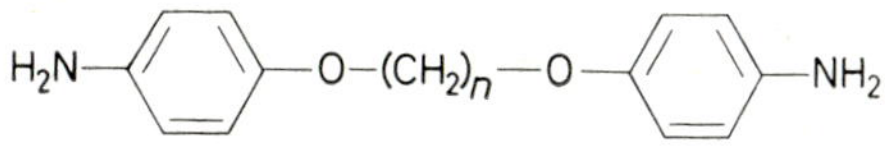


where $n$ for the central $CH_2$ chain may stand for 2 or more, producing pentanes when $n = 5$, or heptanes when it is 7. The hydrogen in the $NH_2$ radical may appear as such in the primary amines or one or both atoms may be replaced by methyl or ethyl groups or other modifications, giving the corresponding secondary or tertiary amines.

**The phenothiazines**

At least three derivatives of chlorpromazine, itself used extensively without retinal complications, have been found to produce pigmentary retinal degeneration

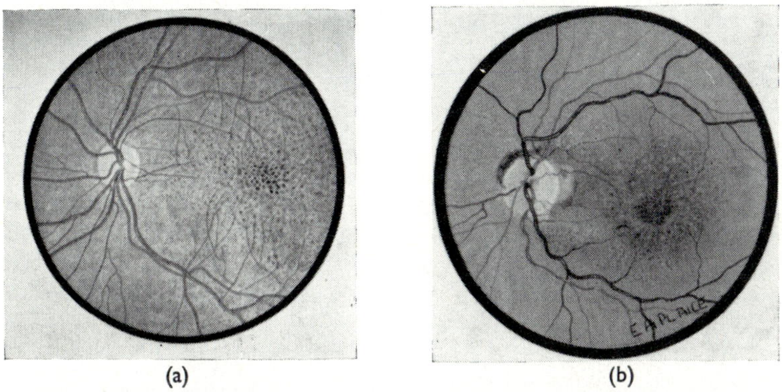


FIG. 163.—Drug-induced retinopathy. (*a*) Phenothiazine retinopathy. Fundus appearances following prolonged use of N.P. 207. (*After Wagner*, 1956.) (*b*) Chloroquine retinopathy. Fundus appearances in a woman aged 53 years treated with chloroquine for over two years. (*Personal observation.*)

in clinical trials (Fig. 163 *a*). Two in particular have given considerable trouble; their relationship to chlorpromazine is seen in the following structural formulae.

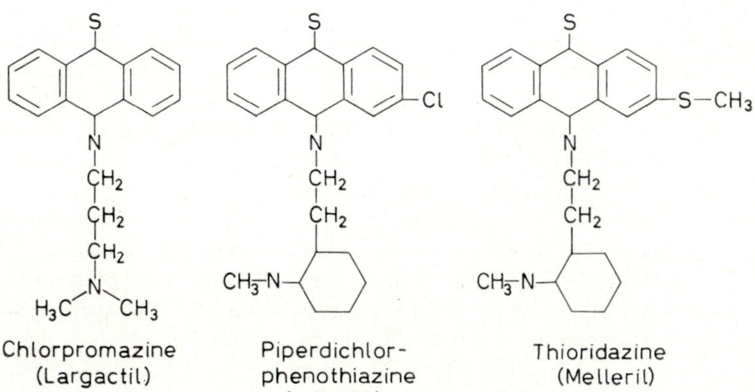

N.P. 207 is the most toxic of these. Ophthalmoscopically visible pigmentary changes without functional disturbances have been observed, but generally considerable restriction of the field and night-blindness are present, whilst central vision fails in some cases. It would appear that there is a direct relationship between dose and lesions, but retinal damage may occur with moderate doses. Observations of this type have been recorded from Switzerland and the United States and the drug has not been marketed by the manufacturers. With Melleril toxic effects are exceptional with clinical doses.

**Chloroquine**

Following the report by Hobbs, Sorsby and Friedman (1959) of five cases of pigmentary degeneration of the retina (Fig. 163 *b*) from the prolonged use of chloroquine for rheumatoid arthritis or lupus erythematosus, a large number of such cases have now been reported. This quinone derivative has a relatively simple chemical structure:

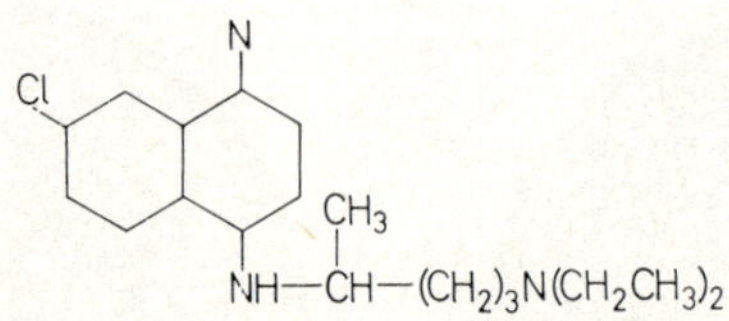


It appears to have been used in larger doses and for longer periods in rheumatoid arthritis, lupus erythematosus and sarcoidosis than in malaria, for which it was first introduced. The retinal complication sets in only after the prolonged use of the drug and is irreversible once ophthalmoscopic changes have developed.

## Experimental Degeneration of the Retina

Five agents or groups of agents have well-established retinotoxic effects in the experimental animal. Two of these, sodium iodate and the diaminophenoxyalkanes, were derived from therapeutic trials; two more, iodoacetate and sodium fluoride, were used experimentally as potential inhibitors of glucose metabolism on which the retina is so dependent. The fifth, diphenylthiocarbazone, is an experimental diabetogenic agent which was found to be retinotoxic. Each of these agents has now a fairly extensive literature.

They all have in common the striking feature that the retinotoxic effect, generally in the rabbit, is achieved by a single intravenous injection of an adequate dose. In all five, both the pigment layer and the neuroepithelium are involved, and attempts at incriminating one or other layer as the seat of the initial lesion with the different agents have not given any convincing results. It is likely that such differences as are seen histologically are determined not by any fundamental differences in action but by such factors as severity and rapidity of the effect. Clinically the five agents give very much the same end result—a pigmentary lesion of the retina often reminiscent of the bone-corpuscle reaction of retinitis pigmentosa, but the extent of the lesion varies somewhat with the different agents (Fig. 164). In the early stages, the reaction may be almost pathognomonic, for the time of onset, the extent of the lesion and the site of the reaction are fairly characteristic. Nonetheless, in many instances these characteristic features are blurred: the overlap is considerable if only because the severity of a lesion varies from animal to animal.

**The individual agents**

*Sodium iodate*

Sallmann in 1933, Vito in 1935 and Kalt in 1937 established that sodium iodate was the toxic component of Pregl's solution. Sorsby in 1941 showed that a single intravenous dose of the order of 25–30 mg./kg. in the rabbit was effective; an unmistakable oedematous fundus reaction, generally limited to the area below the disc, set in within five days, and within a few days more extensive pigmentary degeneration became established all over the fundus (Fig. 164). Liver damage was present only with lethal doses well in excess of the retinotoxic dose.

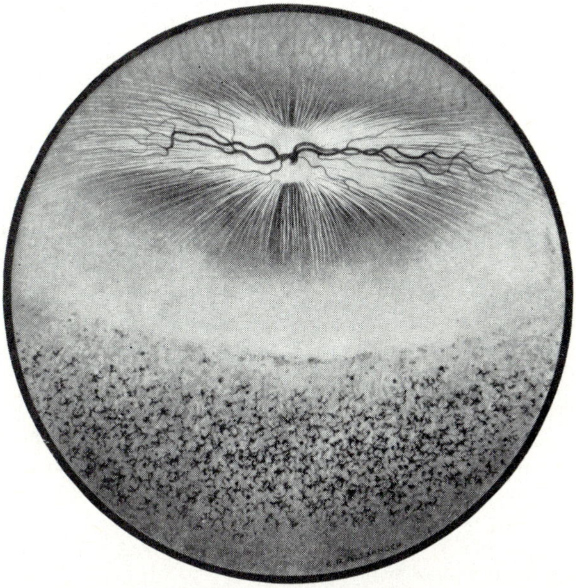

FIG. 164.—Experimental degeneration of the retina in the rabbit. Sodium iodate, dithizone and sodium fluoride give fairly characteristic reactions, but even these are not always readily distinguished from each other, particularly in the later stages.

Histologically the earliest disturbances, seen about two to three days after an injection, are limited to the rods and the pigment layer; oedema and pyknosis soon follow in the other layers of the retina. Extensive disorganization of the retina is generally established within 10 to 15 days. Some observers hold that the rods are the first to be affected; others believe the pigment layer suffers first and most. Electron microscopic studies by Yoshida in 1960 suggest disturbances in the basal part of the rods.

A number of biochemical anomalies have been reported in retinal degeneration induced by iodate, but it is not at all clear that they are initial biochemical disturbances and not merely transient aspects of the breakdown of the tissue.

As to the mode of action of iodate, the following observations are relevant:

(1) Iodate disappears from the blood stream within a matter of minutes. Its action is therefore likely to be of the nature of a "trigger effect" (Sorsby, 1941).

(2) *In vitro* iodate inhibits tissue respiration and glycolysis, but only in

concentrations very much higher than those reached in the intact animal (Auricchio and de Vincentis, 1950).

(3) Apart from sodium periodate and iodine pentoxide, other oxidizing agents tried experimentally have not produced any retinal lesion. Periodate and iodine pentoxide, however, are almost certainly broken down into iodate in the body.

(4) Cysteine and other thiol donors are protective. This is discussed more fully below.

*Sodium iodoacetate*

On the assumption that –SH inhibitors might disturb carbohydrate metabolism, Schubert and Bornschein, in 1951, used intravenous administration of sodium iodoacetate in the rabbit and found it produced retinal lesions similar to that obtained by sodium iodate. They also noted that the electroretinogram was abolished within a few minutes after the injection—a fact also observed by Noell in ERG studies in the same year.

Iodoacetate is much more toxic than sodium iodate and the retinotoxic effect is less constant. A single intravenous dose of 25 mg./kg. in the rabbit gives a mortality of about 20 per cent and fundus lesions in all but a few of the survivors.

Iodoacetate is a powerful thiol group inhibitor; *in vitro* it depresses the production of lactic acid and is a marked inhibitor of glycolysis. The almost instantaneous abolition of the ERG is regarded as interference with the enzyme systems involved in the carbohydrate metabolism of the retina, particularly the Embden–Meyerhof cycle. Electron microscopy suggests that the earliest histological changes are in the outer segments of the rods.

Apart from bromoacetate (an analogue of iodoacetate) no other thiol group inhibitors—some more toxic and others less toxic than iodoacetate—have proved retinotoxic in the intact animal (Sorsby, Newhouse and Lucas, 1957). *In vitro*, many of these agents have profound effects on retinal metabolism. The mode of action remains obscure.

*Dithizone* (*diphenylthiocarbazone*)

This zinc precipitating agent was first employed by Japanese observers in experimental studies on diabetes, on the assumption that the affection might be due to disturbances in the zinc content of the pancreas (in which tissue this metal is present in great quantities). In 1952, Dell'Acqua and Gambassi, and also Grignolo, Butterini and Baronchelli, showed that not only did dithizone produce diabetes, but also a retinal lesion of a particularly severe type.

Dithizone is a highly insoluble and toxic substance. Using adequate solvents, Sorsby and Harding (1962a) have shown that a dose of 30 mg./kg., whilst it killed one out of every three rabbits used, gave a retinal lesion in all survivors, but that hyperglycaemia did not develop in all survivors, and that furthermore only one third of these showed persistence of the hyperglycaemia. The diabetogenic and retinotoxic effects are therefore not linked.

The retinal lesion is most striking and characteristic. Within 24 hours in most cases, and in all cases within 48 hours, an intense retinal oedema becomes apparent, shown by a milk-white reflex from the whole of the fundus. Within the next 48 hours islets of red begin to appear and gradually extend; simultaneously pigment changes begin to appear in the red zones, and by the time the oedema has disappeared—generally within six to eight days—crude pigmentation is widespread. Sometimes the pigmentation takes the form of a rather delicate lacework, but more commonly it is gross and irregular.

This reaction appears to be independent of the actual dose, although in the few instances in which the oedema was not marked the rabbits had received a low dose.

Histologically the intense oedema is reflected in the swelling of the nerve fibre layer. All the layers of the retina are involved in the diffuse process, although the neuroepithelium suffers earliest and most markedly. In severe cases, the end stage is diffuse disorganization of the whole thickness of the retina.

*The diaminophenoxyalkanes*

Following the recognition in clinical screening that a tertiary amine in this series (1:7 di(*p*-dimethylphenoxy) heptane) is retinotoxic, Edge and his co-workers in 1956 and Goodwin and his co-workers in 1957 showed that a primary amine (1:5 di(*p*-aminophenoxy) pentane) gave experimental lesions readily in the cat. Sorsby and Nakajima (1958) found that a single intravenous injection of this agent in the rabbit in a dose of 5 mg./kg. gave consistent retinotoxic results; studying a series of primary, secondary and tertiary amines they showed that retinal damage was mostly limited to the primary amines; neither the phenoxy grouping nor the length of the central carbon chain seemed significant.

A striking feature of the lesion was its high degree of apparent specificity to the retina; doses well below those giving systemic toxicity were effective.

The ophthalmoscopic picture was fairly constant and was similar to that observed with iodate and iodoacetate. Within two to three days there was loss of translucency of the retina, showing itself ophthalmoscopically by an appearance simulating oedema of the retina; some narrowing of the arteries was common and pigmentary proliferation began to set in within five days and tended to progress for the next two to three weeks. The fully developed picture was generally present within 21 days. Histologically the visual cells and pigmented epithelium were most affected.

*Sodium fluoride*

Attempts by several observers to obtain experimental retinal degeneration with fluoride and other inhibitors of glycolysis, apart from iodoacetate and bromoacetate, failed to give any convincing results until it was established that with a sub-lethal dose (50 mg./kg.) some 20 per cent of rabbits developed a characteristic sharply defined ophthalmoscopic lesion within 48 hours and that the incidence rose to 70 per cent if the animals were either fasted for 24 hours or pre-treated with metabolic accelerators (like dinitrophenol), and to almost 100 per cent if treated simultaneously with oxidizing agents (Sorsby and Harding, 1966).

## The nature of the retinotoxic effect

There is no clear understanding of the action of the five agents considered. The following considerations arise.

*The chemical structure of the retinotoxic agents*

Chemically the different retinotoxic agents have little in common and differ but little from allied substances without retinotoxic effect. Thus iodine salts as such are not retinotoxic, and a number of agents structurally similar to diphenylthiocarbazone are innocuous as are most phenoxyalkanes. Sodium fluoride is a highly versatile substance with properties markedly different from the other halogen salts of sodium.

*The biochemical action*

Here, too, there is little to suggest a common basis. Iodate is a powerful oxidizing agent, but other oxidizing agents are not retinotoxic. It is possible that iodate is a thiol group inhibitor, but this is not certain. Iodoacetate is a powerful thiol group inhibitor, but other such agents (apart from the analogue bromoacetate) are without retinal effect. Dithizone has no known effects on enzyme systems and the mode of action of the phenoxyalkanes is equally obscure. Sodium fluoride is an important inhibitor of glycolysis, but other equally significant inhibitors, such as glyceraldehyde, are without effect.

*Potentiating agents*

The potentiating effect of metabolic accelerators and particularly of fasting for 24 hours on the action of sodium fluoride has already been noted. Only iodate shows the same susceptibility, for in the fasted animal subliminal doses of iodate produce retinal lesions. No such potentiation is seen with the remaining retinotoxic agents (Sorsby and Harding, 1962b).

Potentiation of a less limited character is seen with oxidizing agents. The incidence of fluoride lesions in the rabbit is almost 100 per cent when an intravenous injection of potassium permanganate 5 mg./kg. (or of other oxidizing agents, none of which are themselves retinotoxic) is given immediately before the injection of fluoride. This potentiation also applies to iodate and iodoacetate, for subliminal doses become retinotoxic (Sorsby and Harding, 1966).

*Protective procedures*

Protective procedures have been established for sodium iodate but have not been obtained against the other retinotoxic agents. When a single intravenous injection of 50 mg./kg. of cysteine is given immediately before the injection of a retinotoxic dose of sodium iodate there is complete protection. Equally effective protection is obtained from similar pre-treatment with other thiol donors. The lack of protection by these agents against iodoacetate—a known inhibitor of –SH enzymes—is rather paradoxical (Sorsby and Harding, 1962a).

*The –SH level in the retina after the intravenous injection of retinotoxic agents*

The protective effect of thiol donors against iodate suggests the possibility that iodate is retinotoxic by inactivating thiol-dependent enzyme systems. The level of both "soluble" and "total" –SH concentration in the retina falls slightly after an intravenous injection of iodate, but at 16 to 20 hours after injection there was a substantial increase. It is thus possible that iodate acts by denaturation of retinal protein during the first 24 hours after injection, followed by a degeneration of the rods and the pigment layer. Similar, though less marked, disturbances in –SH levels are seen with the remaining four retinotoxic agents, and the protective effect of cysteine against iodate still needs clarification (Sorsby and Reading, 1964, 1966).

*Biochemical and histochemical studies on the degenerating retina*

As already noted, a number of biochemical and histochemical changes have been reported, but there is no convincing evidence that they represent causes of the degeneration rather than effects.

*Vitamin A aldehyde in the function and structure of the retina*

The exclusion of vitamin A from the diet of an experimental animal leads to rapid wasting and death. Several early observers have recorded damage to the rods during such experiments: this, however, has been slight and unconvincing. Dowling and Wald have reported that in the rat vitamin A acid is adequate for the body requirements, but is inadequate for the retina, which can only utilize vitamin A aldehyde. Rats on vitamin A acid remained fit but their retinae showed a degenerative lesion of the retinitis pigmentosa type, a lesion that they found reversible in the early stages by the administration of vitamin A aldehyde.

Using rabbits—in which the ophthalmoscopic changes can be readily followed—Sorsby, Reading and Bunyan (1966) found a fundus lesion developed after seven months of maintenance on vitamin A acid but the appearances suggested not retinitis pigmentosa but the mild functional disturbance described by Lauber in 1910 as retinitis albi punctatus, and the somewhat similar appearances occasionally seen in vitamin A deficiency in man. In these rabbits the electroretinogram showed changes consistent with poor dark adaptation (deficient *b* wave) rather than of retinal degeneration. Histologically the rod layer was essentially intact despite the striking ophthalmoscopic appearances, and the only substantial changes were in the pigment layer. It would therefore appear that in the rabbit at any rate vitamin A aldehyde is indeed essential for the adequate functioning of the pigment epithelium and the visual purple cycle, but the lack of the aldehyde does not influence the rods. On this reading, vitamin A aldehyde deficiency does not rate amongst the causes of experimental degeneration of the retinal neuro-epithelium.

## FOR FURTHER READING

**General Surveys**

Franceschetti, A. and Klein, D. (1950). *Proc. XVIth Int. Congr. Ophthal. London*, p. 158.
— François, J. and Babel, J. (1964). *Les hérédo-dégénérescences chorio-rétinennes.* Paris; Masson.
Sorsby, A. (1963). *Acta Genet. med. Gemell.*, **13,** 20.

**Congenital Anomalies**

*Congenital Stationary Night-blindness*

Bell, Julia (1933). In *The Treasury of Human Inheritance*, Ed. by K. Pearson. Vol. II, Pt. 1. London; Cambridge University Press.

*Retinal Aplasia*

Alström, C. H. and Olson, O. (1957). *Hereditas*, **43,** 1.
Sorsby, A. and Williams, C. E. (1960). *Br. med. J.*, **1,** 293.

*Dominant Macular Cyst*

Remky, H., Rix, J. and Klier, K. F. (1965). *Klin. Mbl. Augenheilk.*, **146,** 473.
Sorsby, A., Savory, M., Davey, J. B. and Fraser, R. J. L. (1956). *Br. J. Ophthal.*, **40,** 144.

*Congenital Sex-linked Pseudoglioma*

Warburg, M. (1966). "Norrie's Disease". *Acta ophthal.* Suppl. 89.
Wilson, W. M. G. (1949). *Canad. med. Ass. J.*, **60,** 580.

*Congenital Sex-linked Retinoschisis*

Gieser, E. P. and Falls, H. F. (1961). *Am. J. Ophthal.* **51**, 1193.
Sorsby, A., Klein, M., Gann, J. H. and Siggins, G. (1951). *Br. J. Ophthal.*, **35**, 1.

**Abiotrophic Disorders**

*The Retinitis Pigmentosa Group*

Bell, Julia (1933). In *The Treasury of Human Inheritance*, Ed. by K. Pearson, Vol. II, Pt. 1. London; Cambridge University Press.

*The Macular Dystrophies*

Sorsby, A. (1940). *Br. J. Ophthal.*, **24**, 469.

— (1957). *Acta genet. Statist. med.*, **7**, 292.

*Choroideremia*

McCulloch, C. and McCulloch, R. J. P. (1948). *Trans. Am. Acad. Ophthal. Otolar.*, **53**, 160.

Sorsby, A., Franceschetti, A., Joseph, R. and Davey, J. B. (1952). *Br. J. Ophthal.*, **36**, 547.

*Choroidal Sclerosis*

Sorsby, A. (1939). *Br. J. Ophthal.*, **23**, 433.

— and Crick, R. P. (1953). *Br. J. Ophthal.*, **37**, 129.

— and Davey, J. B. (1955). *Br. J. Ophthal.*, **39**, 257.

*Dominant Generalized Fundus Dystrophy*

Franceschetti, A., François, J. and Babel, J. (1964). *Les hérédo-dégénérescences chorio-rétiniennes.* Paris; Masson.

Sorsby, A. and Mason, M. E. J. (1949). *Br. J. Ophthal.*, **33**, 67.

*Wagner's Disease*

Ricci, A. (1961). *Bull. Soc. Ophtal France*, 618.

*Retinoblastoma*

Schappert-Kimmijser, J., Hemmes, G. D. and Nijland, R. (1966). *Ophthalmologica*, **151**, 197.

Smith, S. M. and Sorsby, A. (1958). *Ann. hum. Genet.*, **23**, 50.

Vogel, F. (1967). In *Modern Trends in Ophthalmology*—**4**, Ed. by Arnold Sorsby. London; Butterworths.

**Anomalies of Colour Vision**

Kalmus, H. (1965). *Diagnosis and Genetics of Defective Colour Vision.* Oxford; Pergamon Press.

**Tapeto-retinal Dystrophies in Animals**

Graymore, C. N. (Ed.) (1965). *The Biochemistry of the Retina.* London and New York; Academic Press.

Karli, P. (1963). *Progr. Ophthal.*, **14**, 51.

Lasansky, A. and De Robertis, E. (1960). *J. biophys. Biochem. Cytol.*, **7**, 679

Lucas, D. J. (1954). *J. exp. Zool.*, **126**, 537.

Reading, H. W. and Sorsby, A. (1962). *Vision Res.*, **2**, 315.

— — (1964). *Vision Res.*, **4**, 209.

Sorsby, A. Koller, P. C., Attfield, M., Davey, J. B. and Lucas, D. R. (1954). *J. exp. Zool.*, **125**, 171.

**Drug-induced Retinopathy**

Meier-Ruge, W. (1967). *Medikamentose Retinopathie.* Stuttgart; Thieme.

Sorsby, A. (Ed.) (1967). In *Modern Trends in Ophthalmology—4*, pp. 163–166. London; Butterworths.

**Experimental Degeneration**

Dowling, J. E. and Wald, G. (1960). *Proc. natn. Acad. Sci.*, **46**, 581.

Noell, W. (1958). *Am. J. Ophthal.*, **48**, 347.

Sorsby, A. and Harding, R. (1960). *Br. J. Ophth.*, **44**, 213.

— — (1962a). *Vision Res.*, **2**, 139.

— — (1962b). *Vision Res.*, **2**, 157.

— — (1966). *Nature, Lond.*, **210**, 99.

— and Reading, W. H. (1964). *Vision Res.*, **4**, 511.

— — and Bunyan, J. (1966). *Nature, Lond.*, **210**, 1011.

# CHAPTER 10

## THE OPTIC NERVE

## OPTIC ATROPHY

**The sex-limited form (Leber's disease)**

Leber's disease with its abrupt onset, rapid evolution, and essentially stationary course subsequently (with a not infrequent tendency towards some improvement) presents a clinical picture that differs from the abiotrophies in many of the essential features. These clinical incongruities are as puzzling as the difficulties in interpreting the genetic behaviour of the affection.

There is an exceptionally large number of pedigrees on Leber's disease. Some features stand out beyond dispute (Fig. 165 *a* and *b*).

(1) The affection is very much more common in men than in women. The incidence of affected women in pedigrees of Leber's disease varies considerably in pooled pedigrees for different countries. In all probability this arises from the inclusion of a variable number of pedigrees of autosomal dominant optic atrophy —an affection that differs from Leber's disease in both clinical and genetic aspects.

(2) In most sibships there is a tendency for most of the men to be affected.

(3) Likewise, in sibships of affected men there is a tendency for most of their sisters to be carriers.

(4) There is no evidence that a female carrier has an affected father. It appears that transmission is through continuous descent by women, so that the female carrier derives her carrier state from her mother and not her father.

(5) Likewise, and as a corollary, it is accepted that an affected man does not transmit the carrier state to his daughters, nor the affection to his sons. In other words an affected man marks the end of a line of descent.

The fact that the sons of carrier women are affected suggests a simple sex-linked recessive mode of inheritance, and this mode of inheritance has been assumed and is still widely held as applicable to Leber's disease. It is obvious that no such simple mode of inheritance can explain the transmission of Leber's disease, for such an assumption would mean that the grandsons of affected men would be affected—and this is not the case. Transmission by women carriers also fails to explain both the high proportion of affected sons and of carrier daughters (instead of the theoretically expected 50 per cent), nor would it explain readily the fairly high proportion of affected women, unless it is assumed that heterozygous women manifest the affection fairly frequently.

From the practical aspect the significant thing is that it is not the affected man who spreads the pathogenic gene in the population, but his unaffected sister—obviously a matter of importance in advising such patients and their relatives.

The mode of inheritance of Leber's disease fits in with an old pre-mendelian observation which was summed up in the so-called Lössen's law. This stated—in contrast to Nasse's law or Horner's law—that transmission is not by affected men but exclusively through women. Lössen's law was elaborated on findings in

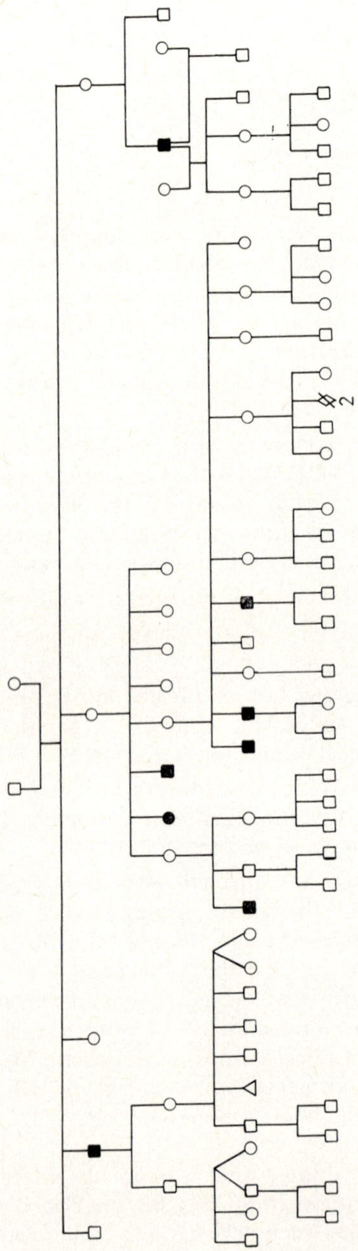


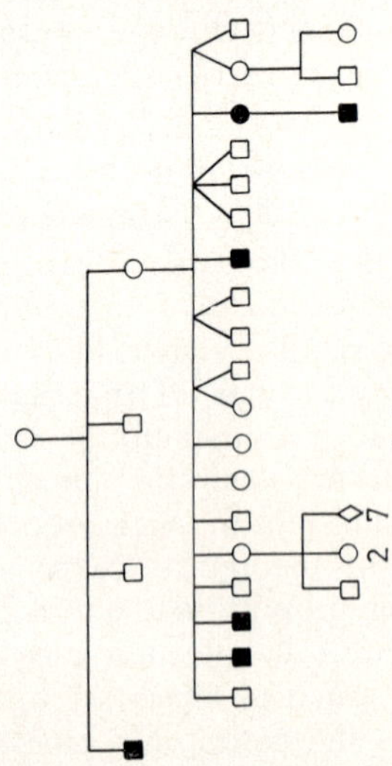


FIG. 165.—Leber's disease. (*a*) Pedigree showing affected sons of unaffected women whose brothers are affected. An affected woman is also seen. (*After Usher*, 1927.) (*b*) Pedigree showing transmission by an affected woman to her son. The son was, however, affected before the mother manifested the disease. (*After Godtfredsen*, 1949.)

haemophilia, wrongly as we now know. In Leber's disease it does, however, apply.

The mode of inheritance seen in Leber's disease cannot be explained on the mechanism of sex chromosomes as understood today, nor on any chromosomal anomaly, for the karyotype is normal both in patients and their mothers. Of the various attempts that have been made to fit the transmission of Leber's disease with present-day genetic theory, the most significant is the one which regards Leber's disease not as a sex-linked affection, but an autosomal dominant with special features. This view, advocated by Komai in 1934, is based on several assumptions—unproven and very largely unprovable.

(1) It is held that the disease is transmitted autosomally, but that the expression is different in the two sexes. It is completely, or almost completely, dominant in men, and completely, or almost completely, recessive in women. Such an assumption, consistent with experimental findings, presents no theoretical difficulties.

But this assumption does not explain the manifestation of the affection in succeeding generations. Such a recessive gene in women should be manifest in 50 per cent of their sons, whilst a dominant gene in men should produce 50 per cent of sons affected and 50 per cent of daughters with an unexpressed gene. These carrier daughters would in turn have 50 per cent of affected sons, that is, an affected man would have affected grandsons. None of these expectations is actually observed.

(2) To overcome these difficulties, Komai postulated that spermatozoa carrying pathogenic genes are less viable than normal spermatozoa. This would explain why affected men do not transmit the affection. Women carriers would remain the only possible source of transmitting the affection, and, as the condition is dominant in men, 50 per cent of the sons should be affected. The considerably greater incidence than 50 per cent observed in pedigrees would, therefore, seem to require yet a further hypothesis.

Other and less probable explanations have assumed cytoplasmic changes in the ovum or the spermatozoon. There is no evidence of any chromosomal anomalies (van Senus, 1963; Rose and Friedmann, 1964). The Lyonization hypothesis has been invoked.

*Japanese cases.*—The complexities of Leber's disease are made still more difficult by the pedigrees recorded from Japan. Here the incidence of affected women is very much higher than in the European cases, and it is possible that the clinical course is also different. It is not unlikely, therefore, that the Japanese cases may represent a different clinical entity.

*Relevance to other forms of optic atrophy*

It would appear that excessive attention has been paid to the Leber type of optic atrophy and its difficult mode of inheritance as the one and only possible variety of abiotrophic optic atrophy. Judging by established data on the retinal abiotrophies, it is not unlikely that several modes of inheritance, and several clinical types of hereditary optic atrophy exist, and little is to be gained by forcing them into one unifying but untenable conception. Both congenital and adult types with dominant inheritance have now been individualized.

**Congenital optic atrophy**

In the past, pedigrees of congenital optic atrophy, and of optic atrophy setting in early in life, were recorded in the literature as examples of Leber's optic atrophy with anticipation. These cases are, however, a distinct clinical entity with a clear-cut mode of inheritance of their own. Some of the confusion in the interpretation of pedigrees of Leber's disease has arisen from failure to isolate these cases into separate categories.

*Dominant congenital optic atrophy*

Fig. 166 shows a pedigree constructed from two independent investigations on the same family after an interval of some 20 years. It shows inheritance over four generations of actually observed cases with two antecedent generations also reputed

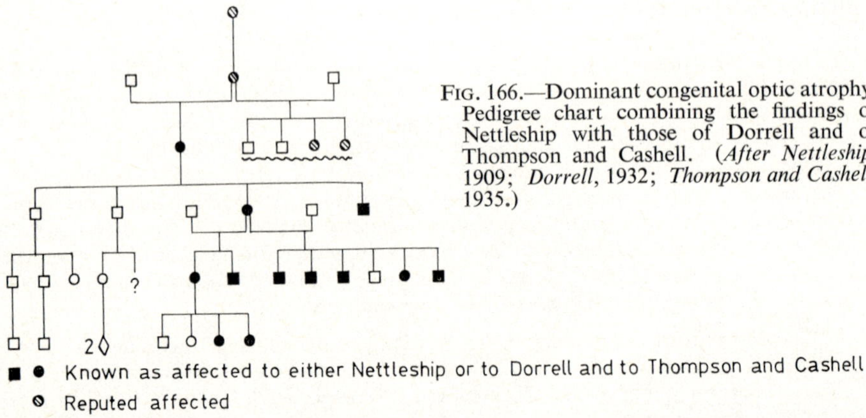


FIG. 166.—Dominant congenital optic atrophy. Pedigree chart combining the findings of Nettleship with those of Dorrell and of Thompson and Cashell. (*After Nettleship*, 1909; *Dorrell*, 1932; *Thompson and Cashell*, 1935.)

affected. Clinically this group differs from Leber's disease not only in its early onset, but also in ophthalmoscopic appearances and in the type of field defect it produces. Ophthalmoscopically, atrophy involving the whole of the disc with atrophic excavation is seen, dead white in colour. The field defect is a peripheral shrinking instead of the characteristic central scotoma of Leber's disease. Nystagmus is common. An outstanding feature is that the affected members are "born with the sight as it is now" and that "none of the affected get either worse or better". Objective evidence of optic atrophy is recorded as early as at the age of 6 months.

The course, is, however, not always mild, for some individuals may be severely affected and some families show a concentration of such severe cases. Trito-anomalies have been a prominent aspect in some families (and has led to the suggestion that such cases are initially retinal in origin). Unusual appearances of the discs are also seen occasionally: in one instance there was glial degeneration filling in the atrophic cup in a man and his son; more frequently the discs are so deeply cupped as to have led to the designation of pseudoglaucoma (Fig. 167).

*Recessive optic atrophy*

A number of sibships have been recorded with severe optic atrophy either of the congenital type, or developing in infancy. The incidence of consanguinity in the more fully worked-out records is high. Fig. 168 *a* and *b* are illustrative pedigrees. In all probability this type is actually congenital, and it is possible that the bulk of these cases were instances of retinal aplasia.

**Post-natal optic atrophy other than Leber's disease**

Whilst most of the cases now recorded as of the dominant or recessive types of congenital optic atrophy are indeed congenital in origin, there is a possibility that

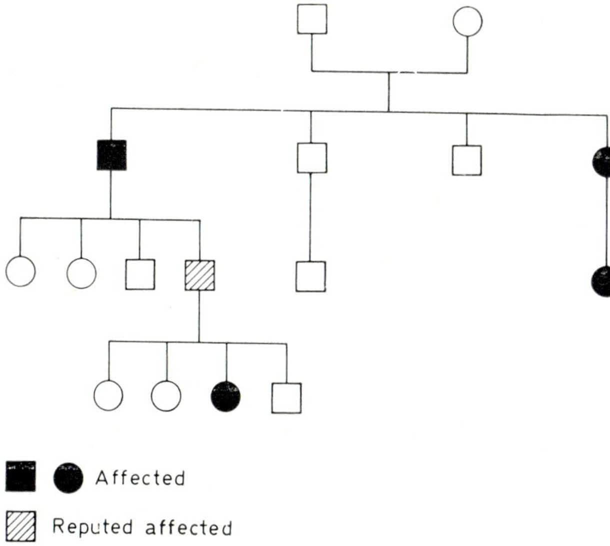


FIG. 167.—Congenital dominant optic atrophy. Pseudo-glaucoma type. (*After Sandvig*, 1961.)

some of them may be optic atrophies acquired early in life, and it is clear that some of the recorded pedigrees of Leber's disease illustrate a dominant—possibly irregularly dominant—hereditary optic atrophy with onset late in childhood, or early adult life. Adequate studies on this type of uncomplicated optic atrophy are lacking, however. Vogt has observed, on two occasions, two elderly sibs with optic atrophy without any other disturbances, and these may well be examples of an abiotrophic optic atrophy with onset late in life.

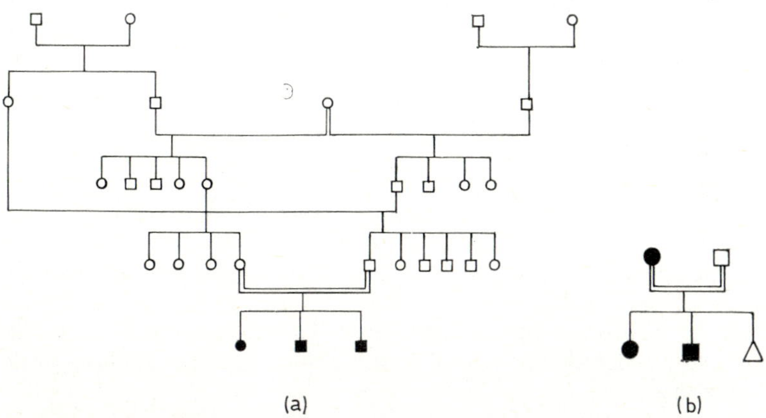


FIG. 168.—Congenital or infantile recessive optic atrophy. (*a*) An affected sibship whose parents were related. (*After Waardenburg*, 1932.) (*b*) An affected sibship, the offspring of an affected mother and a normal father who was her first cousin. (*After Gunn*, 1907.)

## OTHER ANOMALIES

**Pseudo-papilloedema**

At least three distinct types have to be recognized. The commonest is that congenital form of disc in which the physiological cup is absent or minimal and the nerve fibres are crowded together so that they become prominent ("swelling of the disc") and produce an indistinct disc margin, occasionally exaggerated by partially myelinated nerve fibres. Papilloedema may also be simulated by drusen bodies on the disc, whilst veils of epipapillary membrane constitute yet a third variety of pseudo-papilloedema.

*Apparent swelling of the disc*

Familial cases have been recorded by a number of observers. Families thus affected appear to have inherited high hypermetropia, but not all hypermetropes within the family show pseudo-papilloedema. Inheritance over two generations is shown in Fig. 169. Pseudo-papilloedema has also been observed in a father and daughter, the latter showing 1·5 D of myopia.

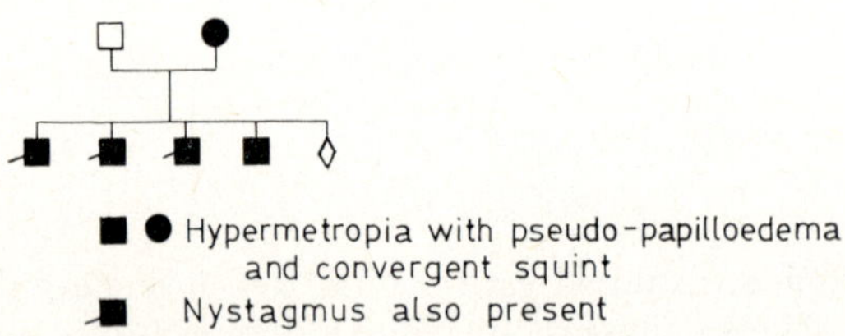


FIG. 169.—Pseudo-papilloedema. Inheritance over two generations. (*After Lambert and McDannald*, 1931.)

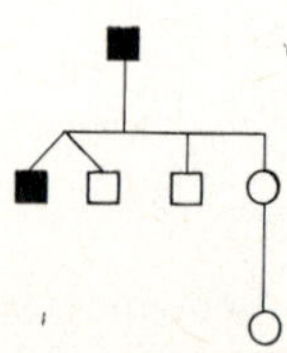

FIG. 170.—Megalopapilla. Inheritance over two generations. (*After Franceschetti and Bock*, 1950.)

*Drusen*

These are usually sporadic, but they have been observed in both regular and irregular dominant forms. They are occasionally associated with other fundus lesions and may be an aspect of tuberose sclerosis.

*Epipapillary membrane*

This has been observed over two generations (Handmann, 1929).

**Crater-like hole in the disc**

There do not appear to be any records suggestive of either dominant or recessive inheritance. Crater-like holes have been observed repeatedly in association with coloboma of the optic nerve, typical and heterotopic crescents, and typical choroidal coloboma. It has also been observed in individuals of families affected with dominant typical colobomatous defects. The exact status of crater-like pits is therefore still undetermined. It is possible that they have nothing to do with typical coloboma.

**Megalopapilla**

A disc substantially larger than normal has been observed over two generations (Fig. 170).

**Rudimentary or absent disc and retinal vessels**

Records in the older literature probably refer to extreme cases of retinal aplasia.

**Coloboma of optic nerve and heterotopic conus**

These anomalies fall into the group of typical colobomatous defects and have already been discussed.

## FOR FURTHER READING

**Leber's Disease**

Bell, Julia (1933). In *The Treasury of Human Inheritance*, Ed. by K. Pearson, Vol. 11, Pt. IV. London; Cambridge University Press.

Lundsgaard, Ruth (1944). "Leber's Disease". *Acta ophthal.*, Suppl. 21.

van Senus, A.H.C. (1963). *Docum. Ophthal.*, **17,** 1.

**Dominant Optic Atrophy**

Kjer, P. (1959). "Infantile Optic Atrophy with Dominant Mode of Inheritance." *Acta ophthal.*, Suppl. 54.

**Drusen**

François, J. and Verriest, G. (1958). *Ophthalmologica*, **136,** 289.

Lorentzen, S. E. (1966). *Drusen on the Optic Disk*. Thesis; Copenhagen.

**Crater-like hole**

Kranenburg, E. W. (1959). *Crater-like Hole in the Optic Disk and Central Serous Retinopathy*. Thesis; Amsterdam.

# CHAPTER 11

## OTHER TISSUES

### LIDS

**The lids proper**

*Epicanthus*

The line of demarcation between the physiological epicanthus of infancy and epicanthus as an abnormal feature is fine. That there is a genetic basis for the marked type of epicanthus is shown by the following observations.

(1) Several observers have recorded concordance as to epicanthus in uniovular twins, and discordance in binovular twins.

(2) Many sibships with epicanthus are on record, with occasional occurrence of consanguinity in the parents.

(3) There are many more pedigrees traced over two or more generations, and in at least one family the possibility of sex-linkage, as opposed to regular or irregular autosomal dominance, emerges (Fig. 171 *a* and *b*).

Epicanthus may be part of the Klein–Waardenburg syndrome—an irregularly dominant affection.

*Blepharochalasis*

Here, too, the line of demarcation between a mild bagginess of the upper lid (epiblepharon) and blepharochalasis is fine. Fig. 172 *a* represents a pedigree for the dominant inheritance of these conditions. Blepharochalasis associated with spasm of the lids and unusual changes in the skin of the lids in some of the patients has been observed as a dominant affection (Fig. 172 *b*); corneal ulceration from inturning lashes was a troublesome complication in some patients.

Hernia of the orbital fat and conjunctiva through the upper lid has been observed in a mother and daughter.

*Elephantiasis*

Elephantiasis of the lids may be part of von Recklinghausen's neurofibromatosis. As such it may be irregularly dominant and the possibility of other tumours elsewhere in the body has to be considered. In different families the same distribution tends to recur.

*Spasm of lids—absence of tarsal plates*

Spasm of the upper lid producing ectropion and lagophthalmos and of the lower lid producing entropion have been observed as dominant affections (Peters, 1915; Usher, 1932).

Lagophthalmos and entropion may be produced by absence of the tarsus in the upper or lower lid respectively. The first of these conditions has been observed in a sibship, and the second in a mother and two children.

*Coloboma*

*Coloboma of the upper lid.*—This is generally associated with other anomalies,

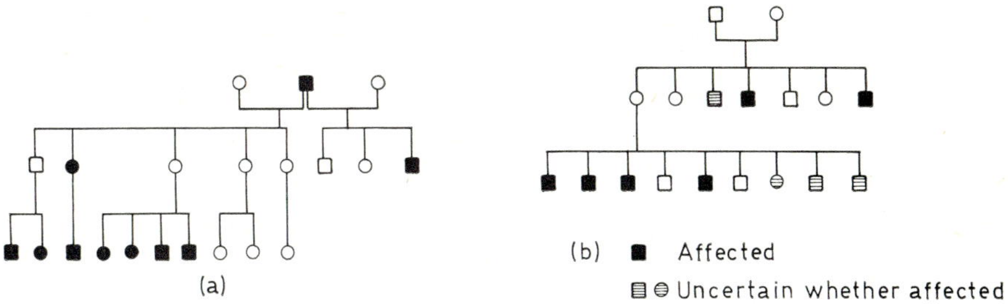


FIG. 171.—Epicanthus. (*a*) Dominant inheritance. (*After Usher*, 1935.) (*b*) Pedigree suggestive of sex-linkage. (*After Brückner*, 1906.)

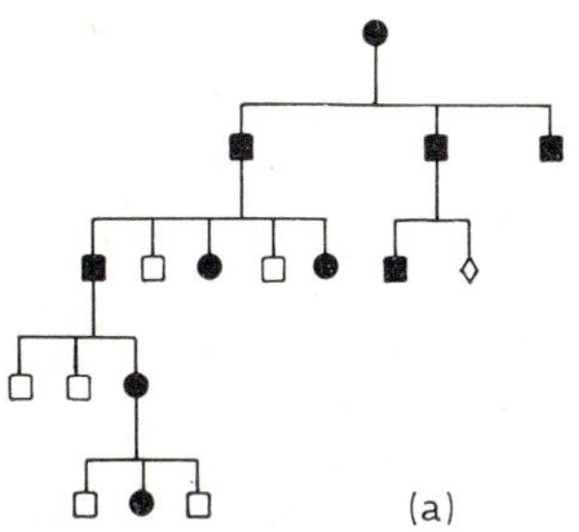


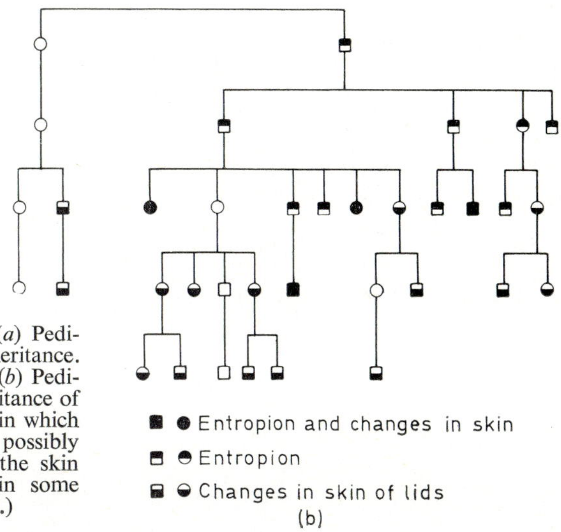


FIG. 172.—Blepharochalasis. (*a*) Pedigree showing dominant inheritance. (*After Franceschetti*, 1930.) (*b*) Pedigree showing dominant inheritance of blepharochalasis in a family in which associated spastic entropion, possibly due to unusual changes in the skin of the lids, was observed in some members. (*After Usher*, 1932.)

both of the globe and of the body as a whole. The condition has been observed in a mother and child, and also in the offspring of a consanguineous marriage.

*Coloboma of the lower lid.*—This is frequent in mandibulo-facial dysostosis.

*Ankyloblepharon*

Partial ankyloblepharon generally affecting the lateral parts of the lids has been observed in one family over four generations. Ankyloblepharon of the medial parts of the lids has been recorded in a pair of twins, and also in a father and six children; in these cases there were abnormally long lower canaliculi (van der Hoeve, 1929; John, 1934). Total ankyloblepharon is, of course, seen in cryptophthalmos.

**Anomalies of the skin of the lids**

Apart from involvement of the palpebral skin in generalized hereditary skin affections and in the Peutz syndrome, some relatively localized hereditary anomalies have been observed.

(1) Dark coloration of the lids with the veins standing out markedly has been observed as a dominant affection over five generations.

(2) Xanthelasmas of the lids have been recorded over two successive generations.

(3) Of the more important generalized skin diseases with a great tendency to involvement of the lids, ichthyosis and xeroderma pigmentosum are both dominant.

**Anomalies of lashes**

*Distichiasis*

Congenital distichiasis has been observed repeatedly as a simple dominant affection (Fig. 173).

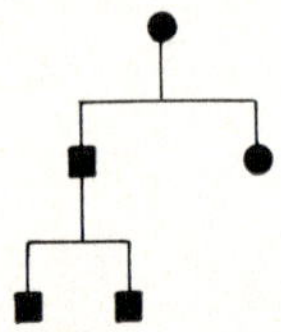

FIG. 173.—Distichiasis. Pedigree showing dominant inheritance. (*After Blatt*, 1924.)

*Tristichiasis*

There are several records of families in which three rows of lashes were inherited over two generations (Darnforth, 1929).

*Congenital deficiency of lashes and intermarginal area*

Madarosis is an aspect of ectodermal dysplasia (p. 241). Twin studies have shown the local defect to be genetically determined.

*Pili torti*

Twisted fragile lashes may give conjunctival irritation. Both dominant and recessive inheritance have been recorded (Appel and Messina, 1942; Gedda and Cavalteri, 1961).

## LACRIMAL APPARATUS

Genetic studies might well help to clarify the relationship of the different clinical types of disturbances in the lacrimal apparatus. Detailed studies are, however, lacking. As yet there is little more than tentative evidence of a genetic basis in some of them.

**Lack of tears**

It is likely that hereditary alacrimia recorded in the older literature was an aspect of systemic disturbances, such as anhidrotic ectodermal dysplasia and the Riley–Day syndrome.

**The lacrimal passages**

*Atresia or congenital absence of all four puncta*

Total absence of all four puncta, with rudimentary indication of the presence of some of them, has been recorded over three generations. A record over two generations with fistula from the sac in the second generation is also available (Fig. 174 *a* and *b*).

*Atresia of the nasolacrimal duct or the nasal openings*

Many sibships, and also the occurrence over two or more generations of congenital dacryocystitis, are on record. Fig. 175 is illustrative of the dominant

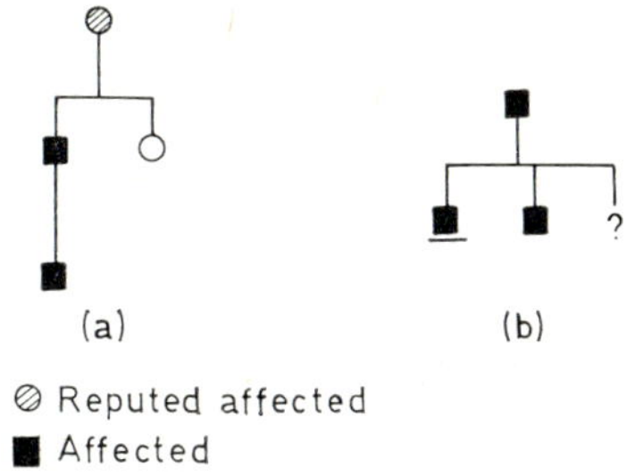


FIG. 174.—Congenital absence of all four puncta. (*a*) Pedigree showing inheritance over three generations. (*After Sorsby*, 1931.) (*b*) Pedigree showing inheritance over two generations. The underlined case showed fistulae at the sac. (*After Town*, 1943.)

transmission. Other pedigrees show dominant or irregularly dominant transmission variability in expression, as shown by the fact that in some affected members of families, the lesion is unilateral and sometimes late in onset, simulating the acquired form of the disorder.

*Elongation of canaliculi*

This may occur as part of the Klein–Waardenburg syndrome.

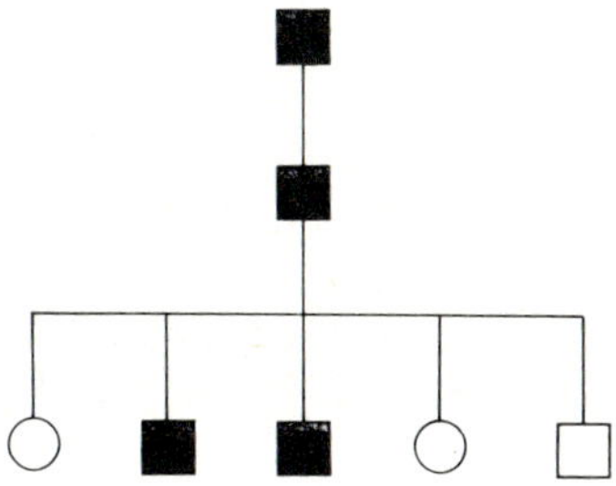

FIG. 175.—Congenital dacryocystitis. (*After François*, 1961.)

**Chronic dacryocystitis**

A striking clinical difference between congenital lacrimal obstruction and chronic dacryocystitis is the sex distribution. The first shows no marked sex difference, whereas the second is largely an affection falling on women.

The evidence for a genetic basis in chronic dacryocystitis is fairly extensive. Figure 176 shows inheritance over four generations. Traquair found that in 11 per cent of his patients admitted for operation a hereditary factor was present. The possibility of congenital lacrimal obstruction—or at any rate some varieties—linking up with chronic dacryocystitis has already been indicated and is further suggested by Figs. 176 *b* and 177.

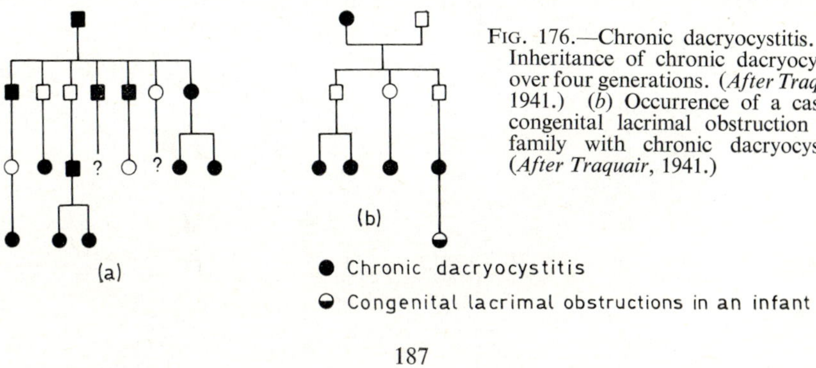


FIG. 176.—Chronic dacryocystitis. (*a*) Inheritance of chronic dacryocystitis over four generations. (*After Traquair*, 1941.) (*b*) Occurrence of a case of congenital lacrimal obstruction in a family with chronic dacryocystitis. (*After Traquair*, 1941.)

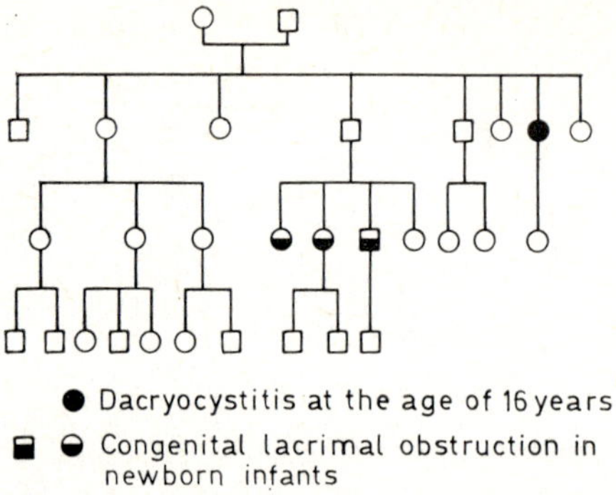


FIG. 177.—Congenital lacrimal obstruction. Occurrence in a sibship whose maternal aunt suffered from chronic dacryocystitis. (*After Traquair*, 1941.)

It is likely that excessive importance has been attached to infection in the aetiology of dacryocystitis, whether of the congenital or adult type. The infection is secondary to stasis, and the underlying condition is presumably some structural anomaly.

## CONJUNCTIVA

### New formations

*Dermo-lipoma*

This has been observed over three generations (Fig. 178).

*Pinguecula*

It is possible that cases of pinguecula are genetically determined, as they have been observed repeatedly in the same sibships late in life and in isolated populations over several generations (Kerkenezov, 1956; Forsius and Ericsson, 1962).

*Pterygium*

The possibility that there is at any rate a hereditary disposition to pterygium is suggested by a number of observations on pterygia in sibships and over two generations. Whether such pterygia are merely a similar reaction to similar environmental exciting factors is, however, not known. It has been observed, obviously as an independent feature, in a family with sex-linked night-blindness and myopia.

*Pigmented naevus*

There is a record of a mother and daughter with pigmented naevus; in the daughter malignant changes supervened (Rosenstein, 1925).

*Epibulbar carcinoma*

This has been observed once in a father and son (Puccioni, 1907).

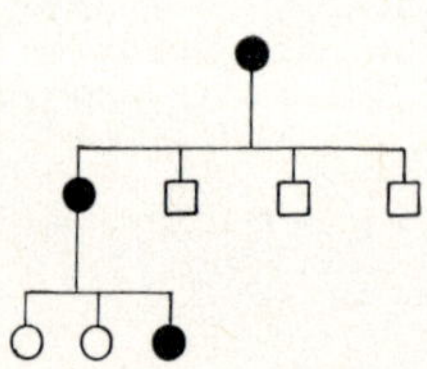

FIG. 178.—Dermolipoma. Inheritance over three generations. (*After Saebø*, 1948.)

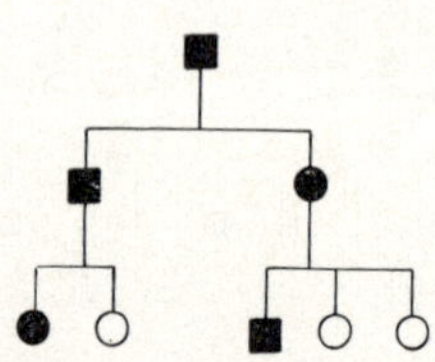

FIG. 179. — Episcleritis fugax. Pedigree showing inheritance over three generations. (*After Heinonen*, 1927.)

**Degenerative changes in the conjunctiva**

Pseudo-membranous conjunctivitis is an outstanding aspect of a dominantly inherited widespread dyskeratosis involving the mucous membranes (*see* p. 228). Keratoconjunctivitis sicca, and also essential shrinking of the conjunctiva and hyalinosis of the conjunctiva, are likewise significant aspects of generalized disorders discussed elsewhere.

**Chalazion formation**

A genetic predisposition is suggested by Lisch (1957) and more emphatically by the family records reported by Collier (1962).

**Telangiectasis**

Telangiectases at the upper fornix may be part of Rendu–Osler disease, whilst conjunctival telangiectases are an aspect of the Louis–Bar disease.

## SCLERA AND VITREOUS

**Episcleritis fugax**

Episcleritis fugax has been observed over three generations (Fig. 179).

**Persistent hyaloid artery**

Generally this would appear to be a developmental rather than a hereditary affection and is confined to one eye, which is frequently highly amblyopic. The occurrence of bilateral persistent hyaloid artery in a man and four of his children, and a unilateral lesion in one, yet another child, has been recorded (Iwanov, 1928).

## FOR FURTHER READING

**Epicanthus**

Usher, C. H. (1935). *Trans. Ophthal. Soc. U.K.*, **55,** 194, 232.
— (1935). *Biometrica*, **27,** 5.

**Anomalies of the skin of the lids**

Waardenburg, J. P. (1963). In *Genetics and Ophthalmology*, pp. 204–236, Ed. by P. J. Waardenburg, A. Franceschetti and D. Klein. Oxford; Blackwell.

**Lacrimal apparatus**

Bischler, V. (1957). *Mod. Probl. Ophth.*, **1,** 584.
Traquair, H. M. (1941). *Archs Ophthal.*, **26,** 165.

SECTION III

# GENERALIZED DISORDERS WITH OCULAR ASPECTS

# CHAPTER 12

## METABOLIC DISORDERS

Mendelian genetics, the development of biochemistry and Garrod's recognition of the "inborn errors of metabolism", with its stress on intermediary products, all date from the first decade of the present century. In recent years automation of chemical analysis has brought rapid advances in the study of the biochemistry of body fluids, tissues and cells, and in consequence many hereditary disorders can now be visualized in terms of biochemical anomalies, themselves often the result of enzyme defects. The rapid accumulation of new data makes all present-day classification highly tentative. For example, it is uncertain how fundamental is the distinction between storage diseases, in which cells are infiltrated with normal or abnormal metabolic products, and the affections in which the biochemical anomalies are mainly reflected in the composition of the blood and urine. Clinically, current classifications are of great value in diagnosis.

### CARBOHYDRATE METABOLISM

Disorders reflected by abnormal blood or urine contents are those of the diabetes group and galactosaemia. The storage diseases are represented only by gargoylism; for the classical carbohydrate storage affections—the glycogenoses—have little importance in ophthalmology.

#### Hyperglycaemia

*Diabetes mellitus*

Clinical diabetes, with its varying degrees of severity, is the fullest manifestation of a gene (or genes) often not fully expressed. It is still not clear whether more than one mode of inheritance is operative and indeed whether environmental factors determine expression. These complexities are still more real in relation to the ocular complications of diabetes, for no adequate studies on the inheritance of diabetic retinopathy and of diabetic cataract are available. The late onset of diabetic retinopathy in diabetes and the lack of response to insulin therapy raise the possibility that the retinal disorder is not genetically determined but is an aspect of environmentally induced vascular lesions as seen in diabetics.

*Wolfram–Tyrer syndrome (juvenile diabetes, optic atrophy, nerve deafness and multiple psycho-neurological disturbances)*

Wolfram in 1938 reported on a sibship of eight, of whom four were affected with juvenile diabetes and optic atrophy. A similar association was noted by Tyrer in 1943 in three out of four offspring of a consanguineous marriage; epilepsy was present in two of the affected sibs whilst the third showed mental and physical retardation. Subsequent reports on similar cases have brought out that the optic atrophy, like the diabetes, generally became obvious in childhood, and that with advancing age the onset of progressive nerve deafness is not uncommon. Less frequent associations are mental deficiency and also a wide range of neurological complications of fairly late onset; these extend from myelopathy to the lesions of the type seen in Friedreich's disease; sideroplastic anaemia is another possible association. The complexity of the clinical appearances warrants an eponymal designation as used here.

The collected literature suggests recessive inheritance and perhaps also a high incidence of diabetes in the ascendants.

A possibly allied syndrome that needs clarification is represented by the cases of juvenile diabetes insipidus with optic atrophy (De Lawter, 1949; Casa, 1955; Raiti, Plotkin and Newns, 1963). The status of the cases recorded by Alström, Hallgren, Nilsson and Åsander (1959) is also not clear: three cases in two related families showed the association of juvenile diabetes, pigmentary degeneration of the retina, adiposity and nerve deafness: mental defect and polydactyly were lacking and two of the patients died at the ages of 32 and 16 years from extensive renal fibrosis. The relationship to dominant optic atrophy and deafness also needs clarification (Ptasinska–Urbanska and Mietkiewicz–Bochenek, 1968).

**Galactosaemia**

In this inborn error of metabolism, an enzyme defect prevents the conversion of galactose into glucose. The accumulated galactose is toxic and distorts normal development. The infant is normal at birth, but does not thrive, physically or mentally. Fatty infiltration of the liver with secondary cirrhosis develops, and the spleen becomes enlarged. The blood and urine show a high content of galactose and albuminuria develops. Opacification of the lens is an important feature and generally develops in the fourth week of life, the opacity being either lamellar or nuclear in type.

The affection is recessive. The early management of such cases is essential, for much damage can be prevented by the exclusion of lactose (as in milk and milk products) from the diet. Reversal of the cataract has been reported.

**Gargoylism**

The histological findings of ballooning and vascularization of the nerve cells in this affection, at first suggested that gargoylism was related to the lipoid disturbances seen in the amaurotic idiocy group. It is clear now that the lipoid changes are secondary and that the primary fault is a metabolic disorder of mucopolysaccharides (or possibly of a mucoprotein) with deposition and storage of a lipoid substance. The widespread skeletal anomalies in this affection are readily understood from the fact that the mucopolysaccharides are particularly important in the development of the skeleton and connective tissues. The corneal lesion is the result of infiltration of the tissue by the polysaccharides and may be so severe as to simulate unresolved interstitial keratitis as seen in congenital syphilis (Fig. 180).

The disproportionate dwarfism, hepato-splenomegaly, mental retardation and the severe corneal opacities constitute the pathognomonic picture of the recessive form of this affection. It has to be distinguished from the Brailsford–Morquio–Ulrich disease, which is also an autosomal recessive disorder, and in which there is no mental retardation. The clinical and biochemical differences of these disorders still need clarification; corneal lesions once regarded as lacking are now known to occur (Maroteaux and Lamy, 1963; Robert and colleagues, 1966). There is also a less common X-chromosomal type of gargoylism characterized by the lack of the corneal complications (Fig. 181*b*).

The difficulties in the clinical differentiation of allied disorders are well shown by the fact that six different types of mucopolysaccharoidosis are now recognized.

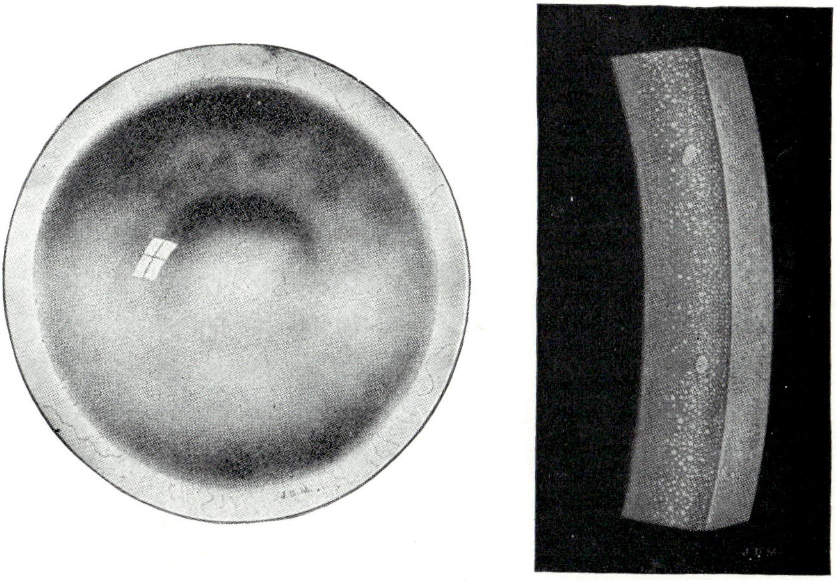

(a) (b)

FIG. 180.—Cornea in gargoylism. (*a*) Face view and (*b*) optical section. The haziness in the face view is seen to be due to yellowish-white deposits in the middle and deeper layers of the cornea. (*After Berliner*, 1939.)

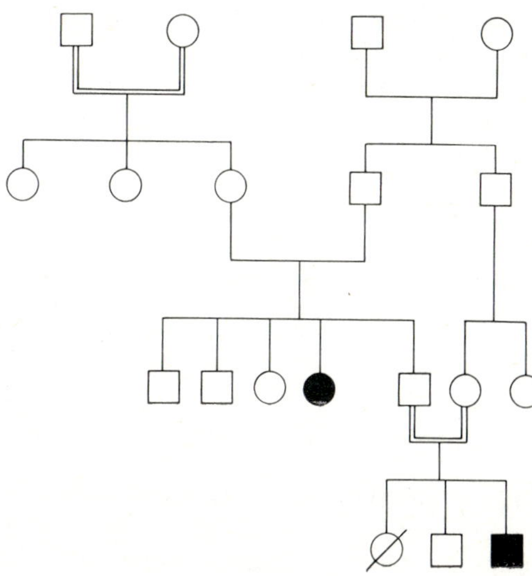

FIG. 181 (*a*).—Gargoylism. Recessive inheritance. (*After François and Rabey*, 1952.)

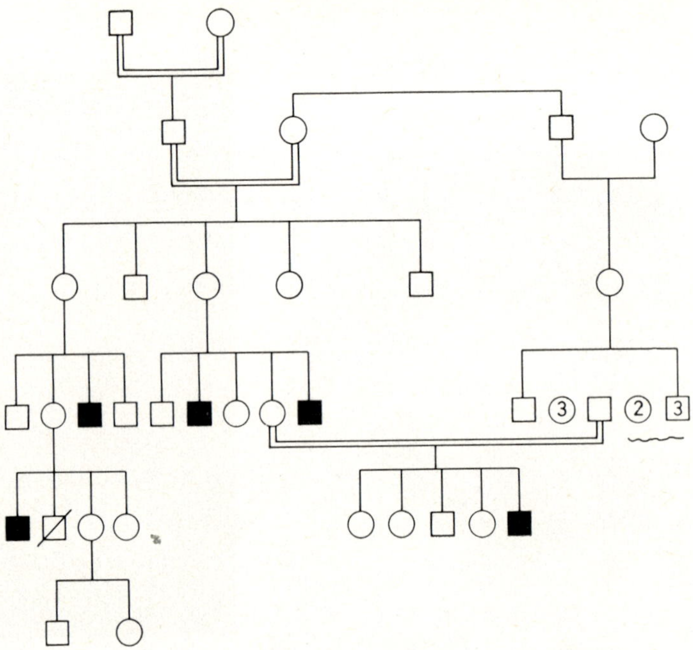


FIG. 181 (*b*).—Gargoylism. Sex-linked inheritance. (*After Bamatter and Lamy*, 1957.)

## FAT METABOLISM

Ocular lesions are prominent in the group of diseases associated with abnormal metabolism of fats—the lipoidoses. In this group storage diseases (Thesaurismoses) are outstanding; they include the ganglioside disturbances in amaurotic idiocy; the sulphatide disturbances in the metachomatic leucodystrophies; the cerebroside disturbances of Gaucher's disease; and the cholesteroses with or without hypercholesterolaemia. In addition to these well-established entities many others with ophthalmological interest have been recorded recently.

Apart from the cholesteroses with hypercholesterolaemia few of the lipoidoses show substantial anomalies in the composition of the blood, the outstanding examples being A-$\beta$-lipoproteinaemia and hypolipidaemia.

## STORAGE DISORDERS

### GANGLIOSIDE DISORDERS

**Infantile amaurotic idiocy (Tay–Sachs disease)**

This affection, which is clinically a clear-cut entity, was at one time mistakenly regarded as exclusively confined to Jews. Histologically the ganglion cells throughout the central nervous system are immensely distended, the nucleus is displaced towards the periphery, stains poorly, and ultimately disappears together with the rest of the cell contents. The ballooned cells become loaded with a ganglioside which normally constitutes a very small fraction of brain gangliosides.

A peculiar vacuolation in the cytoplasm of the lymphocytes appears to be a characteristic finding (Fig. 182).

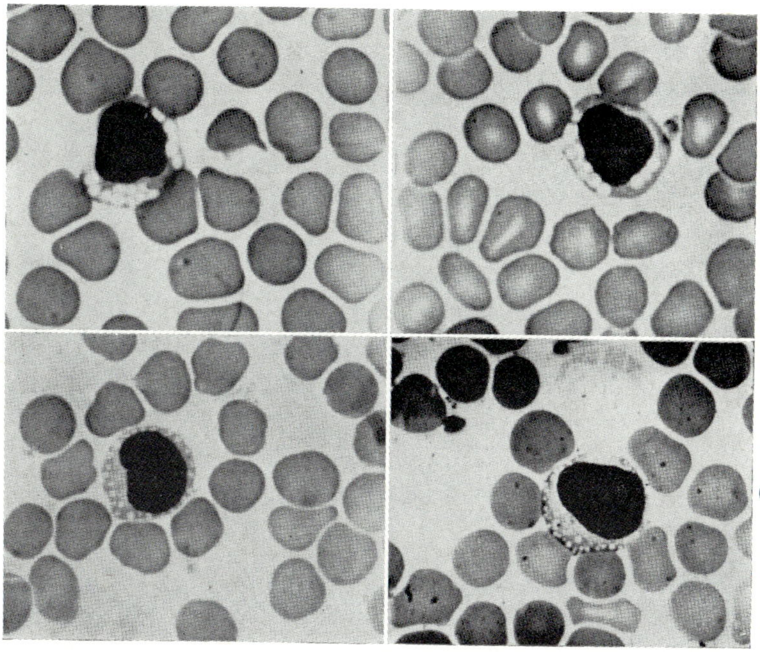


FIG. 182.—(*a*) and (*b*) Examples of vacuolation in the cytoplasm of lymphocytes of two patients with juvenile amaurotic idiocy (1860 ×). (*c*) and (*d*) Examples of vacuolation in the cytoplasm of lymphocytes of two healthy relatives of patients, one a known and the other a presumed carrier. (*c*) Father (1700 ×). (*d*) Sister (1840 ×). (*Reproduced by courtesy of Dr. S. Rayner and the University of Uppsala.*)

The affection has been recorded frequently in several sibs, and there is a high rate of consanguinity in the parents. This would suggest recessive inheritance. There are, however, pedigrees in which the affection has occurred in collateral branches of the family—an unexpected event with rare genes (Fig. 183 *a* and *b*). Direct dominant inheritance does not, of course, arise, as the affection is lethal, generally by the end of the second year of life. The possibility of intermediate inheritance, with the affection as the expression of the homozygous state, cannot be excluded in view of the fact that in families in which Tay–Sachs disease occurs, neurological stigmata are not uncommon. Furthermore, vacuolation of lymphocytes has been recorded in healthy relatives (*see* Fig. 182).

**Juvenile amaurotic idiocy**

This affection, coming on at about the age of 6 years, and running a slower lethal course, differs clinically from the infantile type in lacking the characteristic cherry-red spot at the macula, which in these cases shows pigmentary changes. The pigmentary changes are, however, not confined to the macula, but are seen throughout the whole of the retina, which is highly atrophic histologically. The

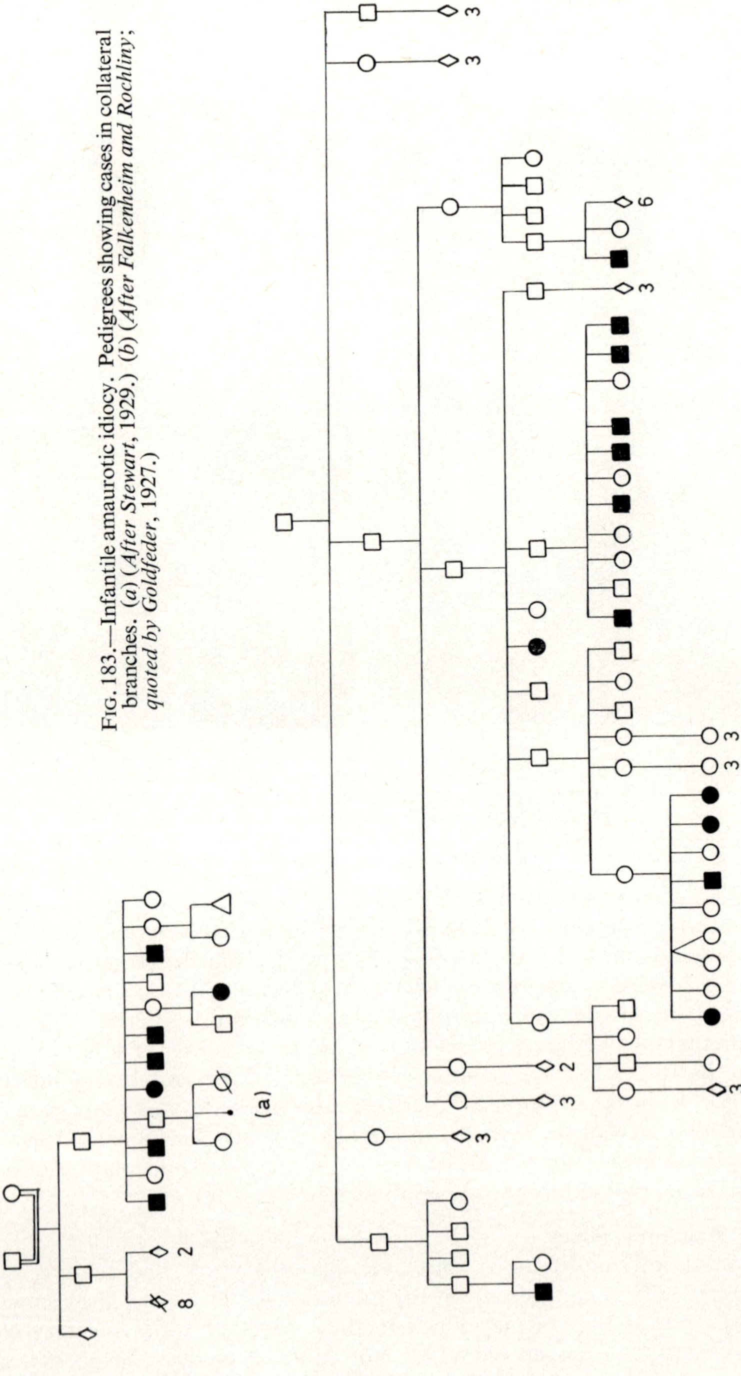


FIG. 183.—Infantile amaurotic idiocy. Pedigrees showing cases in collateral branches. (a) (*After Stewart*, 1929.) (b) (*After Falkenheim and Rochliny; quoted by Goldfeder*, 1927.)

distinction into two types, the macular type (Batten–Mayou disease) and the peripheral type (the Vogt–Spielmeyer disease) is rather tenuous. The chemical identity of the infantile and the juvenile forms of amaurotic idiocy have still to be established, but the vacuolation of lymphocytes is not present. The histological picture is fundamentally similar in the two affections, however.

The mode of inheritance in this group appears to be a simple recessive, as shown by the systematic survey of Sjögren (Fig. 184 *a* and *b*). As in Tay–Sachs disease, there appears to be an increased incidence of mental disorders in heterozygotes.

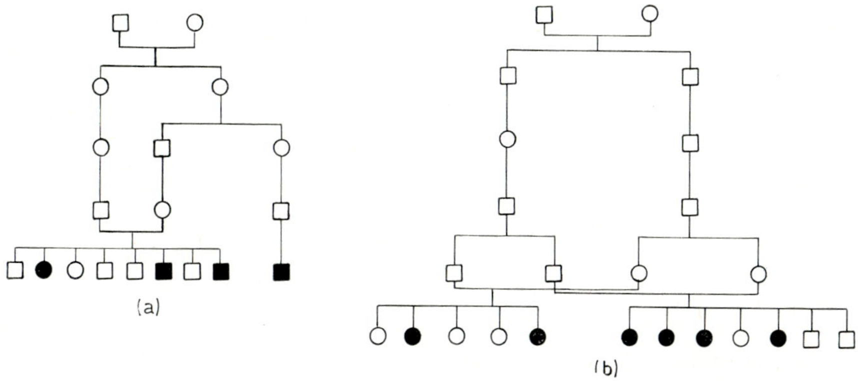


FIG. 184.—Juvenile amaurotic idiocy. Recessive inheritance. Pedigrees showing cases in two collateral branches with common ancestry. (*After Sjögren*, 1931.)

**Other forms**

*Congenital amaurotic idiocy*

This has been recorded in only one family (Norman and Wood, 1941; Brown, Corner and Dodgson, 1954). Its exact status amongst the lipoidoses is not clear.

*Late infantile amaurotic idiocy*

This is a more definite entity which is regarded as an intermediate form between the two classical types. The affection is rare and the literature rather confused from the admission of doubtfully relevant cases, some of which are probably examples of metachromatic leucodystrophy—a sulphatide lipoidosis—in which optic atrophy is fairly common.

*Late juvenile and adult amaurotic idiocy*

These forms, too, are rare and rather ill-defined. Ocular signs are uncommon.

**Relationship of Tay–Sachs disease to Niemann–Pick disease**

There is some evidence that the infantile type of amaurotic idiocy may be part of a systemic lipoid disease extending to the whole of the reticulo-endothelial system in addition to the central nervous system—Niemann–Pick disease. The association of this affection with Tay–Sachs disease has been observed repeatedly in the same infant, and there are records of the appearance of either of these affections within the same sibship (Fig. 185). Chemically Niemann–Pick disease shows infiltration with sphingomyelin, so that it is still a moot point whether

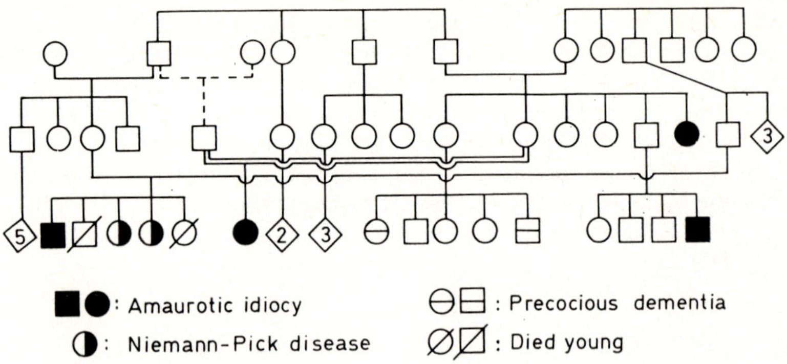


FIG. 185.—Co-existence within a family of Tay–Sachs disease and Niemann–Pick disease. (*After van Bogaert*, 1934.)

Niemann–Pick disease is the visceral form, and Tay–Sachs disease the neurological form of an affection, which when fully developed shows both these components (Norman and colleagues, 1959).

## CEREBROSIDE DISEASES

### Gaucher's disease

*The acute infantile form*

This is a rapidly fatal non-specific cerebral disorder which clinically gives the picture of "decortication" associated with a specific splenohepatomegaly characterized by infiltration with pathognomonic foam cells (Gaucher cells). As in the Niemann–Pick disease the phospholipoid (gluco-cerebroside) is rather different from that seen in the amaurotic idiocy group. Paralytic squint is not uncommon.

*The chronic adult form*

This is a visceral affection without cerebral involvement. In the eye, Gaucher cells are present in the interpalpebral conjunctiva which is thickened and brownish in colour (Fig. 186).

Recessive inheritance probably applies to the infantile form. It is not certain whether the adult form is recessive or irregularly dominant.

## CHOLESTEROL DISORDERS

The affections induced by cholesterol deposition range from xanthelasmata around the eyelids to such lethal disorders as the Hand–Schüller–Christian disease.

### Palpebral xanthelasmata

The incidence increases with age. There is a female excess and there are pedigrees which suggest dominant transmission with incomplete penetrance in men.

### "Arcus senilis"

Here the age factor is even more definite than in palpebral xanthelasmata. When the anomaly occurs relatively early in life, dominant transmission is not unlikely.

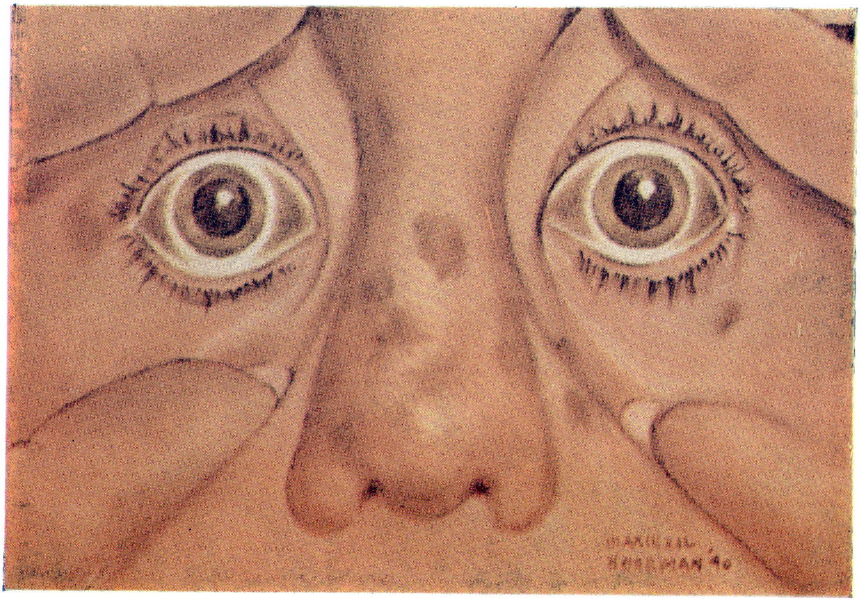

FIG. 186.—Gaucher's disease. Facial appearances. Note pigmentation of skin and sclera. (*After Thannhauser*, 1940.)

[*To face page 200*

**Skeletal xanthomatosis**

These may take the form of isolated eosinophilic granuloma, multiple granulomata or such a specific entity as cranio-hypophysial granulatomatosis—the Hand–Schüller–Christian disease—with its striking triad of multiple lacunar defects in the skull, diabetes insipidus and exophthalmos, the two latter being secondary to a diffuse infiltrating lesion of bone and dura mater around the sella turcica.

There is no convincing evidence as to the genetic status of the Hand–Schüller–Christian disease and there is considerable uncertainty as to its status as a primary lipoidosis. It is suggested that the affection falls within the group of infectious reticulo-endothelioses of which eosinophilic bone granuloma is the mildest and Letterer–Siwe disease the most severe expression, with the Hand–Schüller–Christian disease in an intermediate position.

**Dermochondrocorneal dystrophy**

First recorded by François (1949) in two young sibs, other cases are now known (Jensen, 1958). Xanthomatous nodular deposits in the cartilage and on the skin on the back of the fingers and toes produce deformities and subluxations. Xanthomatous deposits are also seen in the skin at the elbows, nose and outer ear. In addition to these skin and cartilage deposits there are also corneal infiltrates (Fig. 187).

The affection appears to be recessive.

## Other Lipid Storage Disorders

**Hyalinosis of the skin and mucous membranes (Urbach–Wiethe disease)**

Hyaline deposits of lipoid material around the capillaries and in the adjacent connective tissue lead to nodular and hyperkeratotic reactions in the affected tissues, the sites of election in the skin being the face, scalp, neck and extremities, and in the mucosa, the lips, the mouth and larynx. The affection carries a high mortality. In severe cases the face may be scarred as in small-pox and tracheotomy may be needed for laryngeal stenosis. An increase in blood sugar and phosphatide is sometimes present.

The lids may show multiple small nodules, resembling milia and leading to blepharitis with loss of lashes. In the fundus hyaline deposits may give one of the forms of "Tay's choroiditis" (Moynahan, 1966).

The affection is recessive.

**Fabry's disease**

In this generalized skin affection, confined to males, angiomata the size of a pin-head are grouped mainly over the buttocks, scrotum and penis and knees ("bathing suit area"). The overlying skin is rough as indicated by the description of angiokeratoma used by Fabry. There is an associated progressive chronic nephritis which generally sets in at about the age of 20–30 years; abdominal crises severe enough to suggest renal colic are not uncommon.

In the fundi, dilatation of the retinal vessels with microaneurysms are present in about two-thirds of cases. Even more frequent are the appearances of cornea verticillata, whilst the conjunctiva may show a purplish discoloration particularly at the fornices from dilated veins.

The concentration of lipoids in the blood is normal. Histologically the affected tissues show infiltration with glycolipoids.

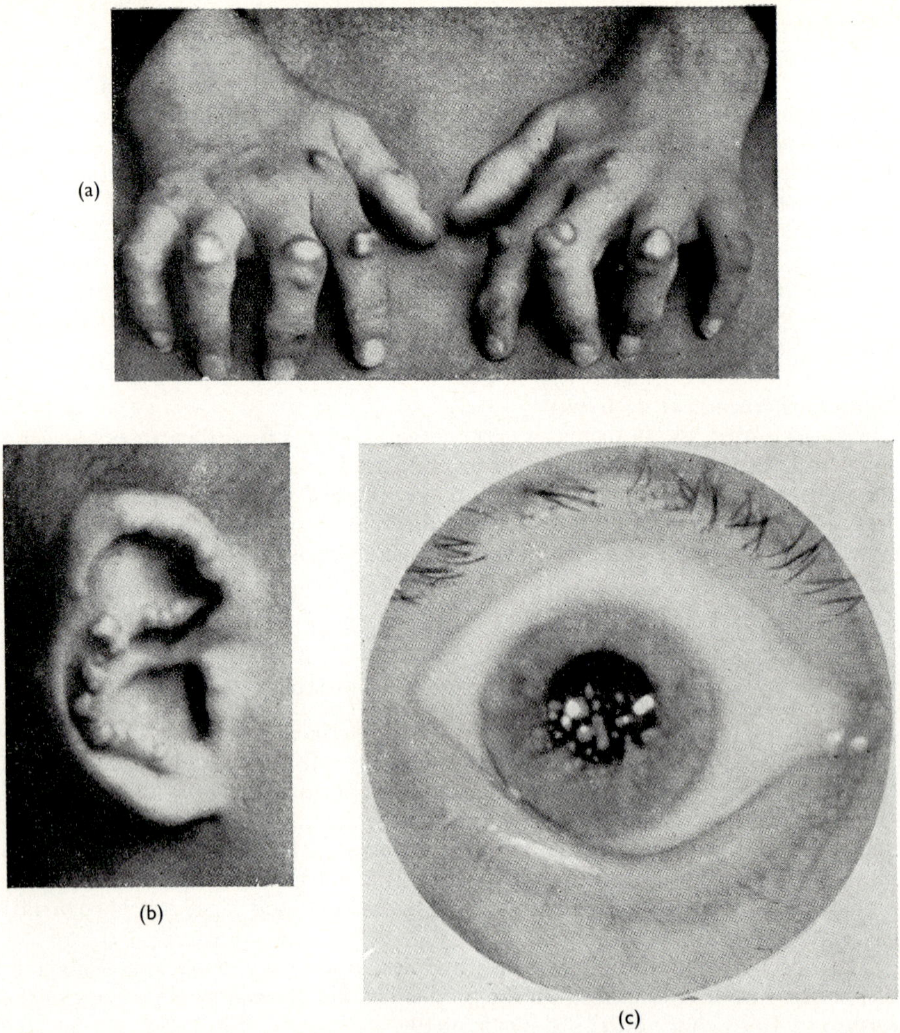


FIG. 187.—Dermochondrocorneal dystrophy. (*a*) and (*b*) Xanthomatous nodules on fingers and on the ear. (*c*) Subepithelial opacities in the cornea. (*After François*, 1949.)

Inheritance appears to be in a sex-linked recessive manner. It has been suggested that cornea verticillata in women is a manifestation of the carrier state.

**Chédiak–Higashi disease**

This affection is characterized by albinism of the oculo-cutaneous type; the lack of pigmentation is not complete, either clinically or histologically but photophobia and nystagmus are present. There are also the following additional features: hepatosplenomegaly and a variable degree of generalized enlargement of the lymphatic glands; anaemia with neutropenia; and skin troubles such as erythema and postular eruptions.

The course of the affection is characterized by a great tendency to generalized infections uninfluenced by antibiotics. A lethal outcome is usual by the age of 12 or so.

The pathognomonic features are cytoplasmic giant inclusions of glycolipoids in the leucocytes and in the myeloid cells of bone marrow (the Steinbrinck–Chédiak anomaly of leucocytes). Subepithelial corneal opacities have been recorded as a possible aspect of the affection.

The affection is recessive (Fig. 188). It has been suggested that carriers can be recognized by mild inclusions in the leucocytes.

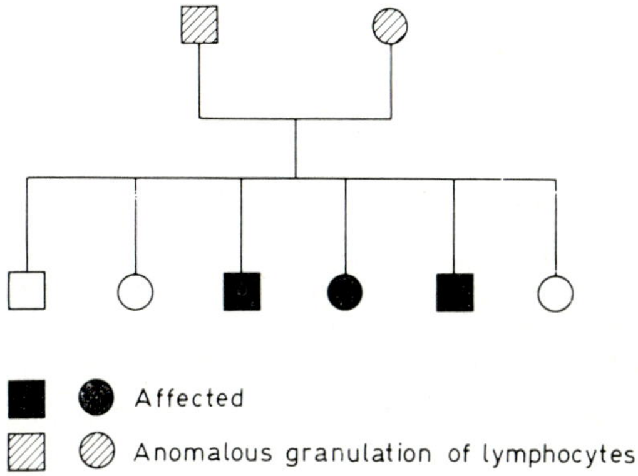


FIG. 188.—Chédiak–Higashi disease. Intermediate inheritance. (*After Bernard and colleagues*, 1960.)

**Refsum's disease**

In addition to congenital "atypical retinitis pigmentosa" there is present chronic progressive polyneuritis leading to paralysis of the limbs and frequently also cerebellar ataxia. Histologically there is cerebral lipoidosis of the amaurotic idiocy type; chemically the fat has been recognized as 3,7,11,15-tetramethylhexadecanoic acid.

The affection is recessive.

## AFFECTIONS WITH ABNORMAL BLOOD LEVELS

**Familial hyperlipaemia**

The hyperlipaemia occurs in episodes during which there is marked elevation of the neutral fats in the blood, so that it becomes milky in appearance. During the attacks there is fever, abdominal pain and hepatosplenomegaly and sometimes also glycosuria. Most cases develop in childhood. Retinal lipaemia may be present and gives the characteristic appearance of the retinal vessels. Fatty corneal infiltrates which do not always clear up may also develop. Transient xanthomata are not uncommon.

Confusion with hypercholesteraemia is possible as the cholesterol content of the blood is often elevated during attacks.

Recessive inheritance is probably the rule, but dominantly inherited cases are also on record.

**Hypercholesteraemia with cholesterinoses**

The ocular aspects of this group are not extensive. Generalized xanthomatosis is a protean disorder which may take different forms, such as those involving mainly the skin tendons, or coronary arteries, heart valves, brain or reticulo-endothelial system.

In about half the cases of cutaneous xanthomatosis, xanthelasma around the lids develop. These constitute only a small proportion of palpebral xanthelasmata seen, but raise the possibility that isolated palpebral xanthelasmata with hypercholesteraemia may represent an abortive aspect of a severe generalized disorder.

Apart from palpebral xanthelasmata, arcus senilis and localized plaques in the conjunctiva may occur in these disorders.

The affection is inherited in a dominant manner. Different families generally show only one or other form of the disorder, although overlaps and abortive forms—including hypercholesteraemia without manifestations—are not uncommon.

**Hypolipidaemia syndrome**

As described by Hooft and his colleagues (1962) in two sisters, there were disturbances in growth, eruptions or a dry skin, nail and dental anomalies and mental retardation in addition to blindness from retinal aplasia. The reduction in the fat contents of the blood were interpreted as due to a deficiency of ATP consequent on faulty metabolism of tryptophane.

**β-Lipoproteinaemia (Bassen–Kornzweig disease)**

Bassen and Kornzweig in 1950 and 1957 recorded the occurrence of atypical retinitis pigmentosa (of the retinal aplasia type), ataxia and also acanthocytosis and steatorrhoea, in addition to the striking finding of absence of β-lipoprotein

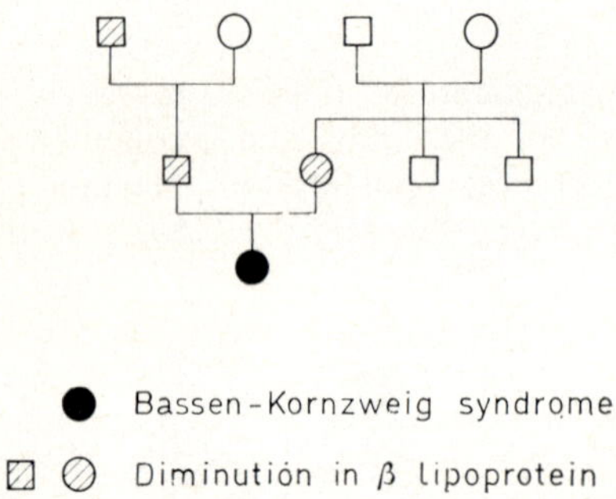


FIG. 189.—A pedigree of the Bassen–Kornzweig syndrome illustrating a biochemical anomaly in carriers. (*After Salt and colleagues*, 1960.)

in the blood serum and some reduction of other fats. Subsequent reports by other observers have suggested that whilst the affection is recessive, the carriers can be identified by a reduction—as distinct from the absence—of β-lipoprotein in the plasma (Fig. 189).

## PROTEIN METABOLISM

With the progressive deciphering of the genetic code a deeper understanding is being reached of the vagaries of protein metabolism as the underlying cause of hereditary disease. Sickle cell anaemia with its characteristic vitreous haemorrhage was the first of the diseases to be recognized as a disturbance in the molecular structure of a tissue, the haemoglobin of the erythrocytes. Anomalies of protein synthesis may underlie such affections as retinitis pigmentosa as is suggested by the experimental data recorded earlier (p. 168). Other disorders, such as albinism, are the result of an enzyme defect in the breakdown of amino acids. Yet other affections are the result of the deposition of normal or abnormal constituents as in hereditary amyloidosis where there is storage of amyloid material, whilst such disorders as the Fanconi syndrome—which is an aspect of several disturbances —are largely the result of transport anomalies.

## MOLECULAR AMINO ACID ANOMALY: HAEMOGLOBINOPATHY

### Sickle Cell Anaemia

In this affection the erythrocytes function normally when exposed to adequate oxygen tension, but they elongate towards a sickle shape when oxygen tension is low. These sickle shaped erythrocytes move slowly with a resultant drop in oxygen tension and a further increase in sickling. In the sickle cell trait these changes are seen only *in vitro;* in sickle cell anaemia they occur clinically and lead to a fatal outcome.

In sickling the haemoglobin (haemoglobin S) carries on the $\beta$-peptide chain two valine residues in place of two glutamic acid residues (in sickling due to haemoglobin C the glutamic acid is replaced by lysine). These molecular mutations are recessive so that the sickling trait is characteristic of the heterozygote and sickle cell anaemia of the homozygote.

Heterozygotes possess some protection against malaria as the *Plasmodium* cannot thrive on haemoglobin S, so that the mutation is advantageous in African negroes in whom the gene is widely scattered.

Retinal haemorrhage leading to dense black scars are not uncommon in sickle cell anaemia (haemoglobin S S) but the most characteristic feature in haemoglobin C disease (haemoglobin S C) is a fan-shaped anomaly in the retina with a great tendency to vitreous haemorrhage, which itself leads to vitreous fibrosis and retinal detachment.

## ESTABLISHED OR PRESUMED AMINO ACID ENZYME DISTURBANCES

### Albinism

Embryologically melanocytes in the skin, mucosa and central nervous system develop from the melanoblasts in the neural crest; the pigment cells in the retina and probably also of the uvea are, however, derived from the outer layer of the optic cup. There is no failure in morphological processes that produce pigment-bearing cells; albinism is the consequence of a failure in the intermediate metabolism of phenylalanine: there is an enzyme block at the cell level which prevents the conversion by succesive stages of tyrosine to melanin.

**Clinical varieties**

There are three sharply contrasted varieties of albinotic disorders.

*Oculo-cutaneous (or generalized) albinism*

This is the classical and commonest form of albinism. No albino is totally devoid of pigment and not all albinoes are equally albinotic. At the one extreme there is the typical albino who is clinically devoid of pigment, and at the other the patient whose hair is straw coloured rather than white and whose iris shows yellow-greenish coloration; the iris does, however, transmit light, so that the eye is red. These are graduations of the same condition, for both types occur within one and the same family, and furthermore many typical albinoes tend to develop some colour later in life.

*Oculo-cutaneous albinism as part of more widespread disorders.*—Chédiak–Higashi disease combines oculo-cutaneous albinism with a glycolipoid disturbance which runs a fatal course (p. 202). Whether high myopia occasionally seen in generalized albinism is incidental or part of a distinct entity is not certain. Deafness is apparently not an associated lesion of the oculo-cutaneous form of albinism.

*Ocular albinism*

The globe only is involved, reproducing the ocular component of generalized albinism. The so-called albinotic fundus is probably a physiological variation unrelated to albinism.

*Cutaneous albinism*

This is a highly complex group, clinically and genetically unrelated to oculo-cutaneous or to ocular albinism. Occasionally the whole of the skin and hair are involved. More commonly there is the piebald pattern: localized vitiligo-like areas, often arranged symmetrically, most frequently on the neck and abdominal extremities. When depigmentation occurs on the forehead it may be associated with a white forelock, which indeed may be the only lesion.

The piebald or patterned type of cutaneous albinism may be associated with deaf-mutism (Margolis, 1962; Ziprkowski and colleagues, 1962). It is also seen with a series of ocular anomalies: blepharophimoses, lateral displacement of the canaliculi, heterochromic iridis and some fundus albinism (the Klein–Waardenburg syndrome)—a symptom complex that recalls the anomalies seen in the offspring resulting from the mating of dappled dachshunds (Sorsby and Davey, 1954).

"Incontinentia pigmenti" is discussed elsewhere (p. 243).

**Inheritance**

*Generalized albinism*

Oculo-cutaneous albinism is concordant in uniovular twins and the recessive character of the affection is shown by a number of well established pedigrees (Fig. 190).

Several difficulties arise in the interpretation of the extensive pedigrees that are available.

(1) The rate of consanguinity is high. This argues in favour of an exceptionally rare condition. Albinism, however, is not so rare as this high rate of consanguinity suggests, though certainly not so common as the extensive literature on the subject implies. The high rate of consanguinity may be an artefact in the older literature, but it has been explained on the supposition that there are several different genes which are capable of producing albinism—an assumption supported by the observation that the two children born to albino parents were both normal (Trevor–Roper, 1952).

(2) The number of affected individuals in pooled pedigrees shows a higher proportion than the theoretical 25 per cent expected. When this pooled material is statistically corrected the theoretically expected percentage is obtained, but it would seem, however, that the expected ratio is not obtained in substantial series of unselected cases.

(3) In the antecedents of albino patients there are frequently partial manifestations suggestive of albinism—such as a great frequency of light-coloured hair, and

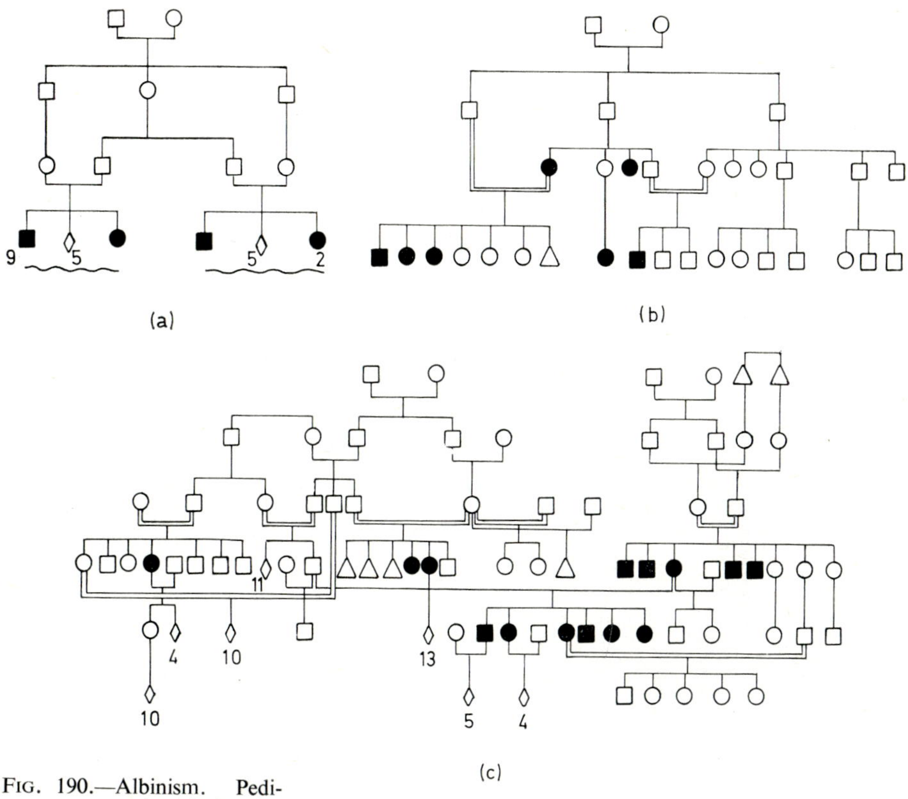


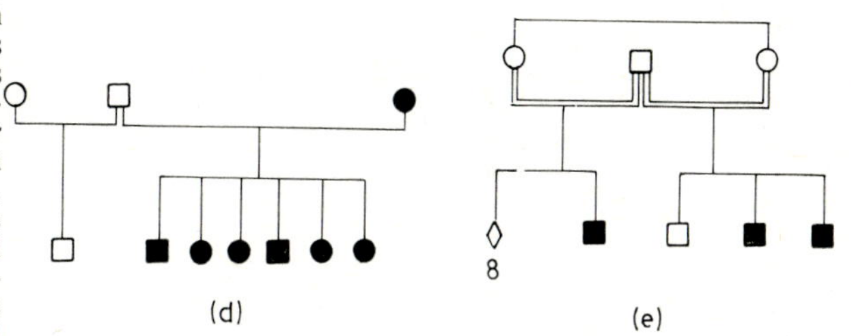


FIG. 190.—Albinism. Pedigrees suggestive of recessive inheritance. (*a*) Albinism in two collateral branches of a family. The parents were all derived from common ancestors. (*After Stainer*, 1913.) (*b*) Albinism in collateral branches. The offspring of parents related in the first and second degree. The assumption of recessive inheritance would explain IV, 9 and also IV, 1–3. To explain IV, 8, one must assume not only that their mother was a carrier, but that she married a carrier. Likewise it is necessary to assume that the same circumstances applied in the case of II, 2. The assumption of irregular dominance would fit this pedigree almost as readily. (*After Tertsch*, 1913.) (*c*) The evidence for recessive inheritance is stronger in this pedigree. (*After Marlow and Faxon*, 1913.) (*d*) This extract from the fourth and fifth generation of the preceding pedigree is particularly convincing in view of the fact that it is known that there is evidence that the unaffected father had affected cousins on both sides of his family. (*After Marlow and Faxon*, 1913.) (*e*) This pedigree is best explained on the assumption that a man and his two cousins, whom he married successively, were carriers. (*After Heidenreich*, 1913.)

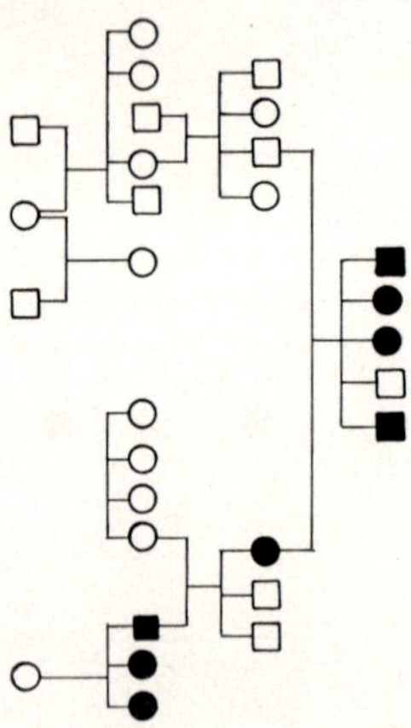

FIG. 191.—Albinism. Pedigree showing dominant inheritance in a Negro family. (*After Pipkin and Pipkin*, 1942.)

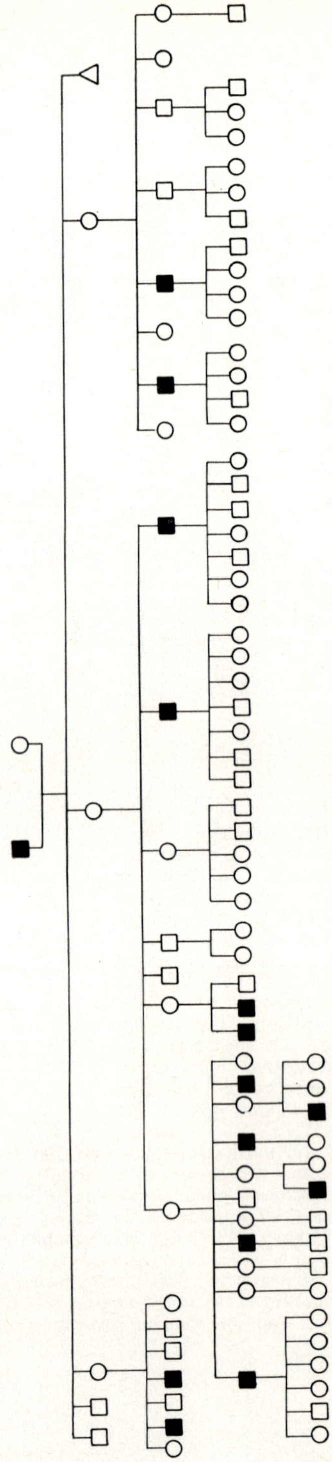

FIG. 192.—Ocular albinism. Pedigree showing sex-linked inheritance. (*After Vogt*, 1925.)

skin. It has been suggested that the recessive gene is not altogether recessive, but shows partial expression in the simplex state.

(4) Dominant inheritance has been seen in some exceptional pedigrees (Fig. 191).

*Detection of heterozygotes.*—Carriers of albinism are said to show abnormal translucency of the iris on transillumination of the sclera. The sign is of limited value as such translucency is frequent in light coloured irides.

*Ocular albinism*

This is inherited in an intermediate sex-linked manner (Fig. 192). The female heterozygote is readily recognized by the fundus appearances (Falls, 1951): small islets of coarse, cocoa-brown pigment clusters towards the periphery with some stippling in the macular areas (Fig. 193). The locus is within measurable distance of that for Xg (Pearce, 1968).

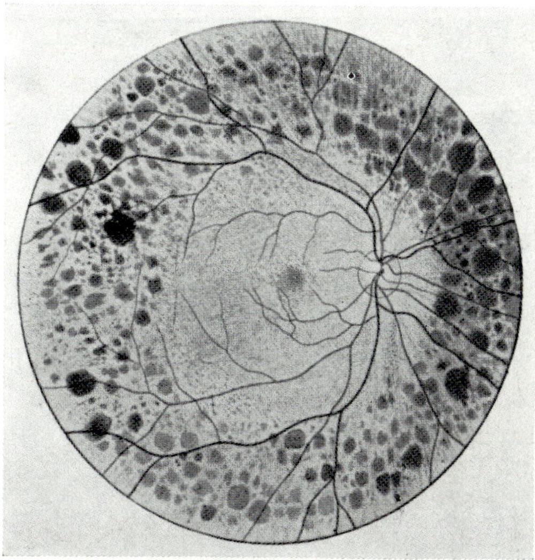

FIG. 193.—The fundus in the female carrier of ocular albinism. An exceptionally heavy degree of pigmentation is seen in this case. (*After Klein*, 1964.)

*Cutaneous albinism*

This is generally dominant (Fig. 194). The Klein–Waardenburg syndrome is irregularly so, and penetrance and expression are rather variable. The corresponding syndrome in animals shows intermediate inheritance. Cutaneous albinism with deaf-mutism is inherited in a sex-linked recessive manner, with deafness possibly indicative of the carrier state (Fried and colleagues, 1969).

## HOMOCYSTINURIA

This affection first recorded by Field and his colleagues in 1962, is apparently not uncommon. It is possible that some 5 per cent of patients with subluxated lenses suffer from this metabolic disorder. The affection resembles Marfan's syndrome in its general skeletal aspects and its congenital subluxation of the lenses. It has additional features, however: mental deficiency is not uncommon, the skin and hair are albinoid in appearance, and hepatomegaly may be present. An outstanding feature is increased viscosity of the blood with a tendency to thrombotic emboli. The pathognomonic aspect is the presence of homocystine in the urine, as shown

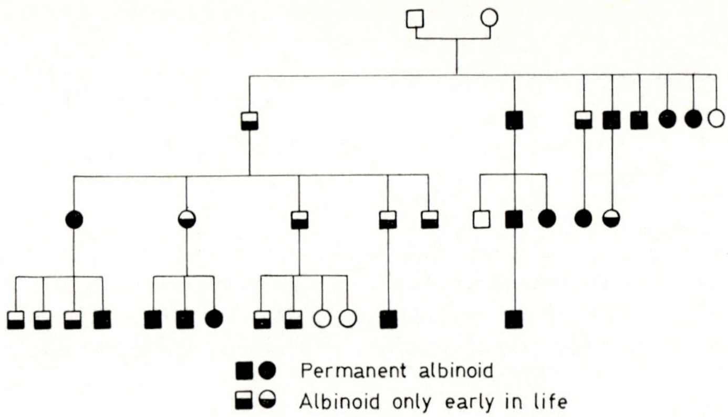


FIG. 194.—Albinoidism. Pedigree showing dominant inheritance. (*After Jablonski*, 1920.)

by chromatography and the nitroprusside test; the plasma shows an increase of metathionine and of homocystine.

The affection is recessive. It is not certain whether carriers can be occasionally recognized by symptomless homocystinuria.

## CYSTINOSIS

This is characterized by the deposition of cystine in the cells of the reticulo-endothelial system (up to 500 times the normal concentration in the spleen) and in the proximal renal tubules and the renal interstitial tissue; there is also increased

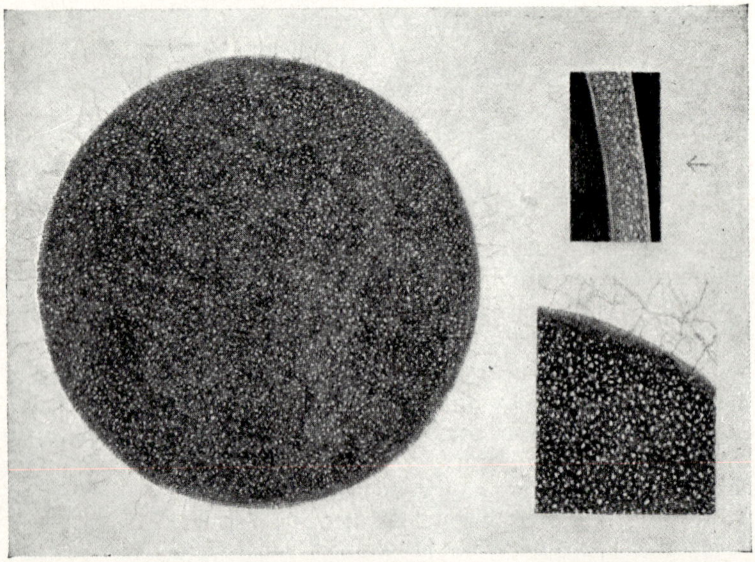

FIG. 195.—The cornea in cystinuria "renal rickets". The cornea is shown in direct illumination with enlargements × 5 and × 25 and in optical section. Cystine crystals are present. (*After Bürki*, 1942.)

cystine concentration in the blood serum. The nature of the metabolic lesion is not definitely known; it is likely to be an enzyme defect in the cells.

The clinical picture is largely determined by the progressive renal dysfunction. There is increasing phospho-gluco-aminoaciduria with loss of electrolytes and the development of renal rickets. Dwarfing is a striking aspect, as is photophobia from the deposition of the insoluble needle-like crystals in the parenchyma of the cornea (seen in some 80 per cent of cases and shown in Fig. 195) and in the conjunctiva. Death in the second or third year of life is common, although some cases follow a milder course.

The affection is recessive. It differs fundamentally from cystinuria—a disturbance in which there is no tissue deposition of cystine.

### Other Anomalies of Amino-acid Metabolism

**Alkaptonuria**

In early cases there are no clinical signs apart from the presence of homogentisic acid, imparting to the urine the characteristic property of darkening on standing. In long-standing cases ochronosis—a bluish-black discoloration of the cartilages—develops, clinically more marked in the ear and nose; chronic arthritis of the osteoarthritic type also develops. The bluish-black discoloration occurs occasionally on the sclerotic, producing web-shaped areas with the base towards the cornea.

This rare disturbance of phenylalanine metabolism is of historical interest in medical genetics. Garrod had recognized the familial distribution of the "inborn errors of metabolism" and, in discussions with Bateson, he came to appreciate that alkaptonuria illustrated mendelian recessive inheritance in human pathology. It is also of interest in that the affection is mimicked in the photographic industry by long exposure to the dust or vapour of quinone (Miller, 1954).

**Tryptophane anomaly**

As already indicated, it is possible that hypolipidaemia syndrome (Hooft) is the consequence of anomalous tryptophane metabolism.

## OTHER PROTEIN METABOLIC DISORDERS

### Lowe's Oculo-cerebro-renal Syndrome

The syndrome develops early in infants who are apparently normal at birth. Mental and physical retardation are usually marked, as is hypotony of the skeletal muscles with absence of tendon reflexes; cataract, buphthalmos and nystagmus are essential components. The renal aspects are pathognomonic: in addition to some proteinuria there is extensive aminoaciduria; there is also diminished blood phosphorus. Osteoporosis is common, as is thermolability with episodes of pyrexia of unknown origin. The affection is confined to boys; and cryptorchism is common.

Inheritance is of the recessive sex-linked type.

### Amyloidosis

Hereditary amyloid disease (as distinct from the disorder of environmental origin), is a dominant affection, generally developing in middle-life. Histologically there is deposition of amyloid material around the blood vessels of different organs throughout the body. Involvement of the kidneys leads to proteinuria whilst an increase of lipoproteins in the serum seems to be an early sign. Ophthalmologically retinal periarteritis with or without extensive dense sheet-like hyaline vitreous opacities—simulating Eales' disease in some cases—are significant (Falls and colleagues, 1955; Andersson and Kassman, 1968).

A variant of hereditary amyloidosis is seen in familial Mediterranean fever—a recessive affection with acute onset in young adults.

### Fanconi Syndrome

The renal failure in cystinosis which leads to renal rickets with phospho-gluco-aminoaciduria, known as the Fanconi syndrome, is not an independent entity but is seen as a terminal event in such diverse affections as chronic porphyria and the glycogenoses. Needle-like crystals in the cornea in a case of the Fanconi syndrome is pathognomonic of cystinosis.

### Gout

Asymptomatic hyperuricaemia occurs in 2 per cent of the population and is five times as frequent as clinical gout in first degree relatives of gouty patients. Polygenic inheritance probably applies. Nothing is known of the hereditary aspects of the ocular manifestations of gout.

## Other Categories

### Copper Metabolism: Hepato-lenticular Degeneration (Wilson's Disease)

The neurological signs include variable spasticity of the limbs and face (intensified by paroxysms) dysarthria, dysphagia and mental changes. The liver damage gives cirrhosis. These changes follow on the deposition of copper in the tissues, the metal being derived from chronic over-absorption from the intestines. Deposition of copper in the kidneys leads to a toxic aminoaciduria; in the cornea it gives the pathognomonic feature of the Kayser–Fleischer ring, and occasionally there is a sunflower opacity in the lens. The corneal lesion is sometimes a pointing sign. The affection is recessive.

### Porphyria Metabolism: Porphyria

The infantile and adult types are distinct affections.

**Infantile erythropoietic porphyria**

The *haem* moiety of haemoglobin is composed of ferro-proto-porphyrin. In infantile porphyria the excessive porphyrin production results in pink-red fluorescing urine and photosensitivity of the skin, with blister formation and subsequent scarring of the exposed skin. Haemolytic anaemia with splenomegaly is an important feature, as is the red colour of the teeth and bones.

Photophobia is almost constant. Less common are keratomalacia and scleromalacia.

Infiltration in the cornea deep to the epithelium and also in the conjunctiva may produce iridescent reflexes.

**Adult hepatic porphyria**

This generally sets in acutely in the third and fourth decades of life. It is probably the result of over-production of porphyrins in the liver. There are episodes of abdominal, neurological and mental disturbance. Barbiturates are particularly liable to precipitate an attack. Transient rectal haemorrhages and exudates, and also retrobulbar neuritis, may occur.

Infantile porphyria is a recessive disorder. The adult form is dominant.

## FOR FURTHER READING


**General Surveys**

McKusick, V. A. (1966). *Heritable Disorders of Connective Tissue.* St. Louis; Mosby.
Milne, M. D. (1966). *Proc. R. Soc. Med.*, **59,** 1157.
Stanbury, J. B., Wyngaarden, J. B. and Fredrickson, D. S. (Eds.) (1966). *The Metabolic Basis of Inherited Disease*, 2nd ed. New York; Blakiston Division of McGraw-Hill.
Thannhauser, S. J. (1950). *Lipoidoses*, 2nd. ed. New York; Oxford University Press.
Woolf, L. I. (1966). *Renal Tubular Dysfunction.* Springfield, Ill.; Thomas.

**Carbohydrate Metabolism**

*Wolfram–Tyrer Syndrome*

Rose F. C., Fraser, G. R., Friedmann, A. I. and Kohner, E. N. (1966). *Q. Jl Med.*, **35,** 385.

*Gargoylism*

McKusick, V. A. (1966). *Heritable Disorders of Connective Tissue.* St. Louis; Mosby.

**Fat Metabolism**

*General Survey*

Anderson, B., Margolis, G. and Lynn, W. S. (1958). *Am. J. Ophthal.*, **45,** 23.

*Amaurotic Idiocy and Allied Conditions*

Bird, A. (1948). *Brain*, **71,** 434.
von Bogaert, L. and Klein, D. (1955). *J. gèn. Hum.*, **4,** 23.
Sjögren, H. (1931). *Hereditas*, **14,** 197.
Slome, D. (1933). *J. Genet.*, **27,** 363.
Videbeck, A. (1949). *Acta paediat.* (*Stockh.*), **37,** 90.
Wyburn-Mason, R. (1943). *Br. J. Ophthal.*, **27,** 193.

*Other Affections*

François, J. (1967). *Ann. méd. Nancy*, **6,** 253 and 375.

**Protein Metabolism**

*Sickle-cell Anaemia*

Welsh, R. B. and Goldberg, M. F. (1966). *Archs Ophthal.*, **75,** 353.

*Albinism*

Fitzpatrick, F. B. and Quevedo, W. C. (1966). In *The Metabolic Basis of Inherited Disease*, 2nd. ed., Ed. by J. B. Stanbury, J. B. Wyngaarden and D. S. Fredrickson. New York; Blakiston Division of McGraw-Hill.

*Homocystinuria*

Carson, N. A. J. (1969). *Br. J. hosp. Med.*, **2,** 439.
François, J. (1967). *Ann. méd. Nancy*, **6,** 254.

*Cystine Storage Disease*

Bickel, H. and Douglas, A. (1952). *Acta paediat.* (*Stockh.*), **42,** Suppl. 90.

**Other Categories**

*Porphyria*

Barnes, H. D. and Boshoff, P. H. (1952). *Archs Ophthal.*, **48,** 567.

# CHAPTER 13

## SOME SYSTEMIC DISORDERS

The ocular aspects of systemic hereditary affections constitute a neglected chapter of genetics. In only a few of these affections are there any systematic studies on the frequency and variability of the ocular lesions.

## SKELETAL SYSTEM

The frequent association of inherited abnormalities of the eye with those of the skeleton has led to various postulates as to the association of the two. The fact that next to the eye the bony system gives the largest number of readily recognized inherited abnormalities is perhaps in itself an adequate explanation.

There is a growing tendency to reduce the multitude of inherited skeletal abnormalities to a few fundamental lesions with a wide range of variation and expression. Some skeletal anomalies are secondary to changes in the bone marrow, others involve mainly the osseous tissue, yet others the periosteum or the epiphysis. For the present a classification into different clinical types is unavoidable.

### Generalized Bone Disturbances

**Osteopetrosis (Albers–Schönberg disease)**

In contrast to fragilitas ossium, there is an excess of osseous tissue, throwing a dense shadow on radiography (hence the name marble bones). This excess encroaches on the cavity of the bone marrow, but consists of remarkably soft bone which tends to fracture (and cut) readily. The adult form of the disease runs a mild course. The infantile form is a severe affection in which abnormal deposits of calcium, dental anomalies, and osteomyelitis, particularly of the jaw, are common. Secondary anaemia is frequent with such compensatory reactions as enlargement of spleen and liver, and death by the age of 10 years is not unusual.

In the infantile form optic atrophy may develop from bony changes at the optic foramina, not always readily detected by radiography. Hydrocephalus with its ocular concomitants has been observed.

The infantile form is recessive. Both recessive and dominant inheritance apply to the adult form.

**Osteitis deformans (Paget's disease)**

It is possible that Paget's disease develops early in life, though it does not lead to symptoms until middle life. The characteristic changes are in the skull, vertebral column and tibiae. Generalized arteriosclerosis is exemplified by skiagrams of the posterior tibial artery, which stands out as a calcified streak.

Retinal arteriosclerosis is frequent; central choroidal sclerosis in its early or late phases is not uncommon. Bilateral grey-brown, or chocolate coloured corneal opacities have been recorded. Optic atrophy, exophthalmos and various palsies have also been noted. The affection is irregularly dominant.

Of late, angioid streaks with and without pseudo-xanthoma elasticum has been reported repeatedly in Paget's disease. As these anomalies, together with widespread arterial changes, constitute the syndrome of elastosis dystrophica, it is possible that Paget's disease may be a variable and unrecognized part of the syndrome.

*Leontiasis ossea*

This affection, in which there may be optic atrophy, various ocular palsies and exophthalmos, is generally regarded as a localized form of Paget's disease. It has been recorded over four generations, developing early in childhood. Angioid streaks have been observed (Barkwin and Eiger, 1956).

**Congenital stippled epiphysis (dysplasia epiphysialis punctata, congenital calcareous or calcifying chondrodystrophy; Conradi's disease)**

In this severe infantile affection there is dwarfing, enlarged immobile joints with flexure contractures, and gastro-intestinal symptoms. The x-ray appearances are striking: multiple chalky deposits at the larger joints sometimes associated with more extensive skeletal anomalies. Ill-defined keratoses of the skin are common, as is congenital cataract which indeed may be a constant feature. Calcification of the heart valves may occur as part of the process of chalky deposition.

The affection is recessive. It generally leads to death by age of 2 or 3 years.

**Léri's pleonostosis**

Mongoloid slanting of the palpebral fissures, and moderate thickening and tenseness of the skin of the lids are common; squint, possibly incidental, has also been observed in this dominant disorder (Rukavina and colleagues, 1959).

**Ankylosing spondylitis**

Ankylosing spondylitis is inherited in a dominant manner in some families. It is not known whether the frequently occurring iritis in this affection is genetically determined.

## Cranio-facial Anomalies

**Oxycephaly (acrocephaly, tower skull)**

This is a composite entity.

*Oxycephaly proper*

There is a characteristic deformity, well shown on x-ray examination which also reveals digital impressions arising from intracranial pressure. Optic atrophy is a common occurrence, frequently preceded by papilloedema. The affection is said to be commoner in males. Most cases are sporadic, but there are records in twins, in sibships and over two and even three generations.

Oxycephaly may be part of a generalized bone marrow disturbance with secondary features. This is seen from the frequent association with generalized bone disturbances, and the repeated observations that oxycephaly may occur in hereditary congenital acholuric jaundice, and also perhaps in hereditary pernicious anaemia manifesting itself early in life.

*Acrocephalo-syndactyly* (*Apert's anomaly*)

The deformity of the skull departs from the classical picture of oxycephaly in that the skull is foreshortened as well as showing the tower deformity. The term acrobrachycephaly is, therefore, more accurate. It is said that only the coronal suture is prematurely closed, allowing growth laterally and vertically, so that there are fewer signs of intracranial compression than in oxycephaly proper.

Apart from the deformity of the skull and the syndactyly at the extremities, other generalized bone defects are not uncommon. Exophthalmos and ophthalmoplegia have been reported repeatedly, and one observation speaks of ectopic lenses.

Genetically, some pedigrees suggest recessive inheritance and others dominance (Fig. 196), perhaps irregular dominance.

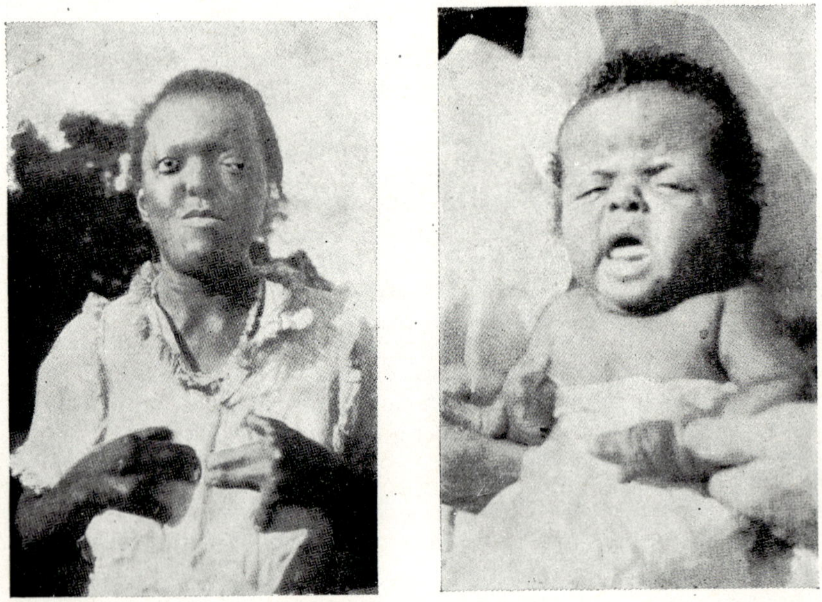

FIG. 196.—Acrocephalo-syndactyly in a mother and daughter. (*After Weech*, 1927.)

*Cranio-facial dysostosis* (*Crouzon's anomaly*)

Here the facial skeleton is also involved. The skull itself approaches the deformity seen in the Apert anomaly, brachycephaly being marked; the facial skeleton shows under-development of the upper jaws, and there is marked prognathism of the lower jaw. Malformation of the nose gives it a hooked appearance suggestive of a parrot's beak. As in oxycephaly proper, divergent squint is frequently present, as also are optic atrophy and exophthalmos.

The dysostosis shows three stages of development: (1) owing to early synostosis the skull assumes its characteristic defect, while the face shows the earliest changes consequent on an undeveloped upper jaw; (2) further deformation of the skull occurs, where it yields at the unfused sutures to the growing brain; (3) compression changes of brain and optic nerve develop.

As with oxycephaly, minor skeletal anomalies elsewhere are not uncommon.

Inheritance is more clearly dominant than in the Apert anomaly (Fig. 197).

The frequency of optic atrophy as a complication in the different branches of the craniostenoses, makes decompression procedures a matter of practical importance.

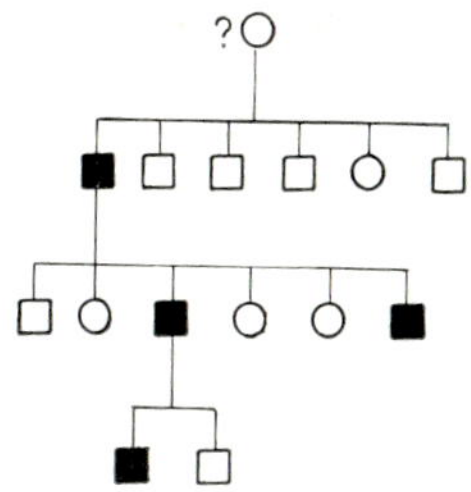


FIG. 197.—Crouzon's anomaly. Dominant inheritance. (*After Günther*, 1933.)

A transition between the Crouzon and Apert anomalies is shown by some cases reported by Vogt. The facial deformity was that seen in the Crouzon anomaly and the syndactyly was suggestive of the Apert anomaly (Vogt, 1933).

**Hypertelorism**

In its minor degrees the condition is not uncommon. Fully marked, the striking appearance of a broad bridge of the nose and a wide interpupillary distance (as much as 85 millimetres) is unmistakable. The wide separation of the orbits is consequent on early ossification of the greater wings of the sphenoid, making them smaller than the lesser wings and so fixing the orbits in the lateral position normal in foetal life. Rarely, cleft face is present, shown minimally at the tip of the nose, and more extensively by cleft palate, or marked furrow in the forehead.

Apart from divergent squint, ocular lesions are uncommon, but optic atrophy has been observed, possibly associated with narrow optic foramina.

There are many records of inheritance over two or more generations.

**Mandibulo-facial dysostosis (Collins–Franceschetti–Zwahlen anomaly)**

Here there is a characteristic facial appearance consequent on an anti-mongoloid lateral downwards slope of the palpebral fissures with a temporal coloboma in the lower lid giving the fissure a triangular form; there is hypoplasia of the facial bones, especially the zygoma and the mandible. There are also malformation of the external and occasionally the middle and inner ears; macrostomia; high palate;

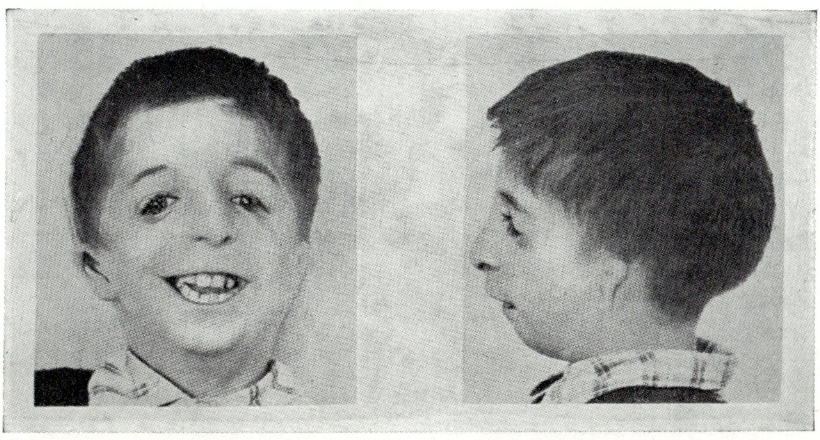

FIG. 198.—Mandibulo-facial dysostosis (Collins-Franceschetti-Zwahlen anomaly). Characteristic facial appearance. (*After Franceschetti and Zwahlen*, 1944.)

blind fistulae between the angles of the mouth and ears; atypical hair growth with tongue-shaped processes towards the cheek; and a possible combination with other and lesser abnormalities. Those fully affected look very much alike, their appearance being somewhat fish-like or bird-like (Fig. 198). Anomalous development of the branchial clefts appears to be the underlying cause.

The affection is probably transmitted as an irregular dominant, the gene having occasionally a lethal effect. Expression is variable (Fig. 199).

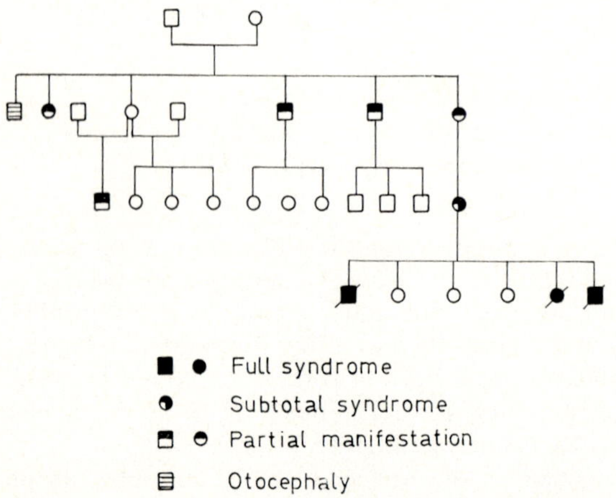


FIG. 199.—Mandibulo-facial dysostosis (Collins-Franceschetti-Zwahlen anomaly). Pedigree showing dominant inheritance with variable expression. (*After Debusmann. Quoted by Franceschetti and Klein*, 1949.)

**Progressive hemiatrophy of the face (Romberg)**

The genetic status of this bizarre affection with its complete and incomplete forms is uncertain. The disorder is of ophthalmic interest as various ocular anomalies may occur, such as ptosis, ectropion, lacrymation, exposure conjunctivitis, endophthalmitis and squint. To all these, secondary factors may contribute, but in addition primary defects have been reported, such as Horner syndrome, Argyll Robertson pupil, heterochromia of the iris and heterochromic cyclitis (Ioannides, 1965).

## DIGITAL ANOMALIES

**Apical dystrophy with coloboma of the macula**

Apical dystrophy of hands and feet is a dominant affection. The terminal phalanges and the nails are rudimentary or lacking. The hands and feet are distinctly stump-like. This anomaly, together with changes in the thumb, which in extreme cases leads to doubling of thumbs, has been observed as a dominant affection over three generations, all affected members also showing bilateral macular colobomas (Fig. 200); and in two of them a renal anomaly of the agenesis type was present. Possibly allied bony anomalies were observed in two sibs with coloboma of the macula (Phillips and Griffiths, 1969).

**Brachydactyly**

The many varieties of brachydactyly may arise from shortening of the metacarpals, of the middle phalanges, or of the terminal phalanges. In the more severe anomalies stature is generally shortened. Most of these anomalies are probably inherited dominantly. Microcornea has been observed in a father and son, both brachydactylous and of short stature (Tizzard, 1933).

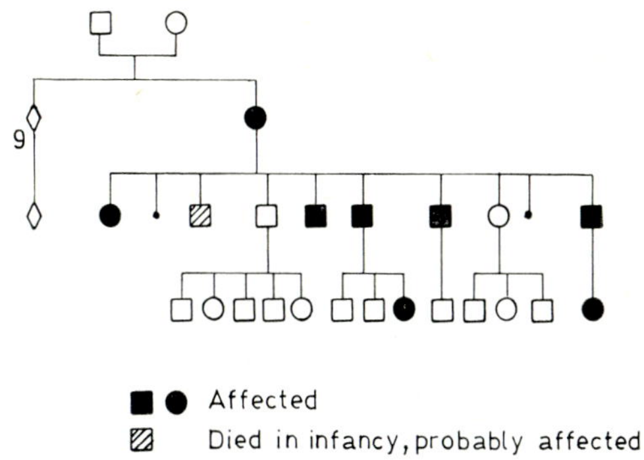


FIG. 200.—Apical dystrophy with macular coloboma. Pedigree showing dominant inheritance. (*After Sorsby*, 1935.)

**Lobster hand and aniridia**

Aniridia has been observed in a member of a family with dominantly inherited lobster hand and foot. The aniridic patient himself did not have the skeletal anomaly (Savin and Sorsby, 1934).

**Syndactyly**

No clear-cut associations are established. Syndactyly has been observed in the Laurence–Biedl syndrome, alternative or in association with polydactyly. In two families on record, syndactyly and night-blindness with fundus albi-punctatus has been noted. It is not known whether these cases represent a fortuitous association of two distinct anomalies—as is suggested by the dissociation of the two affections in some of the individuals.

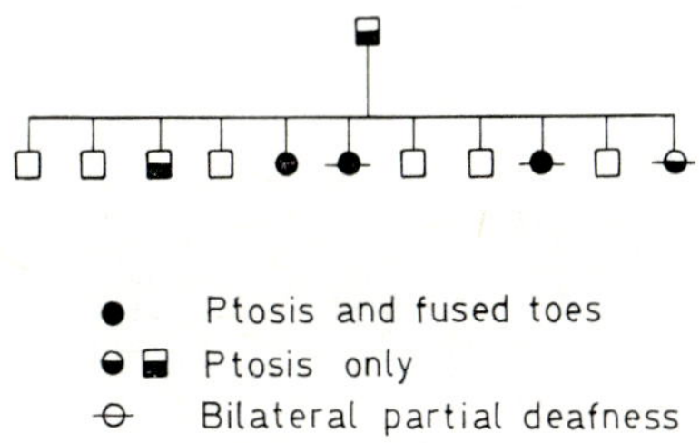


FIG. 201.—Ptosis with fused toes. Pedigree suggestive of dominant inheritance. (*After Walsh*, 1947.)

Syndactyly has been observed with microphthalmos. Syndactyly in association with aniridia has also been noted. In one family it has been observed with ptosis (Fig. 201).

**Polydactyly**

The association of polydactyly with retinitis pigmentosa, frequently noted in the literature, probably represents incomplete observations of the Laurence–Biedl syndrome.

**Other affections**

A number of anomalies have been recorded as occurring together and such cases have been described under the designations of dysmorphia oculo-mandibulo-facialis (Hallermann–Streif anomaly and its variant such as dyscephaly oculo-mandibularis facialis—François), oculo-auricular dysplasia (Goldenhar anomaly), dysplasia oculo-vertebralis (Wyers and Thier), oculo-dental-digital dysplasia (Meyer–Schwickerath), and dysmorphia cervico-oculo-facialis (Franceschetti and

Klein). It is not at all clear that they constitute clinical entities and in none of these is there any evidence of a genetic background.

The allied syndrome of hypoplasia of the mandible (microgenia) with glossoptosis (Pierre Robin anomaly) is better established. It carried diverse ocular defects, but not consistently. Its genetic status is uncertain.

## CENTRAL NERVOUS SYSTEM

### THE HEREDITARY ATAXIAS

Friedreich's ataxia and Marie's ataxia, though they have some features in common, are genetically distinct, and they differ greatly in their ocular complications.

**Friedreich's spinal ataxia**

The classical ocular feature in Friedreich's spinal ataxia is nystagmus. This may develop early or late and is generally only present when the eyes are deviated from the primary position. Abducens palsy, ptosis and the Argyll Robertson pupil are rare complications, whilst optic atrophy, though uncommon, is probably not particularly so in the late stages. It is possible that optic atrophy may occur only in some families (Fig. 202 *a*), whilst in a few families retinitis pigmentosa, generally atypical, has been recorded (Fig. 202 *b* and *c*). It has been suggested that Leber's

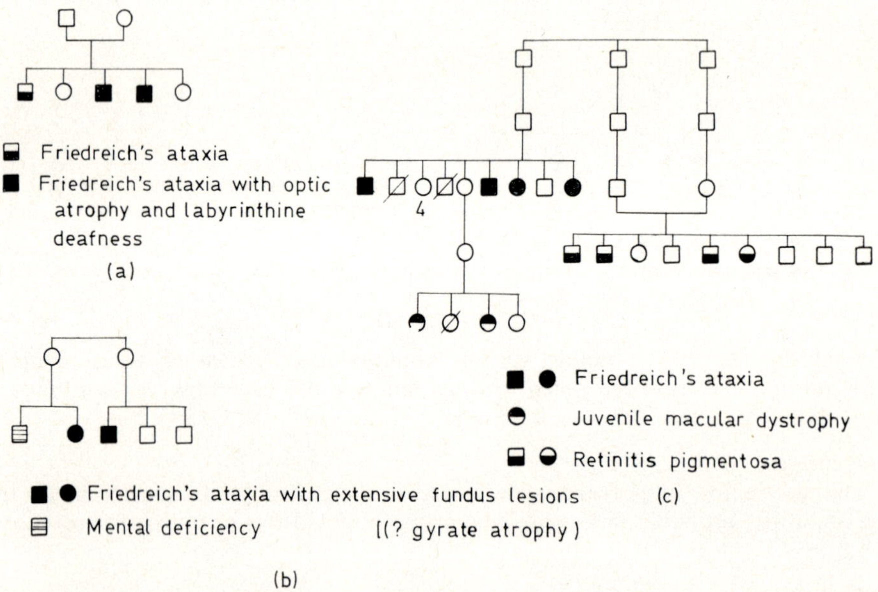


FIG. 202.—Friedreich's ataxia with ocular lesions. (*a*) Pedigree showing optic atrophy and labyrinthine deafness. (*After van Bogaert*, 1948.) (*b*) Pedigree showing two affected members with extensive fundus lesions (? gyrate atrophy). (*After de Mello. Quoted by Franceschetti and Klein*, 1948.) (*c*) Extract from the "Glaser" pedigree showing the occurrence of either retinitis pigmentosa or juvenile macular dystrophy with Friedreich's ataxia. (*After Franceschetti and Klein*, 1947.)

disease, which so frequently carries minor neurological stigmata, is an intermediate form between the type of Friedreich's ataxia with optic atrophy and the Marie type of ataxia in which optic atrophy is common—a view difficult to maintain on genetic grounds.

Friedreich's ataxia with its early onset is generally recessive. There are, however, a number of families in which the affection was dominant.

**Marie's cerebellar ataxia**

Primary optic atrophy is common in this condition. Palsies of the extra-ocular muscles and internal ophthalmoplegia are not infrequent, but nystagmus is exceptional. Retinitis pigmentosa as an associated condition is also rare, although perhaps more common than in Friedreich's ataxia (Fig. 203 *a*).

The later onset of Marie's ataxia, and its generally dominant course, form a sharp contrast to Friedreich's ataxia. Recessive cases are, however, known and there are also cases with an infantile onset in which the affection appeared to be recessive (and was associated with progressive external ophthalmoplegia, Fig. 203 *b*).

There are many intermediate forms between the clearly spinal and the clearly cerebellar type and fundus anomalies have been observed in these cases too (Fig. 203 *d*). The spino-cerebellar ataxia of Sanger Brown is dominant. A type resembling disseminated sclerosis with characteristic exacerbations of retrobulbar neuritis is also dominant, whilst the type in which there is transition from ataxia to spasticity appears to be recessive.

The "complicated optic atrophy" recorded by Behr in children, who showed optic atrophy in addition to cerebrospinal symptoms, has been regarded as a transition between Leber's optic atrophy and Marie's ataxia, but neither its clinical nor its genetic status is clear (Fig. 203 *c*).

In the Marinesco–Sjögren syndrome (p. 246) cerebellar ataxia is an outstanding feature.

## Paralytic Affections

**Hereditary spastic diplegia**

The older literature contained case reports of ocular lesions, especially optic atrophy and pigmentary fundus changes, in association with diplegias. It would appear that these refer to ill-defined clinical entities classified by symptoms. Amongst these must have figured *hereditary spastic diplegia* which is a definite entity and appears to be recessive. The ocular lesions are nystagmus, and, less frequently, optic atrophy and various ocular palsies including pupil anomalies.

**Stationary congenital facial paralysis (oculo-facial paralysis; congenital paralysis of sixth and seventh nerves; Moebius's syndrome)**

The mask-like face, the inability to close the eyelids completely, the lack of lateral ocular movement, and the occasional atrophy of the tongue, constitute a characteristic picture. Sometimes it is part of a more widespread and ill-defined systemic disorder of uncertain genetic status (status Bonnevie–Ulrich). The affection has been observed in sibs.

**Progressive bulbar palsy**

Ocular lesions are uncommon in this complex group of affections. When present they are striking. The orbicularis palpebrarum is involved in the wide-

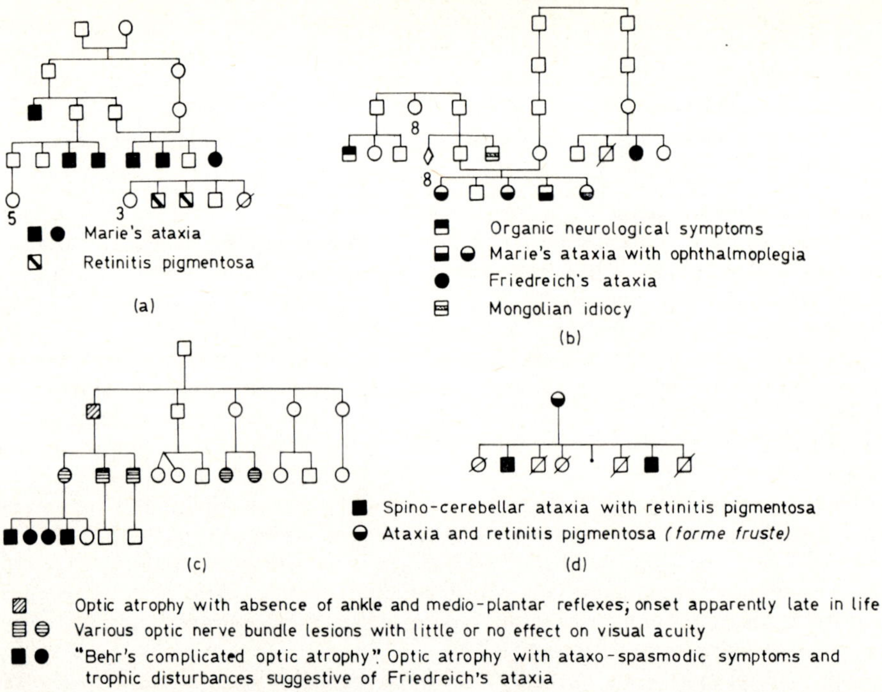


FIG. 203.—Marie's ataxia and allied conditions with ocular complications. (*a*) Pedigree showing Marie's ataxia with retinitis pigmentosa. (*After Franceschetti and Klein*, 1941.) (*b*) Pedigree showing the uncommon recessive form of Marie's ataxia which had two further unusual features, infantile onset and progressive external ophthalmoplegia. (*After Franceschetti, de Morsier and Klein*, 1945.) (*c*) Complicated optic atrophy as recorded by Behr in children with cerebrospinal symptoms. Pedigree showing relationship to simple optic atrophy. (*After van Bogaert*, 1948.) (*d*) Pedigree showing occurrence of retinitis pigmentosa in a family with spino-cerebellar ataxia. (*After Zonca. Quoted by Franceschetti and Klein*, 1948.)

spread paralysis of face, palate and pharynx, with consequent inability to close the lids fully. The affection has been observed in sibships, but also over two generations. In some families there is an associated ophthalmoplegia but these cases are puzzling as the ophthalmoplegia is apparently myogenic. Oculo-pharyngeal dystrophy (p. 248) may perhaps also belong to this group.

### Progressive interstitial hypertrophic neuritis

Ocular signs are sluggish response of the pupil to light; this is frequent, and a fully developed Argyll Robertson pupil is not uncommon. The affection is generally recessive, but may be inherited in a dominant manner. Its relationship to neurofibromatosis is questionable.

## THE DEMYELINATING DISEASES

### Disseminate sclerosis

The genetic status of disseminate sclerosis is still undetermined. The affection has been noted in sibs, as also in uniovular twins. Generally the family history is, however, negative, except that not infrequently there is a history of nervous or mental disease. Iridocyclitis, too, is probably not uncommon both in those affected and in their relatives (Fig. 204).

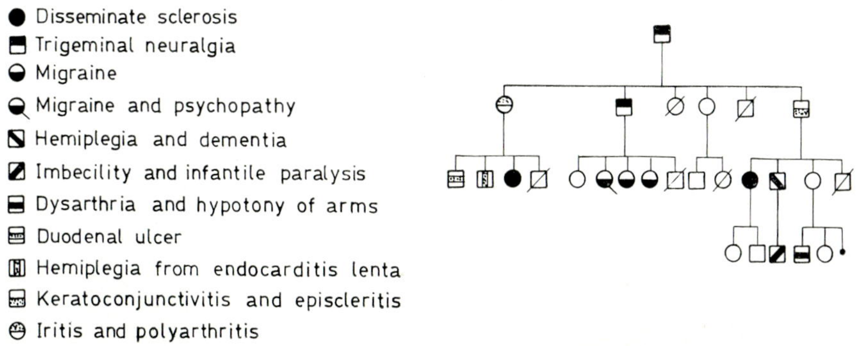


FIG. 204.—Disseminate sclerosis. Pedigree of two cases in collateral branches of a family. (*After Curtius*, 1933.)

**Neuromyelitis optica**

Here, too, most cases tend to be sporadic, but evidence of a genetic basis for the affection is derived from the fact that the disease has been observed in uniovular twins. One such pair developed neuromyelitis optica at 24 and 25 years of age respectively, and both died blind in the acute phase of the affection (McAlpine, 1938).

**"Schilder's disease"**

Schilder's disease is a complex of several disorders of which juvenile metachromatic leucodystrophy and the Pelizaeus–Merzbacher disease are outstanding. The first of these affections has many of the features of infantile amaurotic idiocy. Palizaeus–Merzbacher disease is sex-linked and its infantile form, with its cortical blindness, runs a severe and lethal course. Cerebral blindness tends to come on from involvement of the occipital lobes, though no part of the optic tract itself may be involved. Optic neuritis is uncommon, but papilloedema may occur from increased intracranial pressure.

## THE DYSKINESIAS

**Hepato-lenticular degeneration (Wilson's disease)**

In this recessive metabolic disorder, discussed elsewhere, the Kayser–Fleischer ring may be a pointing sign.

**Myoclonic epilepsy**

Nystagmus is frequent in this rare affection (*see* p. 64).

## THE MUSCLE DYSTROPHIES

Of the many varieties of hereditary muscle disturbances only a few have ocular complications.

### Myotonia congenita (Thomsen's disease)

In this clearly dominant affection the orbicularis muscle may be involved, producing difficulty in closing the lids. Cataract is lacking in this affection, and this constitutes a striking point in the differential diagnosis from myotonia dystrophica.

### Myotonia dystrophica

In myotonia dystrophica the extra-ocular muscles do not appear to be involved, Tonic pupils are common, but the outstanding ocular lesion is a characteristic punctate cortical cataract (Fig. 205). Minimal lens changes are almost constant,

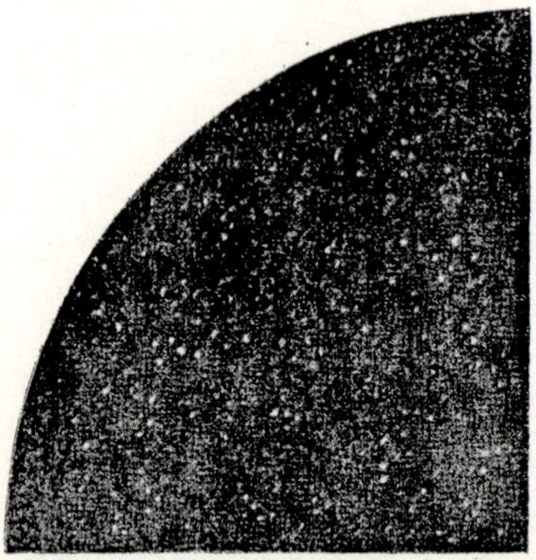

FIG. 205.—Myotonia dystrophica. Appearances of lens opacities. Face view and optical section. (*After Bücklers*, 1938.)

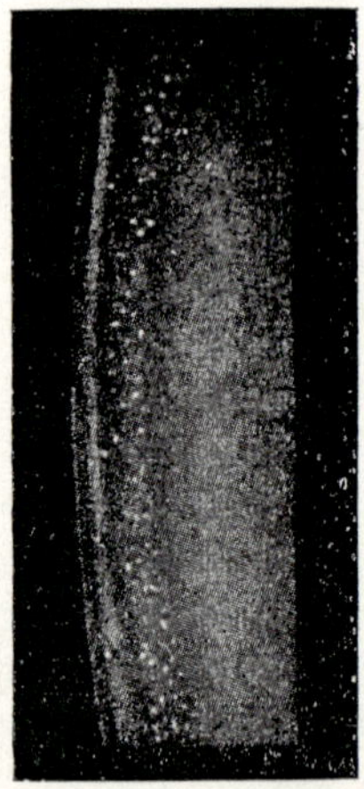

and fully developed cataract, which may come on very rapidly, is present in probably 30–40 per cent of patients. The affection is dominant, though possibly irregularly so. Fleischer holds that the affection increases in severity with succeeding generations and that in a generation in which it appears fully developed further transmission becomes impossible.

## OTHER AFFECTIONS

### Syringomyelia

If the concept of syringomyelia is extended to include status dysraphicus, dominant inheritance is obvious (Fig. 206). The concept of status dysraphicus is based on the reading that syringomyelia represents faulty closure at the midline of the neural canal, and that syringomyelia is the extreme form of a disturbance which minimally shows various other aberrations of midline development.

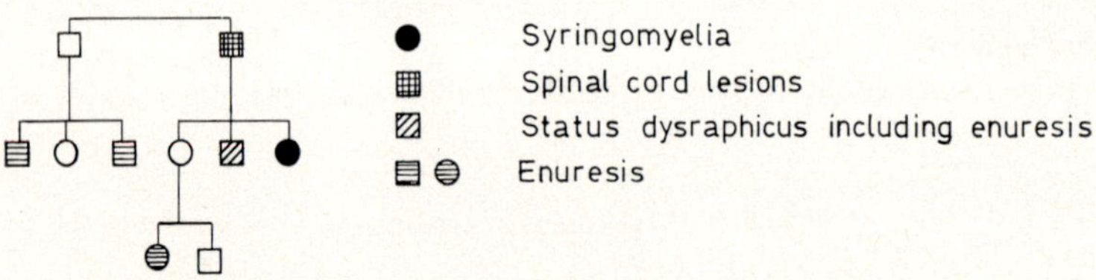


FIG. 206.—Syringomyelia as an aspect of status dysraphicus. Pedigree. *After Bremer*, 1926.)

**Tonic pupils**

Most cases are sporadic, but Adie's syndrome has been observed both in sibships and over two generations, sometimes in incomplete form.

**Word blindness**

Generally sporadic, there are several observations of the anomaly over two generations, and even over three generations.

**Torticollis**

Congenital muscular torticollis is usually sporadic, but it has been seen as a concordant feature in uniovular twins and there are pedigrees showing its occurrence over two generations.

**Deaf-mutism or deafness in fundus lesions**

Retinitis pigmentosa is not infrequently observed at schools for deaf-mutes. In consecutive pedigrees of recessive autosomal retinitis pigmentosa deaf-mutism, or deafness, figures with an incidence of about 10–22 per cent (Usher's syndrome).

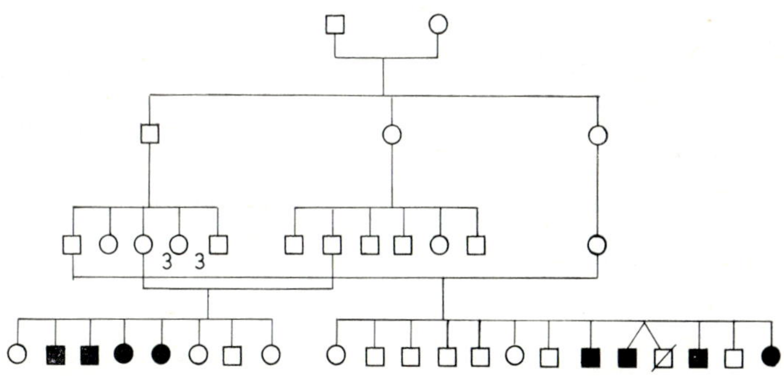


FIG. 207.—Retinitis pigmentosa and deaf-mutism. Pedigree showing the occurrence of the two affections together in two related sibships, both the offspring of first cousin marriages. (*After Usher*, 1914.)

The fortuitous association of two recessive genes is a possible but unlikely explanation. The essentially parallel course of the two affections suggests a monofactorial basis (Fig. 207). The gene is distinct from that for deaf-mutism only, as can be seen from Fig. 208.

Deafness of deaf-mutism is also seen at blind schools in children suffering from macular lesions, presumably of the Stargardt type (Amalric, 1960). It is also a feature of the syndromes with retinal aplasia listed in Table X.

**Mental deficiency (oligophrenia)**

Mental deficiency is a component seen in many or the syndromes with ocular involvement such as the Hallgren syndrome, the Marinesco–Sjögren syndrome, the Sjögren–Larsson syndrome, the Cockayne syndrome and in sex-linked pseudoglioma. It is also seen in some apparently isolated ocular lesions, such as congenital optic atrophy, some cases of retinitis pigmentosa, anophthalmos, and possibly in other ocular anomalies. The better established associations are as follows.

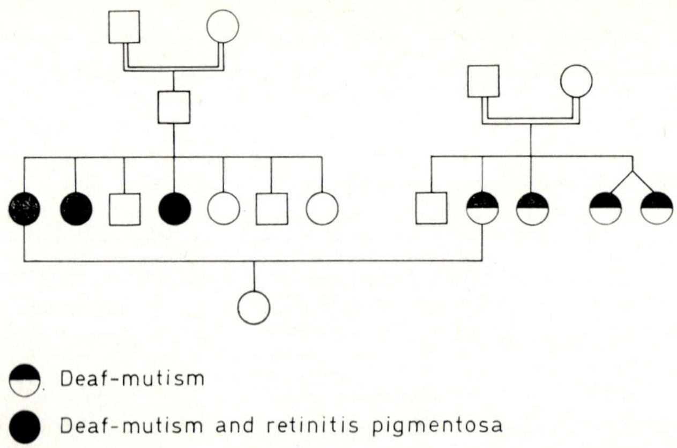


FIG. 208.—Deaf-mutism and retinitis pigmentosa. Recessive and independent inheritance of the two affections. (*After Lindenov*, 1945.)

*Mental deficiency with microphthalmos*

Mental deficiency is present in about 50 per cent of cases of microphthalmos and anophthalmos. In a detailed field survey Sjögren found that most cases were sporadic. In seven families only males were affected, and in two families only females. Two of the families with only males affected showed sex-linked pseudoglioma.

*Mental deficiency with cataract* (Sjögren, 1935)

It is unlikely that the association is fortuitous. Inheritance is recessive. The relationship of this group to the Marinesco–Sjögren syndrome and the Sjögren–Larsson syndrome still requires elucidation.

*Mental deficiency with retinitis pigmentosa*

According to Julia Bell, about 4 per cent of all cases of retinitis pigmentosa show mental deficiency. When this combination occurs other mental anomalies are likely to be seen in the remaining members of the family (Fig. 209).

*Mental deficiency with retinal aplasia*

This occurs occasionally in both the recessive and dominant varieties.

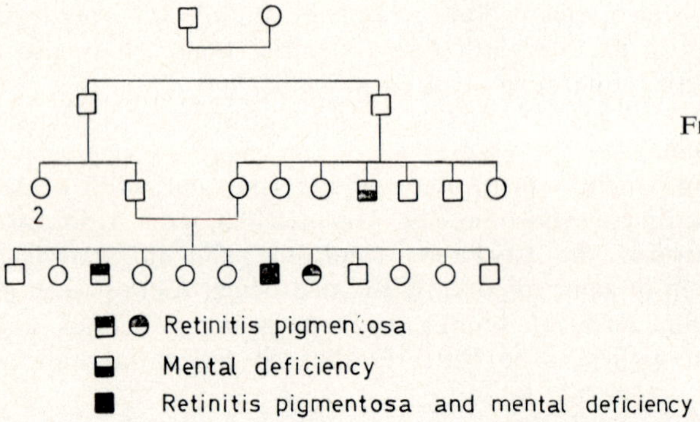


FIG. 209.—Retinitis pigmentosa with mental deficiency. Pedigree. (*After Usher*, 1914.)

### The Genetic Factor in Neurological Affections of Environmental Origin

In many of the genetically determined affections of the central nervous system there is ample evidence that environmental disturbances such as trauma or intercurrent disease may precipitate, or aggravate, the disease. This is, of course, an example of the interaction between genetic and environmental factors. Another aspect of fundamentally the same process is seen in affections generally regarded as exclusively environmental in origin; some of these affections occur more frequently in certain families than in others. Fig. 210 shows the frequent occurrence of

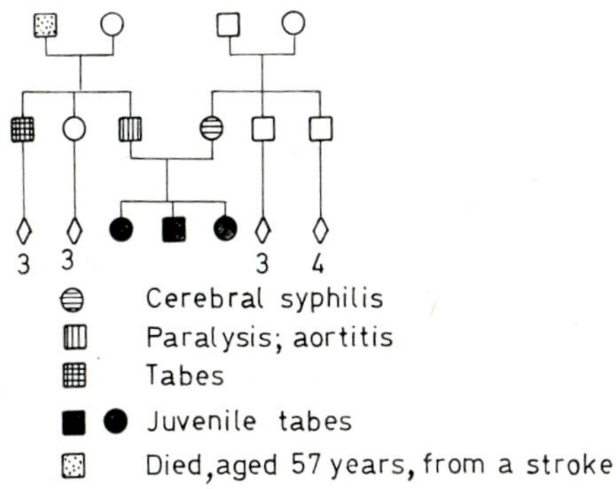


Fig. 210.—Occurrence of syphilis of central nervous system in a family. Pedigree. (*After Curtius and Schlotter*, 1934.)

syphilis of the central nervous system in one particular family. In such and similar pedigrees a genetic predisposition to environmental pathogens may be assumed. The occasional occurrence of congenital syphilis in only one of a pair of dizygotic twins suggests the same genetic predisposition to the pathogen.

## OTHER SYSTEMS

### Skin and Mucosa

**Xeroderma pigmentosum**

In xeroderma pigmentosum conjunctival and corneal involvement are not uncommon, and photophobia may be intense. At any particular point there may be a succession of erythema, pigmentation, atrophy and tumour formation, though the different stages need not develop successively.

The affection is recessive and carries a high mortality. Conforming to the rarity of the disease, consanguinity in parents is high. It has been suggested that in the heterozygous state the skin is freckled.

**Ichthyosis**

This is a complex disorder, generally recessive, but not uncommonly sex-linked. Dominant or irregularly dominant inheritance may also occur (the reputed Y chromosomal inheritance of this affection is mythical). Ichthyosis is an aspect of the Sjögren–Larsson syndrome and occasionally of the Refsum syndrome.

The lids may be involved in the skin disturbance, and this may lead to corneal lesions secondary to the hyperplasia and inflammatory reaction of the conjunctiva. The cornea, however, may be involved primarily in the dermatosis and this has no very characteristic form: it has been described variously as bluish white dots immediately in front of Descemet's membrane, as refractive nodules in the epithelium, superficial stroma and endothelium, and also as ring opacities. It is possible that ichthyosis with corneal lesions constitutes a distinct entity (Savin, 1956; Jay, Blach and Wells, 1968).

**Acne rosacea**

Dominant inheritance is seen occasionally. It is not known whether corneal complications are seen more often in such families.

**Hereditary benign intra-epithelial dyskeratosis**

In a large isolate of mixed Indian, Negro and Caucasian origin in North Carolina, 75 out of an estimated 350 descendants of a woman born in 1834 were affected by an anomaly locally known as Red Eye and regarded as a birthmark. There was a foamy, gelatinous pseudo-membraneous conjunctival thickening situated mainly in the interpalpebral zone and generally horseshoe-shaped. There were also associated changes in the buccal mucosa, taking the form of either a delicate lace-pattern or a diffuse shaggy white area on the cheek mucosa. Photophobia was common, as was corneal vascularization. Histologically both the conjunctiva and the buccal mucosa showed epithelial hyperplasia with necrobiotic cells (Witkop and colleagues, 1960; von Sallmann and Paton, 1960). A report on an unrelated family in Philadelphia has come from Yanoff (1968).

**Dystrophic epidermolysis bullosa with shrinking of the conjunctiva**

Most cases are sporadic, but the association has been observed in two sisters, the offspring of consanguineous parents (Fig. 211). Corneal involvement led to

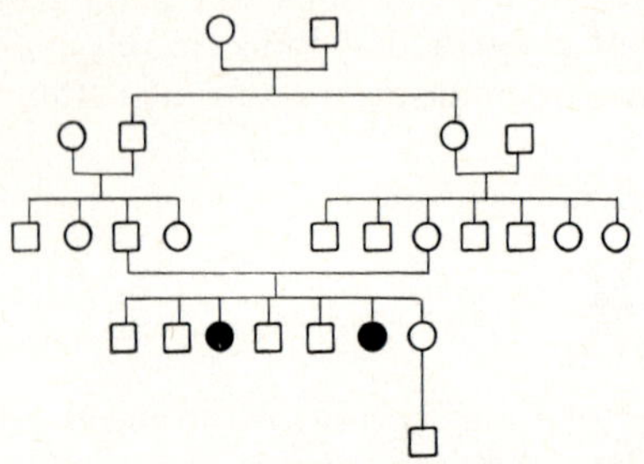

FIG. 211.—Epidermolysis bullosa. Pedigree suggestive of recessive sex-linkage. (*After Sorsby, Fraser Roberts and Brain*, 1951.)

blindness in one sister, and to grossly defective vision in the other. Both showed extensive deformities of the hands from scarring.

**Multiple telangiectasia**

In this dominant affection cutaneous and mucosal capillary angiomas develop in childhood and increase in severity and number. They give a characteristic appearance when situated at the upper conjunctival fornix. Some cases may perhaps represent the carrier state of the Louis–Bar syndrome.

## DENTAL ANOMALIES

**Microphthalmos and dental anomalies**

Actual records are few. The anomalies were rather different in the families recorded by Brailey and by Wolff (Fig. 212).

**Lamellar cataract with hypoplasia of dental enamel**

This has been recorded as dominantly inherited by Nettleship and by Harman. Early deaths from fits are not uncommon (Fig. 213).

**Pre-senile cataract with hypoplasia of dental enamel**

In two other pedigrees of Nettleship this was also observed as a dominant anomaly.

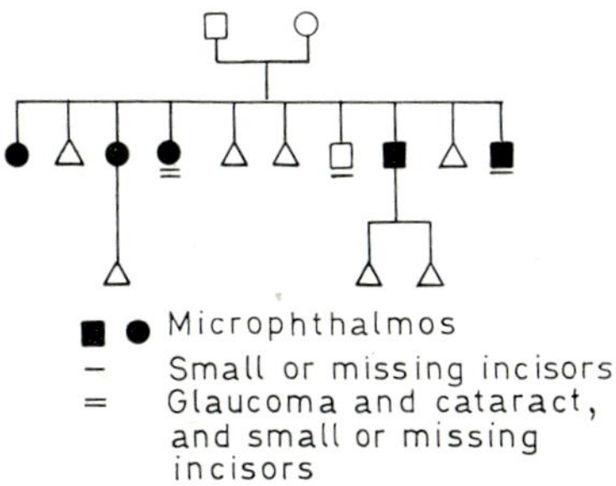


FIG. 212.—Microphthalmos with dental anomalies. Pedigree suggestive of recessive inheritance. (*After Wolff*, 1929–30.)

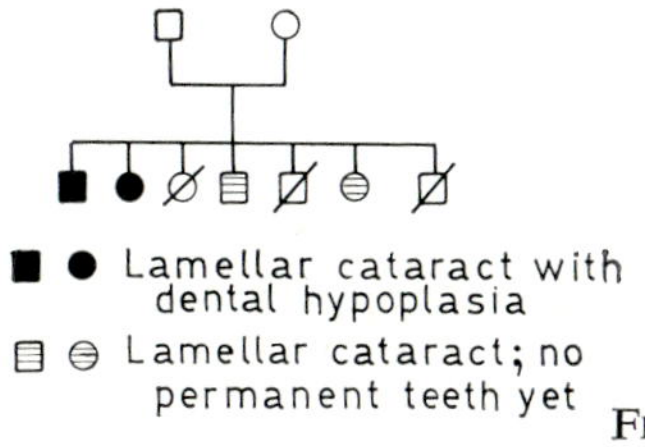


FIG. 213. — Lamellar cataract with hypoplasia of dental enamel. Pedigree showing an affected sibship. (*After Harman*, 1910.)

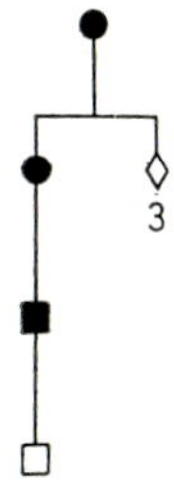


FIG. 214.—Hypertrophy of gums with dental defect and recurrent corneal lesions. Pedigree showing dominant inheritance. (*After Rutherford*, 1931.)

**Hypertrophy of the gums with dental defect and recurrent corneal lesions**

In one family this was observed as a dominant affection (Fig. 214).

## THE ALLERGIC DISEASES

The dominant inheritance of allergic sensitivity is well established (Fig. 215). It is not known whether purely ocular allergy constitutes a distinct genetic type.

**Angioneurotic oedema**

Dominant inheritance is the rule, and in different families selective localization such as to the glottis—with fatal consequences—or in different viscera or areas of skin are frequently seen. An area once affected tends to show recurrent attacks. Almost any part of the body may be involved. Exclusively palpebral angioneurotic oedema does not appear to have been observed as a specific genetic type.

Angioneurotic oedema may be part of generalized allergic sensitivity, so that in some families angioneurotic oedema alternates with other forms of allergy.

**Migraine**

Dominant inheritance in migraine is well established (Fig. 216). As women appear to be affected twice as frequently as men, the possibility of dominant sex-linked inheritance arises.

In one family with twelve affected members ophthalmoplegic migraine was inherited as a dominant (Fig. 217).

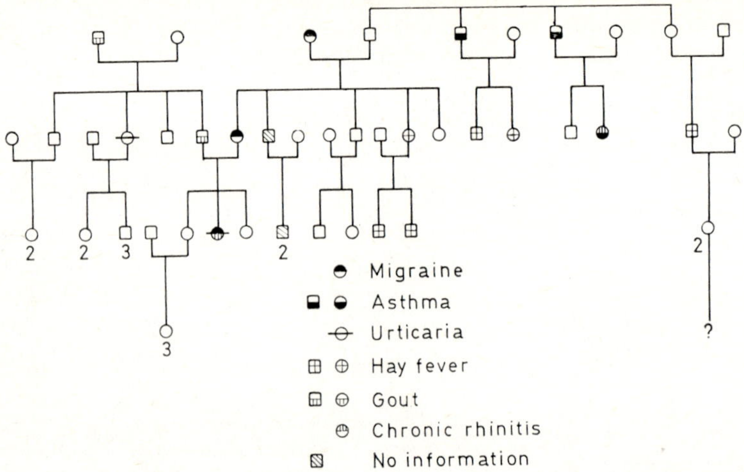


FIG. 215.—Allergy. Pedigree showing dominant inheritance and clinical range of manifestations. (*After Julia Bell*, 1933.)

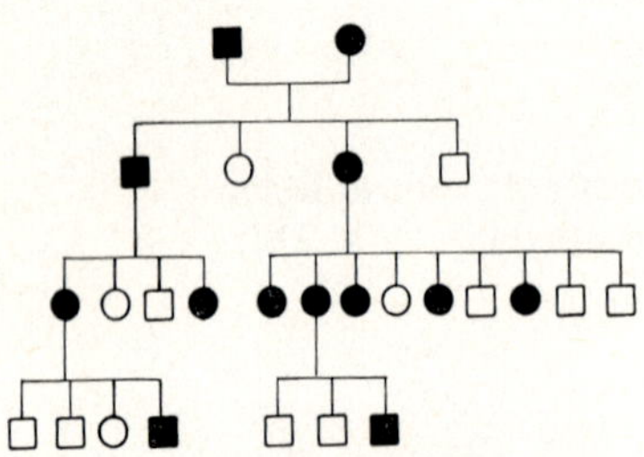

FIG. 216.—Migraine. Pedigree showing dominant inheritance. (*After Unger. Quoted by Julia Bell*, 1933.)

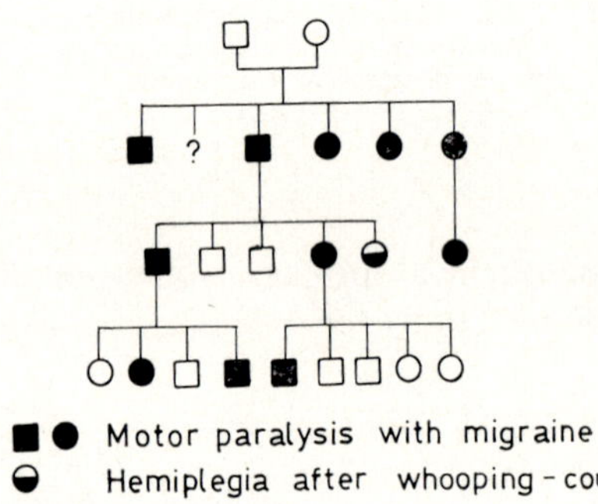


FIG. 217.—Ophthalmoplegic migraine. Pedigree showing dominant inheritance. (*After Clarke*, 1910.)

## BLOOD DISEASES

### Haemophilia

This sex-linked affection does not seem to carry any special ocular aspects. It has, however, considerable significance in ophthalmology as it has been used for determining linkage with colour anomalies, also inherited as a sex-linked recessive.

### Acholuric jaundice

This irregularly dominant affection with its increased fragility of erythrocytes is of significance as bone anomalies are not uncommon, and there is the possibility that some cases of oxycephaly are secondary to acholuric jaundice.

### Rh haemolytic disease

Optic atrophy in addition to widespread neurological disturbances is not uncommon in this severe affection. The recognition that the erythroblastosis arises from iso-immunization to an Rh antigen has been a landmark in the prevention of genetically determined disease.

**Polycythaemia vera**

The violet discoloration of the conjunctiva, and the characteristic fundus appearance in polycythaemia vera give a special ophthalmological interest to this irregularly dominant affection.

**The leukaemias**

The exact genetic status of this group, and its relationship to neoplasms, are still undetermined. It is also not known whether the ocular changes are incidental, or constitute a special genetic type.

*Sickle cell anaemia* and *acanthrocytosis* have been discussed under metabolic disorders (pp. 204 and 205). *Thalassaemia*—a haemoglobinopathy allied to sickle cell anaemia—is of interest in that bony changes, which include skull anomalies and mongoloid features, are common.

## Other Affections

**Hyperthyroidism**

The occurrence in sibships is well established. The affection appears to be dominant, variably expressed and largely sex-limited to women (Fig. 218), with environmental factors as precipitating causes.

Bartels holds that, genetically, hyperthyroidism is only one aspect of thyroid disturbances generally, for simple goitre and myxoedema often occur in families with hyperthyroidism.

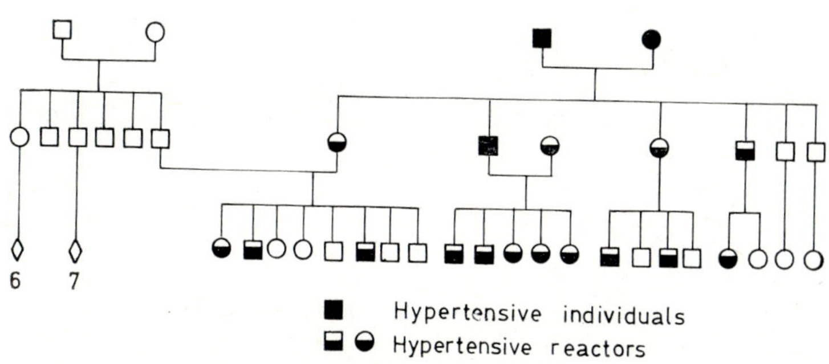


FIG. 218.—Vascular hypertension. Pedigree showing presumed dominant inheritance, expression being either clinical hypertension or induced hypertensive reaction. (*After Hines*, 1937.)

**Vascular hypertension**

The possible inheritance of hypertension is complicated by the fact that the condition is excessively common. There is, however, good evidence that dominant inheritance is probably the rule (Fig. 218). This may apply to many of the arterial degenerative lesions including coronary atheroma. Whether ocular complications constitute a special genetic type or are incidental to all hypertensive patients is not known.

## FOR FURTHER READING

**Skeletal Anomalies**

*General Surveys*

Becker, P. E. (Ed.) (1964). *Humangenetik*, Vol. II. Stuttgart; Thieme.

Waardenburg, P. J., Franceschetti, A. and Klein, D. (1961). *Genetics and Ophthalmology*, Vol. 1, pp. 301–411. Oxford; Blackwell.

Walsh, J. B. (1957). *Clinical Neuro-Ophthalmology*, 2nd ed. Baltimore; Williams and Wilkins.

*Cranio-facial Anomalies*

Tridon, P. and Thiriet M. (1966). *Malformation Associées de la tête et des extrémités.* Paris; Masson.

**Central Nervous System**

*General Surveys*

Franceschetti, A., François, J. and Babel, J. (1963). *Les hérédo-dégénérescences Chorio-rétiniennes*, pp. 1035–1076. Paris; Masson.

Pratt, T. C. (1967). *The Genetics of Neurological Disorders.* London; Oxford University Press.

Walsh, J. B. (1957). *Clinical Neuro-Ophthalmology*, 2nd ed. Baltimore; Williams and Wilkins

*The Muscle Dystrophies*

Klein, D. (1958). "La dystrophy myotonique (Steinert) et la myotonie congenitale (Thomsen) en Suisse." *J. gén. Hum.*, Suppl. 7.

Maas, O. (1947). *Msch. Psychiat. Neurol.*, **113,** 79.

Thomasen, E. (1948). *Myotonia* (Vol. 17, *Opera ex Domo Biologiae Hered. Human Univer. Hafniensis*). Copenhagen; Munksgaard.

*Adie's Pupil*

Waardenburg, J. P. (1963). In *Genetics and Ophthalmology*, Vol. II, p. 1154, Ed. by J. P. Waardenburg, A. Franceschetti and D. Klein. Oxford; Blackwell.

*Word Blindness*

Hallgren, B. (1950). "Specific Dyslexia." *Acta psychiat. neurol. scand.*, Suppl. 65.

*Torticollis*

Isigkheit, E. (1931). *Arch. orthop. Unfall-Chirurg.*, **30,** 459.

Pfandler, U. (1952). *J. gén. Hum.*, **1,** 169.

*Deaf-mutism in Retinitis Pigmentosa*

Bell, Julia (1963). In *Treasury of Human Inheritance*, Ed. by K. Pearson, Vol. II, Part 1. Cambridge University Press.

*Mental Deficiency and Ocular Anomalies*

Roberts, J. A. F. (1937). *Br. med. J.*, **2,** 1213.

Sjögren, T. (1950). *Conf. Neurol.*, **10,** 293.

— (1956). *Acta genet.*, **6,** 80.

— and Larsson, T. (1949). "Microphthalmos with or without Coincident Oligophrenia." *Acta psychiat. neurol. scand.*, Suppl. 56.

# CHAPTER 14

## SYNDROMES

Studies of disturbances confined to one organ, or to one system, are a characteristic reflection of the present-day attitude in medicine, for they fit in well with the findings by pathologists and physiologists. The syndromes—and these have been described in increasing numbers in recent years—run counter to these conceptions, for they bring together a mass of apparently disconnected anomalies. Attempts to explain syndromes as disturbances in relatively ill-defined systems—such as the reticulo-endothelial system—do not solve many difficulties. Nor is the embryological approach of attempting to explain syndromes in terms of disturbances in ectodermal or mesodermal tissues always successful, for more than one embryonic layer is generally involved. The concept of status dysraphicus with its postulate of a failure in midline development, is a refinement of the embryological approach and is at best only of limited application. The search for metabolic disorders has probably been the most successful of such attempts.

Genetics has provided another possible approach in stressing the pleitropic action of genes, so that a combination of bizarre anomalies becomes less unintelligible. The variable expression of such genes does, moreover, help to explain both incomplete syndromes—the *formes frustes*—and the frequent observation of apparently unrelated disturbances in collateral branches. Even so, it is not easy to see why club-foot, or cleft palate and such-like anomalies, should be recorded so frequently in relatives of patients with various syndromes, the components of which have apparently no obvious relationship to such anomalies. But this excess may be largely illusory, since comparative data from equally detailed searches in the general population are not available.

Since syndromes cannot, by definition, be classified by organs or systems, nor—except in a few cases—on the basis of a metabolic disorder, nor, as yet as the result of anomalous effects of particular genes, the embryological approach, with all its limitations, has some value, but is becoming increasingly inadequate and burdensome. For these reasons the classification adopted here follows essentially a clinical pattern.

### MULTI-SYSTEMIC CONGENITAL AND INFANTILE SYNDROMES

**The Laurence–Moon–Biedl syndrome**

In the pentad of obesity, hypogenitalism, mental deficiency, polydactyly, and retinal dystrophy of the retinitis pigmentosa type, the ocular changes are almost constant, whilst some of the other components may be lacking. The retinal dystrophy itself may take the form of typical retinitis pigmentosa, a macular lesion with pigmentary disturbance such as seen in juvenile amaurotic idiocy, a combination of retinitis pigmentosa and macular dystrophy, or the appearances of retinal aplasia. Of the many subsidiary features—such as atresia ani, syndactyly and various skeletal anomalies, ataxia and possibly also diabetes—congenital deaf-mutism is significant, and may perhaps appear as a variant to the retinal dystrophy (Fig. 219).

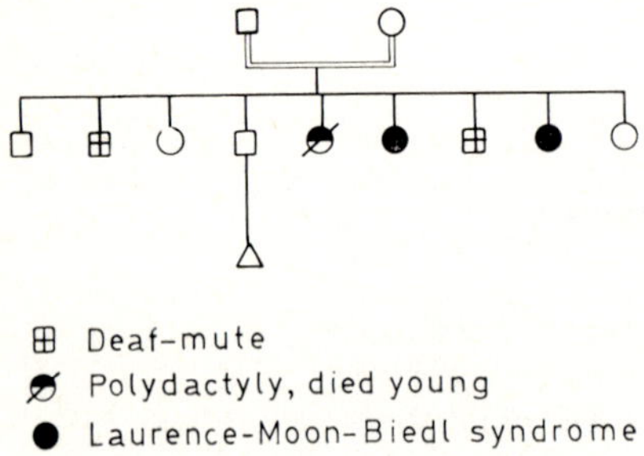


FIG. 219.—Laurence–Moon–Biedl syndrome. Pedigree showing deaf-mutism in an affected sibship. (*After Burn*, 1950.)

The rate of consanguinity in the Laurence–Biedl syndrome is high; as no case of direct transmission of the syndrome is known, and as the affection has been recorded in sibships, the recessive character of the affection is beyond doubt (Fig. 220). Earlier attempts to explain the apparently disconnected components

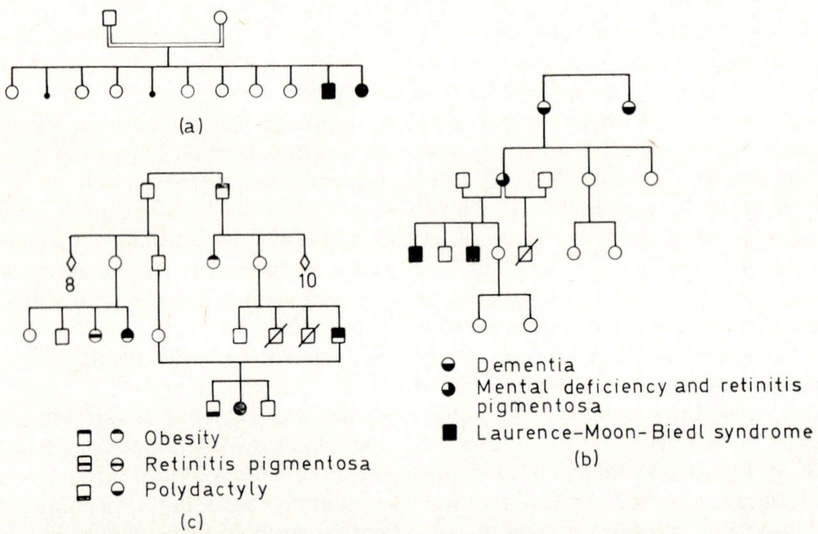


FIG. 220.—Laurence–Moon–Biedl syndrome. Pedigrees. (*a*) Recessive inheritance. (*After Sorsby, Avery and Cockayne*, 1939.) (*b*) and (*c*) Partial manifestation of the syndrome in ascendants. ((*b*) *After van Bogaert and Borremans*, 1936; (*c*) *After Laborne*, 1944.)

of the syndrome on the basis of two or more genes must be regarded as untenable, and the fact that partial—and frequently only minimal—manifestations are observed in the ascendants, cannot be taken as proving the transmission of a dominant gene responsible for some features in addition to a recessive gene responsible for others. The most likely reading is that which sees the affection as the result of a recessive gene in the duplex state, and the partial manifestations in ascendants as the expression of the gene in the simplex state. There is an excess of males, presumably due to sex limitation in the manifestation of the gene.

**Down's syndrome (mongolian idiocy)**

The dwarfed stature, mongolian facies, seborrhoeic skin, large tongue, and mental defect, constitute a characteristic syndrome. Minor anomalies are present in the skull.

A characteristic subcapsular cataract is frequently present, and in about one-third of patients there is high myopia. Brushfield spots (speckled iris) are almost always present.

The affection, the first to be recognized as due to a chromosomal anomaly (commonly trisomy 21), has been recorded in sibships. Most mongolian idiots are born to ageing mothers.

**Retinal atrophy, progressive infantile deafness, mental deficiency and progeria-like traits (Cockayne)**

Dwarfism with disproportionate growth of slender limbs, a skin sensitive to light and showing scarring and pigmentary changes, in addition to gross mental deficiency corresponding to a mental age of 3–4 years, give a striking picture in which deafness and the typical findings of retinal aplasia with subsequent cataract formation are also present. Spasticity is not uncommon in older children.

Unlike progeria, the affection shows normal blood lipoid levels. Recessive inheritance is likely.

**Cystic fibrosis of the pancreas**

In this complex affection there is involvement of the sweat glands, the salivary and lacrymal glands, the mucous-secreting glands and of the pancreas, i.e. a series of exocrine glands. The characteristic consequent changes are increased concentrations of sodium chloride, increased viscosity of mucous secretions (hence the older name of mucoviscidosis) and also diminution of the trypsin content of the duodenal fluid. In addition, there are also present fairly typical physical findings—general, alimentary and pulmonary in character: the child shows malnutrition, steatorrhoea, moderate to severe emphysema and frequent attacks of bilateral bronchopneumonia.

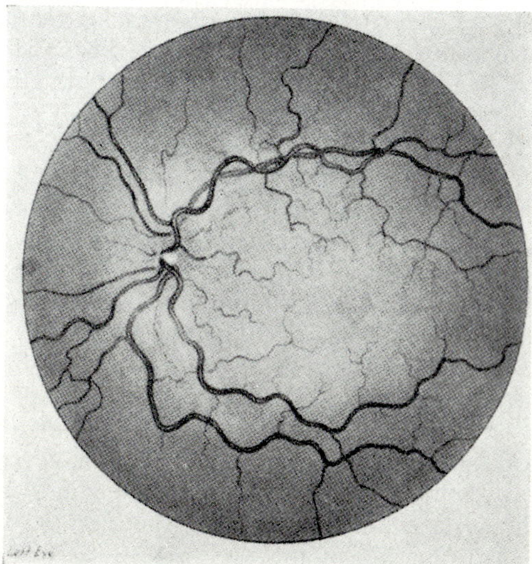

FIG. 221.—The fundus in cystic fibrosis of the pancreas. Note the venous distension and the cystic macular lesion. (*After Bruce, Denning and Spaller*, 1960.)

Fundus findings are common in all cases with moderate to severe pulmonary involvement, and they range over papilloedema, venous distension and tortuosity, retinal haemorrhages and cystic changes at the macula (and possible also "macular hole") (Fig. 221).

The affection is steadily progressive. Survival beyond early adult age is exceptional. Surviving males are sterile; spermatogenesis is apparently normal and transport of spermatozoa may be at fault owing to diminished water and electrolyte secretion. Cystic fibrosis is a recessive disorder of considerable frequency, possibly as high as 1:1,000 of live births.

**Familial autonomic dysfunction (dysautonomia, Riley–Day syndrome)**

"Congenital alacrymia" and "congenital neuroparalytic keratitis" appear to be part of a more widespread syndrome, probably recessive in character and involving various autonomic functions. The affected infants show retarded development and do not thrive. There is difficulty in swallowing and there are frequent bouts of respiratory infection or aspiration pneumonia with exaggerated febrile response. There is excessive sweating with a tendency to dehydration. The neurological symptoms include indifference to pain—including corneal hypoaesthesia—hyperflexia, labile hypertension and postural hypertension. Lack of tears on crying may be a striking feature. The corneal complications may be relatively slight leading to corneal scarring of no great significance, or the eye may be lost from perforation of a centrally placed corneal ulcer. Inflammatory reactions need not be marked.

**The syndrome of fragilitas ossium, otosclerosis and blue sclerotics**

A large number of proper names have been attached to this syndrome, such as Eddowes, Adair–Dighton, Lobstein, van der Hoeve and others.

The bluish sclera is the most constant feature, and is always present; fragility of bone is present in rather more than half the cases, whilst otosclerosis is seen in about 25 per cent of those over 25 years of age. The penetrance of the different components therefore varies considerably. Expression within the same family varies slightly, but varies considerably as between different families. Subsidiary features of the syndrome are a somewhat characteristic deformity of the skull—there is a high occipital region, a markedly curved parietal region, and a rather broad base; dental defects; minor abnormalities of the extremities; a slender bone system throughout the body, markedly transparent to x-rays; and laxity of joints. Defective calcification, possibly based on a disturbance of calcium and phosphorus metabolism, appears to be the underlying pathological condition.

The affection is transmitted in a dominant manner, with a variable distribution of the individual components (Fig. 222). A possibly sex-linked form characterized by recurrent corneal ruptures has been recorded (Stein and colleagues, 1968).

**Arachnodactyly (Marfan's syndrome)**

The designation of arachnodactyly suggests a merely localized abnormality of hands and feet; this is, however, part of a particularly generalized disturbance. Poor musculature and joint ligaments, poor development of subcutaneous fat, spinal anomalies, dolichocephaly, slender development of bones, particularly in the extremities, increased stature, congenital heart lesions, progressive dilatation of the aorta ending in aortic regurgitation or in thoracic or abdominal aneurysm, and malformation of the ears, are all seen in addition to the important ocular

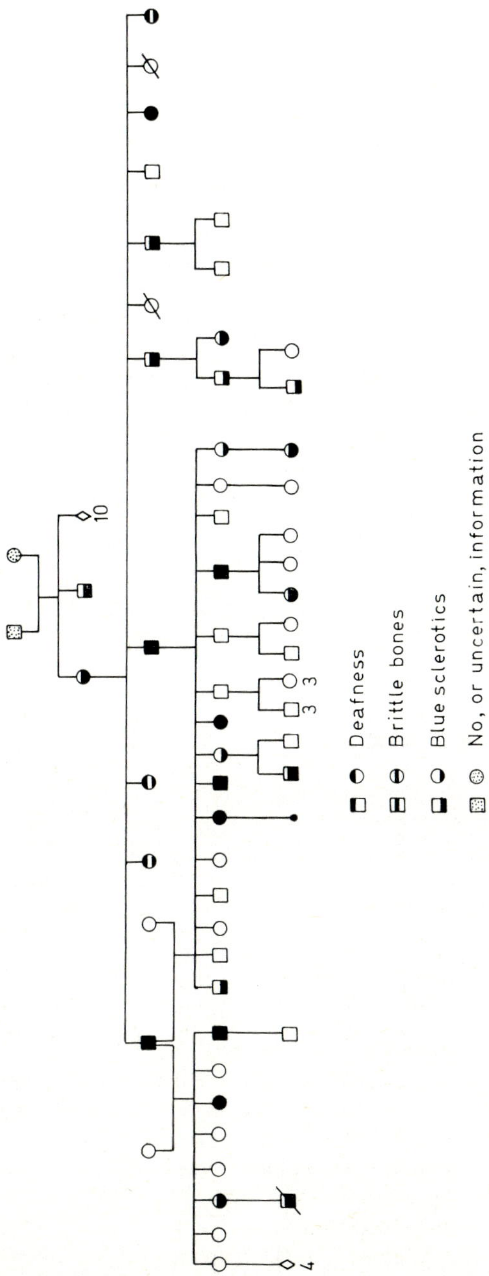


FIG. 222.—Fragilitas ossium. Pedigree showing dominant inheritance and variable expression. (*After Seedorff*, 1949.)

lesions. These, in turn, though most commonly in the nature of subluxation of the lens with tremulous iris, frequently show other features. Coloboma of the lens, opacities of the lens, buphthalmos, megalocornea, high myopia or high hypermetropia, miotic pupils, deep anterior chamber, macular coloboma and even colour-blindness have all been recorded. Amongst the rarer general disturbances are fissure of the face or of the palate, macroglossia, syndactyly, hypogenitalism or hypergenitalism, and spina bifida.

Apart from the skeletal anomaly, which is characteristic, poor development of fat is rather more common than congenital subluxation of the lens. The other anomalies are all seen less frequently.

It is generally accepted that Marfan's syndrome is a mesodermal disturbance. The ocular lesions are regarded as secondary to embryonic changes in the fibro-vascular tunic of the lens, or in the suspensory ligament which may, perhaps, be of mesodermal origin.

Abortive forms without eye complications and serious systemic disorders are exceptional (Abraham Lincoln is illustrative) but generally a patient affected with arachnodactyly is a frail individual. There is a heavy mortality in childhood, particularly in the more severely marked cases. Some pedigrees suggest that the condition might be recessive, but the rate of consanguinity is not high, and it is more likely that only dominant inheritance comes into consideration. Direct inheritance of the more severe defects is not likely to be frequently observed, owing

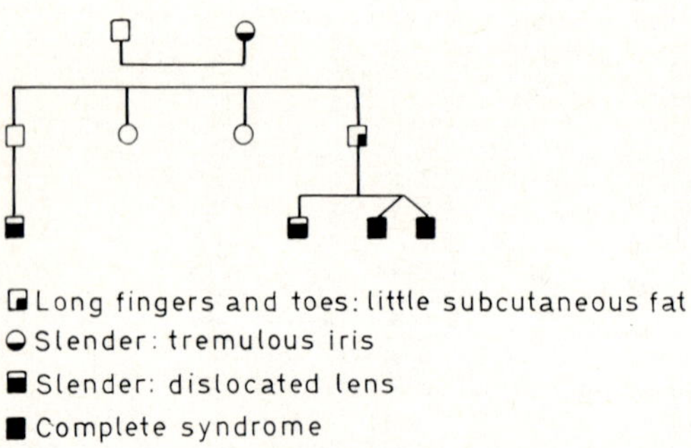


FIG. 223. — Arachnodactyly. Pedigree showing dominant inheritance and variable expression. (*After Becker*, 1935.)

to the high mortality of affected individuals. It becomes more obvious when the less marked cases are studied (Fig. 223).

**Brachydactyly with spherophakia (Marchesani)**

This disorder is less well established than Marfan's syndrome, of which it is the opposite in many respects. Stature is short; hands and feet are short and broad; the musculature and subcutaneous fat are well developed; and there is brachycephaly rather than dolichocephaly. The ocular abnormality is essentially spherophakia, which produces an index myopia; the lens is also small; ectopia and secondary glaucoma are not uncommon.

The condition has been observed in the offspring of first cousins, but the exact genetic status is still undetermined. In the original family, recorded by Marchesani, the possibility of dominant inheritance arose. Intermediate inheritance with full manifestation in homozygotes is likely (Fig. 224).

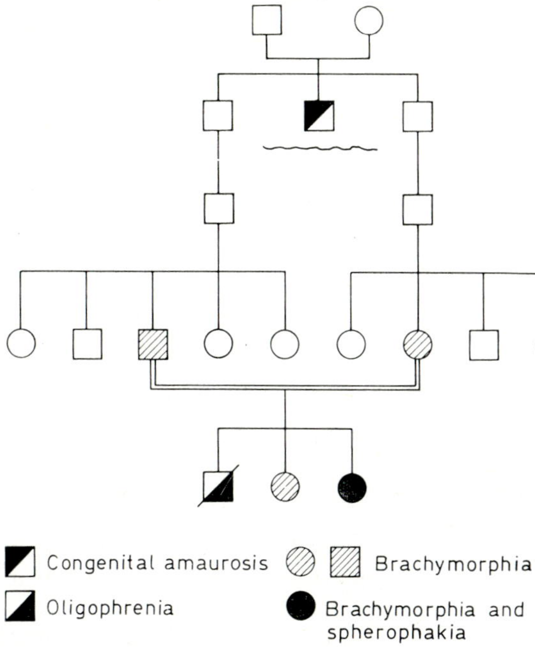


FIG. 224.—Brachydactyly with spherophakia. Possibly intermediate inheritance. (*After Stadlin and Klein*, 1948.)

**Ehlers–Danlos syndrome**

Marked hyperelasticity of the skin (which in extreme cases can give the bizarre picture of a man picking up with his teeth the skin of his shoulder), and equally marked hyperlaxity of the joints with consequent extreme mobility, are the outstanding features of the Ehlers–Danlos syndrome. In addition, there is ready fragility of the skin and the blood vessels, so that mild trauma may cause marked haematomas and pseudo-tumour formations calling for differentiation from haemophilia. The affection is dominant but with variable expression; it is possible that the homozygous state is necessary for full expression (Fig. 225). A sex-linked form has been recorded (Beighton, 1968).

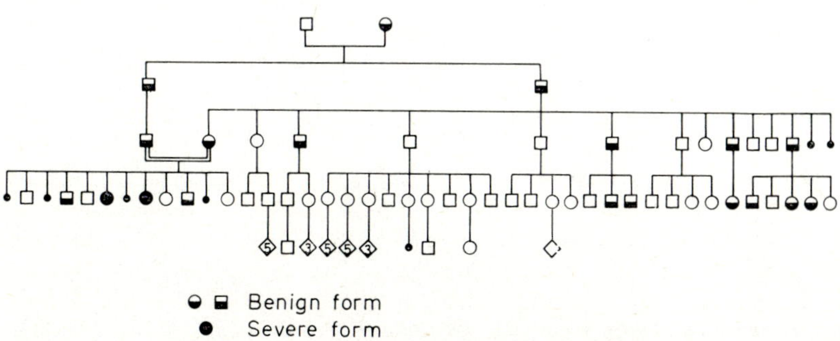


FIG. 225.—Ehlers–Danlos syndrome. Dominant inheritance with variable penetration and manifestation. (*After Johnson and Falls*, 1949.)

The ophthalmological interest of the affection is the ready tendency to complications from trauma including operative procedures. In addition, keratoconus, subluxation of the lens, blue sclera—as in fragilitas ossium—and angioid streaks—as in pseudo-xanthoma elasticum—have all been observed and regarded as secondary to weakness of the mesodermal tissues: choroidal haemorrhages have also been noted.

The nature of the affection is not clear. It is said to be due to failure in the organization of collagen with a stable collagen "wickerwork". The occurrences of angioid streaks and of blue sclerotics suggests some relationship to both elastosis dystrophica and to fragilitas ossium. There is apparently a high incidence of prematurity (as defined by a birth weight of less than 5½ lb.) in affected individuals; this is regarded as the consequence of premature rupture of the foetal membranes, which share in the increased fragility of the tissues (Barabas, 1966).

## SYNDROMES WITH PROMINENT LESIONS OF THE SKIN OR MUCOSA

### Elastosis dystrophica (Grönblad syndrome)

The association of angioid streaks with pseudo-xanthoma elasticum was first recognized in 1929 by Grönblad. Subsequently Prick and also Urbach and his associates have shown that elastic tissue degeneration involves the systemic arteries with secondary hypertension. The term elastosis dystrophica was suggested by Böck. Calcinosis of the skin is not uncommon and gastro-intestinal haemorrhage—sometimes fatal—may occur. In one family (Fig. 226 *b*) central choroidal sclerosis appears to have replaced angioid streaks.

The possibility that osteitis deformans also falls into this group has already been indicated, but angioid streaks appear to be relatively uncommon in osteitis deformans, whilst pseudo-xanthoma elasticum would appear to be exceptional.

The frequency with which the components of the syndrome are associated is not well known; the association of angioid streaks with the skin lesion is probably

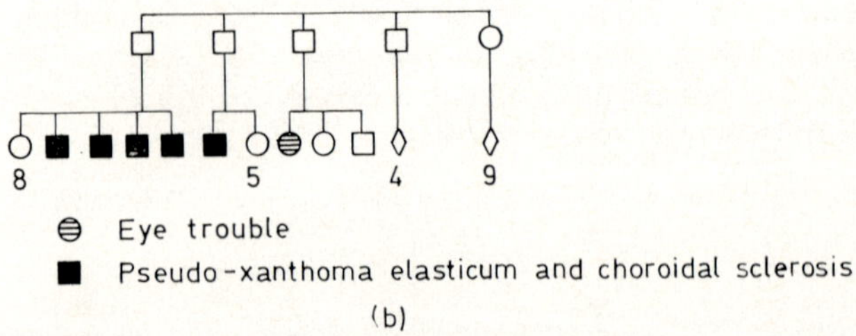


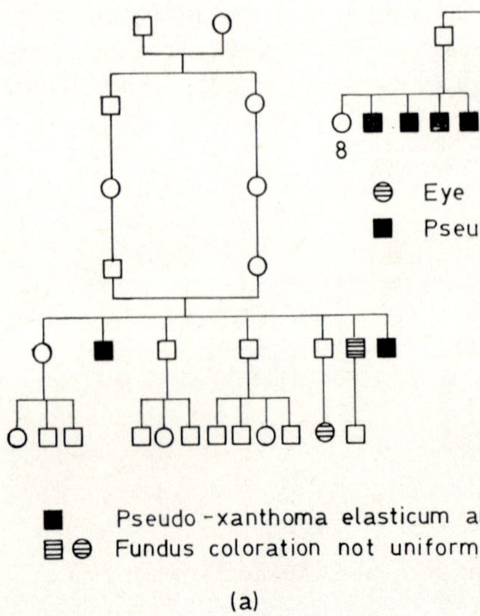


FIG. 226.—Elastosis dystrophica. (*a*) Pedigree suggestive of recessive inheritance. (*After Hartung*, 1932.) (*b*) Pedigree recording choroidal sclerosis instead of angioid streaks. (*After Anderson*, 1948.)

very close, but it is uncertain how frequently the serious retinal complications of angioid streaks occur, nor how common are the other features of the disorder.

The mode of inheritance is probably recessive (Fig. 226 *a*), although there is some evidence that there might be a dominant form.

In contrast to true xanthomatous changes of the skin, there is no evidence of any lipoid disturbance.

**Congenital anhydrotic ectodermal dysplasia**

In the fully developed and generally sex-linked form (Fig. 227 *a*), the individual shows characteristic features: he is toothless, or deficient in teeth; he is intolerant to heat owing to deficient or absent sweat glands; the skin shows fine, pale scanty hair; and the facial appearance may be more or less characteristic from prominence

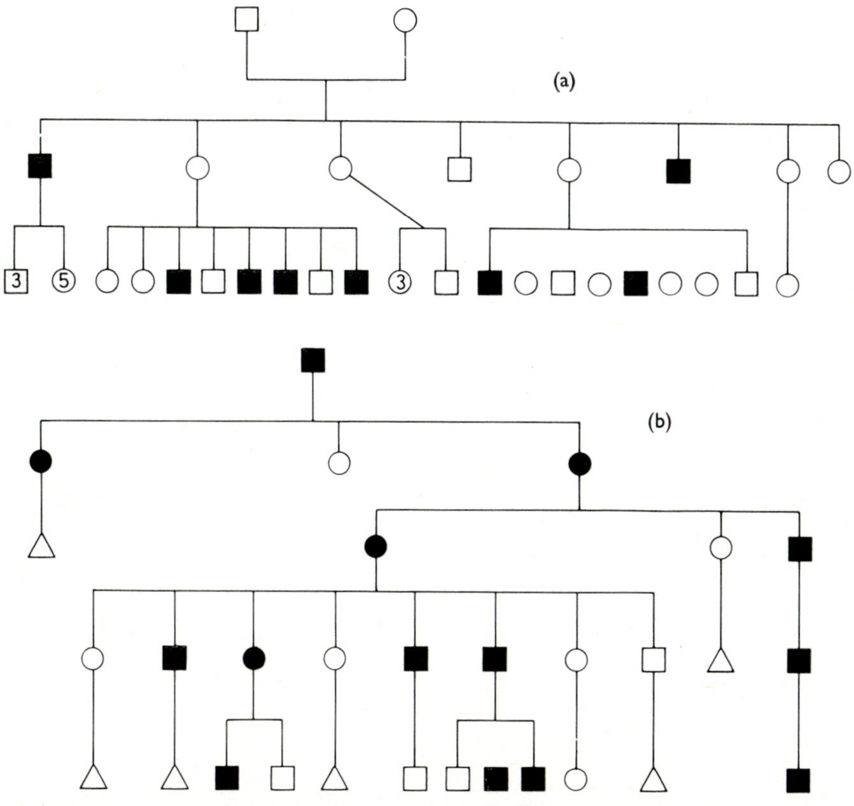


FIG. 227.—Anhydrotic ectodermal dysplasia. (*a*) Recessive sex-linked inheritance. (*After Gibbs*, 1915, 1916.) (*b*) Dominant inheritance. (*After Helweg-Larsen and Ludvigsen*, 1946.)

of the superciliary arches and of the chin associated with a saddle nose and thickened lips. Chronic rhinitis and ozaena are frequent. Stature is affected. The lacrymal glands may be lacking with a consequent inability to weep, but a tendency to excessive weeping has also been recorded. In the less complete form, inherited in a dominant manner (Fig. 227 *b*), microphthalmos has been observed (Fig. 228).

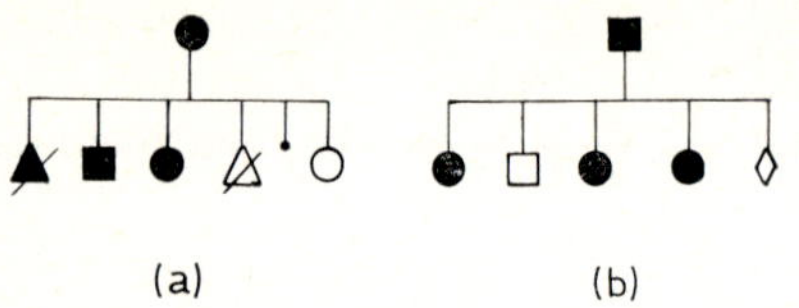


FIG. 228.—Congenital anhydrotic ectodermal dysplasia with microphthalmos. (*After Moon*, 1876–7, *quoted by Cockayne*, 1933.)

## Rothmund's syndrome

Skin changes are observed early in infancy and may perhaps be present at birth. These changes are those seen in poikilodermia of the Zinsser–Thomson type. Early on there is a reticulated appearance of the skin taking on a reddish hue. Subsequently telangiectases appear, and later on yellowish scars which tend to scale. Normal skin encircled by such yellowish scar tissue acquires a characteristic areolated appearance. The skin on the hands and feet is pliable and thin as tissue paper. Cataract develops early and other ocular anomalies, such as microcornea may be present. General development is affected, but not always markedly

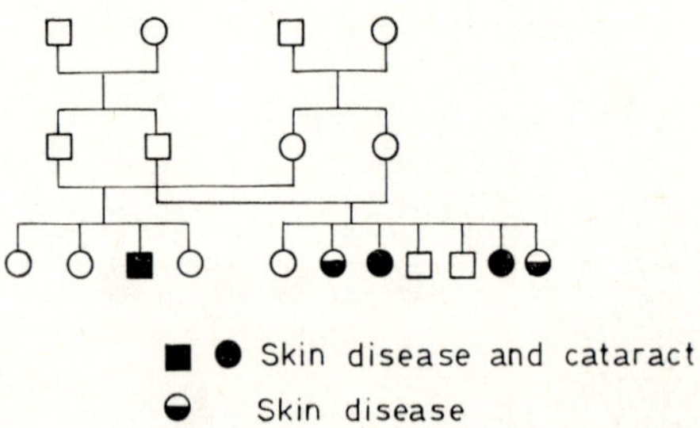


FIG. 229.—Rothmund's syndrome. Pedigree showing recessive inheritance. (*After Rothmund*, 1868.)

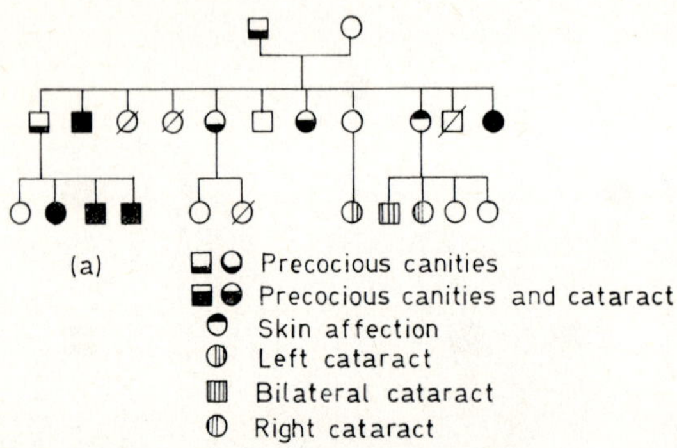


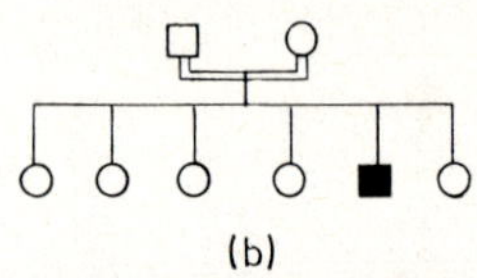


FIG. 230.—Werner's syndrome. (*a*) Pedigree showing dominant inheritance. (*After Krebs, Hartmann and Thiebaut*, 1930.) (*b*) Pedigree showing recessive inheritance. (*Personal observation. Royal Eye Hospital No.* 0/8875.)

so. Marked shortness of stature is common, aplasia of the bones, especially of the phalanges, may occur, and sexual under-development not infrequent. The affection is compatible with long life and reproduction.

The condition is uncommon, and appears to be recessive (Fig. 229).

## Werner's syndrome

This is a more widespread disturbance, but does not become fully obvious until about the age of 20–30 years. Stature is markedly affected. Greying of hair sets in at about the age of 20 years, when cataract, atrophy of muscles and subcutaneous fat, huskiness of voice from characteristic and bizarre changes in the vocal cords, diffuse arteriosclerosis, osteoporosis, joint deformities, and ulcers on the feet, all begin to make their appearance, producing the characteristic picture of "progeria of adults". Hypogenitalism is present, and the skin changes—a progressive scleropoikilodermia of the Arndt–Jaffe type—are essentially in the nature of an atrophic and thin skin tightly drawn over the underlying tissue. Telangiectases and pigmentation are not marked. Proptosis is not uncommon.

Recessive inheritance (Fig. 230 *b*) is probably the rule, although in some families irregular dominance may apply (Fig. 230 *a*).

**Keratoconjunctivitis sicca syndrome (Sjögren)**

Most recorded cases are sporadic and there is a marked female excess. The affection has been recorded in familial concentration (Lisch, 1937; Coverdale, 1948) as possibly dominant; its mucosal features recall the Plummer–Vinson syndrome which is a more definitely dominant affection.

## SYNDROMES WITH PROMINENT PIGMENTARY CHANGES

**"Incontinentia pigmenti" (Bloch, Sulzberger)**

In this ectodermal syndrome Bloch found that the melanin pigment of the skin behaves "incontinently"; it is not retained by the melanoblasts, but passes into the corium and its chromatophores. Clinically the changes in the skin are a striking feature.

A macular or vesicular eruption sets in generally within a few days after birth, and tends to recur, ultimately becoming widespread over the body and tending to be arranged in lines and whorls. During attacks of fever and other general disturbances pigmentation in the skin eruption develops and tends towards a linear or racemose pattern; occasionally the pigmentation occurs without preceding inflammatory reactions.

Other features of the affection are brittle nails, absence or malformation of the teeth, and alopecia; congenital heart disease, mental deficiency, and spastic paraplegia have all been noted. Almost all—if not all—patients reported have been girls, and familial concentration is not uncommon. The mode of inheritance, however, is obscure. It is possibly dominant with very variable manifestation.

Ocular lesions have been noted in about one-fifth of the reported cases. Nystagmus, squint, cataract, optic atrophy, and macular dystrophy have all been seen, but the commonest complication is a massive anomaly of the whole of the globe of the endophthalmitis or pseudoglioma type.

Franceschetti and Jadassohn have recorded cases they designate as dominantly inherited reticular pigmentary dermatosis and separated by them from the incontinentia pigmenti syndrome. The validity of this distinction is uncertain.

**Pigment-fleck polyposis (Peutz)**

In this dominantly inherited disorder, there is polyposis of the colon or rectum and occasionally in the stomach or nasopharynx. Associated with this are melanin or *cáfe-au-lait* spots on the face, mainly around the orifices (mouth, nose and lids), but sometimes also on the conjunctiva and buccal mucosa.

**Other affections**

Chédiak–Higashi disease and the Klein–Waardenburg syndrome have been discussed under albinism (p. 206).

# PREDOMINANTLY NEUROLOGICAL SYNDROMES

## THE PHAKOMATOSES

As already indicated (p. 4) the phakomatoses occupy an intermediate place between the abiotrophies and the hereditary tumours. Genetically determined minimal blemishes of the skin and possibly also in the central nervous system are present at birth or in early infancy in the whole group; some of these blemishes may grow and even become malignant. This characteristic led Van der Hoeve to suggest the genetic name of phakomatoses (φακοσξ = mother spot). Four clinically distinct types are recognized.

### Neurofibromatosis

The constant features in neurofibromatosis are subcutaneous nodules, tumours along the nerve trunks, and pigmentary changes in the skin. Rather less commonly psychic troubles, anomalies of bone, and endocrine disturbances are also seen. The ocular aspects of neurofibromatosis cover a wide range: neurofibromatosis may involve almost any part of the eye so that neurofibromas may be seen in either the lids, orbit, optic nerve, and in the individual structures of the eye, such as any part of the uveal tract, the retina, the conjunctiva, episclera, sclerotic, and even the cornea. Buphthalmos may arise owing to neurofibromatosis of the ciliary nerves. Multiple small tumours or cysts may be seen in the retina.

The affection appears to consist clinically of two distinct types. In one, malignant degeneration of tumours is common, and in the other it is exceptional. As many pedigrees show irregular dominance, the gene is not fully penetrant, and, moreover, the expression is variable. Some intrafamilial regularity is not uncommon. Inheritance of iris tumours is shown in Fig. 231 *a*, whilst Fig. 231 *b* shows bilateral optic atrophy in both members of a uniovular twin.

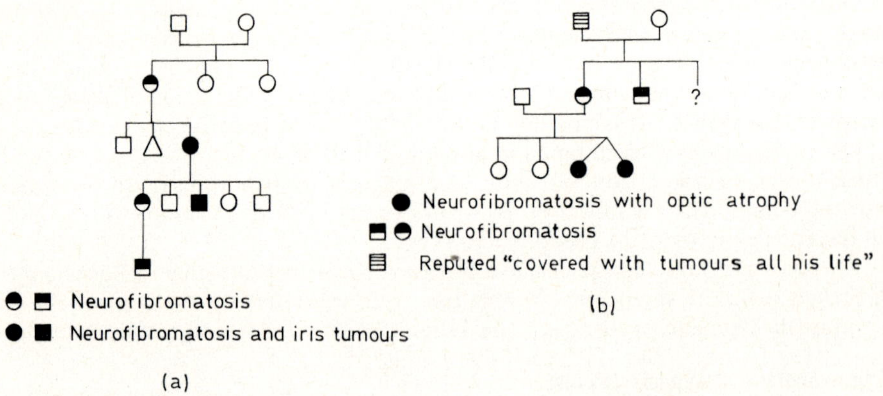


FIG. 231.—Neurofibromatosis. (*a*) Pedigree showing dominant inheritance of neurofibromatosis over four generations, with iris tumours over two generations. (*After Waardenburg. Quoted by van der Hoeve*, 1932.) (*b*) Pedigree showing bilateral optic atrophy in a uniovular twin in a family with neurofibromatosis. (*After Dresner and Montgomery*, 1949.)

### Tuberose sclerosis

The range of manifestations in individual patients extends from adenoma sebaceum alone, to adenoma sebaceum associated with epilepsy but no mental change; adenoma sebaceum associated with symptoms of cerebral tumour; and visceral tumour alone; retinal tumours may be associated with any of these types. Cerebral calcification is not uncommon. A family history of psychopathy is frequent. The affection is dominant and the range of manifestations is brought out in Fig. 232. It would, therefore, seem that whilst the penetrance of the gene is high, expression is particularly variable.

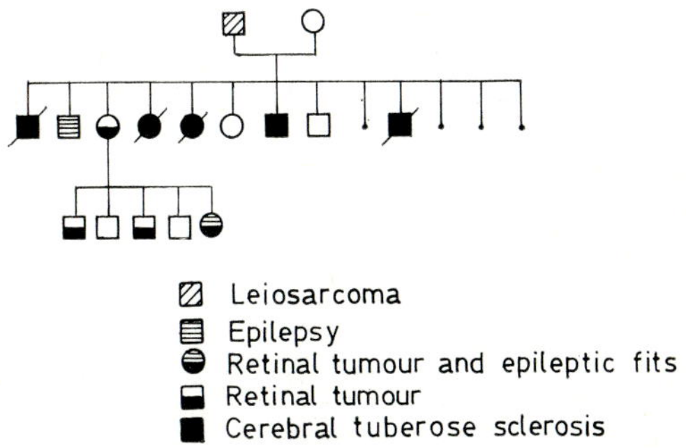


FIG. 232.—Tuberose sclerosis. Pedigree suggestive of dominant inheritance and variable expression. (*After van der Hoeve*, 1940.)

## Lindau's syndrome

Angiomatosis of the retina with its characteristic picture is now recognized as part of the Lindau syndrome. Calcification in the cerebellum or cerebrum is not uncommon. Cysts and tumours in the cerebellum, spinal cord, pancreas and kidney and other organs are also seen.

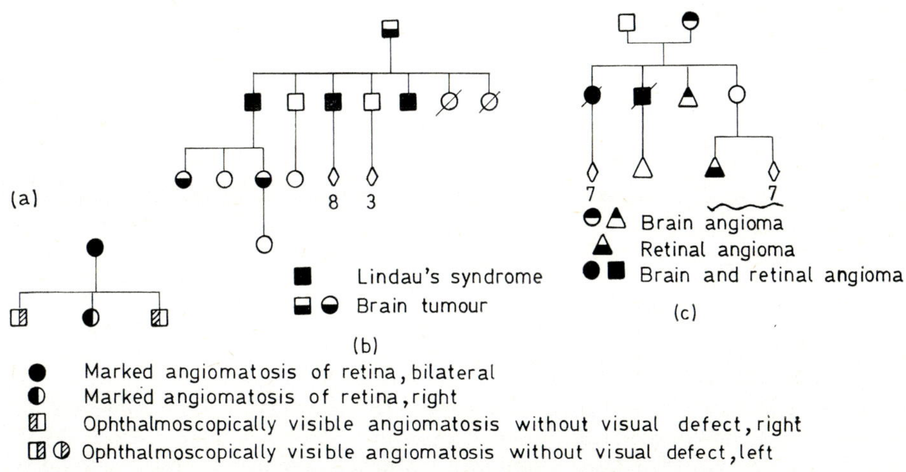


FIG. 233.—Lindau's syndrome. Pedigrees suggestive of dominant inheritance and variable expression in: (*a*) Angiomatosis of retina. (*After Staz*, 1941.) (*b*) Brain and retinal angioma. (*After Möller*, 1929.) (*c*) Brain and retinal angioma. (*After van der Hoeve*, 1932.)

It would appear that the affection is dominant with variable expressions in the different members affected (Fig. 233 *a*, *b* and *c*).

## Sturge–Weber syndrome (cephalo-facial angiomatosis)

Typically there is naevus flammeus of the face, largely following the distribution of the fifth nerve on one side, together with unilateral buphthalmos and calcification in the cerebrum shown by x-ray. Localized ipsilateral skull anomalies are common, as is mental deficiency. Epilepsy and hemiplegia may occur. Buphthalmos may be replaced by chronic glaucoma, or glaucomatous optic atrophy without rise in tension.

It is likely that mono-symptomatic forms are not uncommon, so that angioma of the choroid or buphthalmos may be the only aspect of the affection. On the other hand there are also observations of angiomas in the cerebellum and spinal cord, raising the question whether the fundamental lesion is not one of capillary angiomatosis and, as such, the relationship with haemangiomatosis of the Lindau syndrome becomes close.

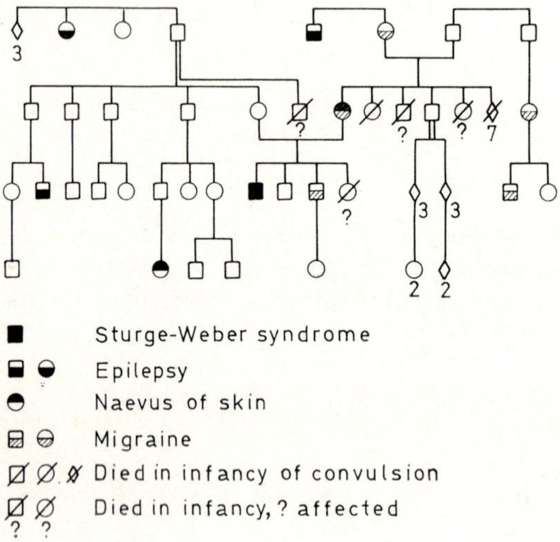


FIG. 234.—Sturge–Weber syndrome. Pedigree suggestive of dominant inheritance and variable expression. (*After Koch*, 1940.)

The affection is probably dominant, with different members of the families showing somewhat different lesions corresponding to the site of the capillary angiomas (Fig. 234).

## SYNDROMES WITH ATAXIA

**Ataxia-telangiectasia (Louis–Bar)**

The telangiectases in this infantile form of cerebellar ataxia appear to have a seat of election at the conjunctiva, although extensive cutaneous telangiectases on the face and elsewhere are also prominent. Chronic recurrent upper respiratory infections (with a deficiency of $\gamma$-A-globulin) are also prominent, as are dwarfism and infantilism. Mental defect is not uncommon. Few patients have survived beyond the second decade.

The affection is recessive and it is possible that the conjunctival telangiectases are indicative of the carrier state.

**Congenital spino-cerebellar ataxia, dwarfing, mental deficiency and congenital cataract (Marinesco; Sjögren)**

This bizarre combination is a well defined clinical entity and is inherited in a recessive manner (Fig. 235).

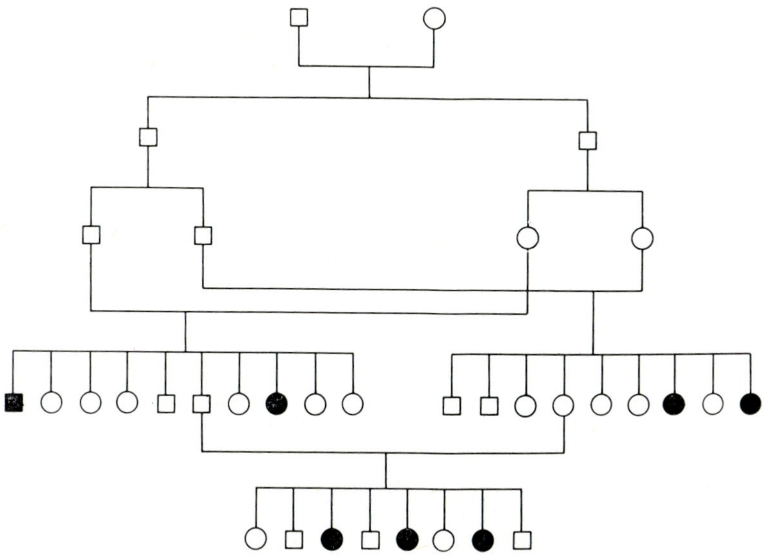

FIG. 235.—The Marinesco–Sjögren syndrome. Recessive inheritance. (*After Sjögren*, 1950.)

**Retinitis pigmentosa, vestibulo-cerebellar ataxia and mental deficiency (Hallgren)**

Hallgren (1958, 1959) has drawn attention to the familial existence of ataxia and mental deficiency in addition to the classical association of retinitis pigmentosa and congenital deafness. The affection is clearly recessive.

**Hereditary spastic ataxia with central retinal lesions and vestibular defects**

This has been observed in four members over three generations in a Swedish family (Bergstedt, Johansson and Muller, 1962) and, judging from incomplete reports in the older literature, it is likely that it constitutes a clinical entity.

**Ataxia as a component of other syndromes**

As already noted, ataxia may occur in the Refsum syndrome (p. 203), and in the Bassen–Kornzweig syndrome (p. 204).

## SYNDROMES WITH SPASTICITY

**Oligophrenia, congenital ichthyosis, spastic disorders and fundus lesions (Sjögren and Larsson)**

To the established association of ichthyosis with mental deficiency, Sjögren and Larsson in 1957 added the spastic disorders of the type seen in Little's cerebral palsy and occasional fundus lesions recorded as macular in type (but apparently more correctly described as retinal aplasia).

The affection is recessive, and a non-specific aminoaciduria has been recorded.

**Spasticity as a component of other syndromes**

This still requires elucidation. It has already been noted that spasticity is an aspect of the Cockayne syndrome (p. 235).

## OTHER SYNDROMES

### Oculopharyngeal dystrophy

The occurrence of progressive dysphagia ("vagus-glossopharyngeal paralysis") in families with hereditary ptosis of late onset was noted in a French Canadian family by Taylor in 1915. Barbeau, who has traced this family, and a number of others reported since, to an isolate near Quebec has established its dominant character in a pedigree showing 249 affected members (Barbeau, 1967).

*Formes frustes* are not uncommon. Often these are associated external ophthalmoplegias or more widespread anomalies reminiscent of dystrophic myotonia, such as flattening of the facial features and impaired mobility of the masticatory muscles and of the limb girdles. Prostigmin tests are negative. Histologically there is a great loss of muscle fibres and much atrophy in the remaining muscles, the changes being most marked in the extra-ocular muscles. Errors in immunoglobulin katabolism (a significant evelation of both IgA and IgG) as recorded in myotonic dystrophy have also been found in this disorder.

The affection has also been recorded in Sweden.

### Familial nephrophtisis with retinal aplasia

The juvenile form of this renal affection described by Fanconi in 1951 is probably recessive. An associated retinal aplasia has been recorded in several sibships (Senior, Friedmann and Braudo, 1961; Løken and colleagues, 1961).

### Polycystic kidneys and basilar aneurysm

Both these affections have hereditary forms, possibly dominant. The association of the two disorders has been described repeatedly in sporadic cases. It is not known whether such cases constitute a genetic entity.

### Alport's syndrome

The ocular aspects of this presumably dominant syndrome of glomerulonephritis and nerve deafness are not negligible. Lenticonus, lens opacities and drusen on the disc have all been noted (Gregg and Becker, 1963; Brownell and Walter, 1964; Friedburg, 1968).

### Nephroblastoma (Wilms' tumour), aniridia and genital anomalies

It is believed that this apparently sporadic syndrome is not an aspect of dominant aniridia; the aniridia in the reported cases has been sporadic (DiGeorge and Harley, 1966).

### Progeria

In the classical form as described by Hutchinson in 1886 and Gilford in 1904, the dwarfed stature, wrinkled atrophic skin and scanty greying hair, aptly described by the designation of *Nanism type sénile*, a number of associated defects may be present. Death from cardiovascular complications generally occurs before adult life, and possibly often in infancy. Recessive inheritance is likely. Various ocular anomalies have been reported as occasional occurrences.

## FOR FURTHER READING

### General

Cockayne, E. A. (1933). *Inherited Abnormalities of the Skin and its Appendages.* London; Oxford University Press.

McKusick, V. A. (1966). *Heritable Disorders of Connective Tissue*, 3rd ed. St. Louis; Mosby.

Obal, A. (1967). "Syndrome mit Augenbeteilung." In *Der Augenartz*, Ed. by K. Velhagen, Vol. VII, p. 905. Leipzig; Thieme.

Timm, G. (1961). "Missbildungssyndrome mit Beteilung der Augen." In *Der Augenartz*, Ed. by K. Velhagen, Vol. IV, p. 518. Leipzig; Thieme.

**Multi-systemic Congenital and Infantile Syndromes**

*The Laurence–Moon–Biedl Syndrome*

Bell, Julia (1958). In *The Treasury of Human Inheritance*, Ed. by L. S. Penrose, Vol. II, Pt. III. London; Cambridge University Press.

Cockayne, E. A., Krestin, D. and Sorsby, A. (1935). *Q. Jl Med.* (N.S.), **4,** 93.

Sorsby, A., Avery, H. and Cockayne, E. A. (1939). *Q. Jl Med.* (N.S.), **8,** 51.

*Down's Syndrome*

Lowe, R. F. (1949). *Br. J. Ophthal.*, **33,** 131.

*Cockayne's Syndrome*

Macdonald, W. B., Fitch, K. D. and Lewis, J. C. (1960). *Pediatrics*, **25,** 997.

*Cystic Fibrosis of the Pancreas*

Bruce, G. M., Denning, C. R. and Spaller, H. F. (1960). *Archs Ophthal.*, **63,** 391.

Lobeck, C. C. (1966). In *The Metabolic Basis of Inherited Disease*, Ed. by J. B. Stanbury, J. B. Wyngaarden and D. S. Fredrickson. New York; Blakiston Division of McGraw-Hill.

*Riley–Day Syndrome*

Boruchoff, S. A. and Dohlman, C. H. (1967). *Am. J. Ophthal.*, **63,** 523.

Howard, R. O. (1967). *Am. J. Ophthal.*, **64,** 392.

Yatsu, F. and Zussman, W. (1963). *Archs Neurol.*, **10,** 459.

*Syndrome of Fragilitas Ossium, Otosclerosis and Blue Sclerotics*

Bell, Julia (1933). In *The Treasury of Human Inheritance*, Ed. by K. Pearson, Vol. II, Pt. III. London; Cambridge University Press.

McKusick, V. A. (1966). *Heritable Disorders of Connective Tissue*, 3rd ed. St. Louis; Mosby.

Seedorff, K. S. (1949). *Osteogenesis Imperfecta* (Vol. 20, *Opera ex Domo Biologiae Heredit. Human. Univ. Hafniensis*). Copenhagen; Munksgaard.

*Arachnodactyly*

McKusick, V. A. (1966). *Heritable Disorders of Connective Tissue*, 3rd ed. St. Louis; Mosby.

*Brachydactyly with Spherophakia*

Rosenthal, J. W. and Kloepfer, H. W. (1956). *Archs Ophthal.*, **55,** 28.

*Ehlers–Danlos Syndrome*

McKusick, V. A. (1966). *Heritable Disorders of Connective Tissue*, 3rd ed. St. Louis; Mosby.

**Syndromes with Prominent Lesions of Skin or Mucosa**

*Elastosis Dystrophica*

Grönblad, E. (1940). In *Modern Trends in Ophthalmology—1*, Ed. by F. Ridley and A. Sorsby. London; Butterworths.

McKusick, V. A. (1966). *Heritable Disorders of Connective Tissue*, 3rd ed. St. Louis; Mosby.

Berlyne, G. M., Bulmer, M. and Platt, R. (1961). *Q. Jl Med.*, **30,** 201.

*Congenital Anhydrotic Octodermal Dysplasia*

Cockayne, E. A. (1933). *Inherited Abnormalities of the Skin and its Appendages*, p. 218. London; Oxford University Press.

Spira, L. (1947). *Acta med. scand.*, **127,** 197.

*Rothmund's Syndrome*

Franceschetti, A. (1953). *Dermatologica*, **106,** 129.

Taylor, W. B. (1957). *Archs Dermatol.*, **75,** 236.

*Werner's Syndrome*
Epstein, C. J., Martin, G. M., Schultz, A. L. and Motulsky, A. (1966). *Medicine*, **45**, 177.

**Syndromes with Prominent Pigment Changes**
"*Incontenintia pigmenti*"
Francheschetti, A. and Jadassohn, W. (1954). *Dermatologica*, **108**, 1.

**Predominantly Neurological Syndromes**
*Neurofibromatosis*
Davis, F. A. (1940). *Archs Ophthal.*, **23**, 735, 957.
François, J. (1947). *Bull. Acad. r. Med. Belg.*, **12**, 477.

*Tuberose Sclerosis*
Koch, F. L. P. and Walsh, M. N. (1939). *Archs Ophthal.*, **21**, 465.

*Lindau's Syndrome*
Larson, C. A. (1957). *Acta genet. Statist. med.*, **7**, 341.
Melmon, K. L. and Rosen, S. W. (1964). *Am. J. Med.*, **36**, 595.
Usher, C. H. (1935). *Trans. ophthal. Soc. U.K.*, **55**, 183, 228.

*Sturge–Weber Syndrome*
Alexander, G. L. and Norman, R. M. (1960. *The Sturge–Weber Syndrome*. Bristol; Wright.
Larmande, A. M. (1948). *La Neuro-Angiomatose encephalo-faciale*. Paris; Masson.

*Ataxia-telangiectasia (Louis–Bar)*
Border, E. and Sedgwick, R. P. (1958). *J. Paediat.*, **21**, 526.
Guttman, L. (1963). *Acta neurol.*, **8**, 318.

*Marinesco–Sjögren Syndrome*
Alter, M., Tabert, O. R. and Croffhead, G. (1962). *Neurol. (Minneap.)*, **12**, 836.
Garland, H. and Morhouse, D. (1953). *J. Neurol. Neurophysiol. Psychiat.*, **16**, 110.
Marinesco, G., Draganesco, S. and Vasilia, D. (1931). *Encéphale*, **26**, 97.
Sjögren, T. (1943). *Acta psychiat. neurol. scand.*, Suppl. 27.
— (1947). *Acta psychiat. neurol. scand.*, Suppl. 46.
— (1950). *Conf. Neurol.*, **10**, 293.
Todorov, A. (1965). *J. Gén. hum.*, **14**, 197.

*Sjögren–Larsson Syndrome*
Sjögren, T. (1956). *Acta genet. Statist. med.*, **6**, 80.
— and Larson, T. (1957). "Oligophrenia in Combination with Congenital Ichthyosis and Spastic Disorders." *Acta psychiat. neurol. scand.*, Suppl. 13.

*Oculo-pharyngeal Dystrophy*
Barbeau, A. (1967). *Second International Congress of Neuro-genetics and Neuro-ophthalmology*. Abstract No. 176. The Hague; Excepta Medica Abstract Series, No. 154.
Murphy, S. F. and Drachman, D. B. (1968). *J. Am. med. Ass.*, **203**, 1003.

## BIBLIOGRAPHY

The lists "For Further Reading" at the end of each chapter generally give key references to the chapters as a whole and to the classified subjects shown in these lists. Most carry extensive bibliographies.

Of the two subjoined lists, the first gives the general works on ophthalmic genetics, and the second references to individual points in the text that carry a named and dated entry in brackets, e.g. (Alström and colleagues, 1959).

### GENERAL WORKS


Bell, Julia (1933 *et seq.*). In *The Treasury of Human Inheritance*, Vol. II (Nettleship Memorial Volume), Ed. by K. Pearson and later by L. S. Penrose. Pt. I: Retinitis pigmentosa and allied diseases. Pt. II: Colour-blindness. Pt. III: Blue sclerotics and fragility of bone; The Laurence–Biedl syndrome. Pt. IV: Hereditary optic atrophy. Pt. V: On some hereditary structural anomalies of the eye and on the inheritance of glaucoma. Cambridge University Press.

Franceschetti, A. (1930). "Die Vererbung von Augenleiden." In *Kurzes Handbuch der Ophthalmologie*, Ed. by F. Schieck and A. Brückner, Vol. I, pp. 630–855. Berlin; Springer.

— and Klein, D. (1955). "Les affections génétiques en ophtalmologie." *Encyclopedie Medico-chirurgicale*, Vol. Ophtalmologie. Paris. 21400 A10-21400 D 10.

François, J. (1958). *L' hérédité en Ophtalmologie*. Paris; Masson. (English translation: *Heredity in Ophthalmology* (1961). St. Louis; Mosby.

Gütt, A. (Ed.) (1938). "Erbleiden des Auges." In *Handbuch der Erbkrankheiten*, Vol. 5. Leipzig; Thieme.

Howe, L. (1921). "A Bibliography of Heredity Eye Defects." *Bulletin No. 21*, Carnegie Institution of Washington. Eugenics Record Office. Cold Harbour.

Klein, D., and Franceschetti, A. (1964). "Missbildungen und Krankheiten des Auges." In *Humangenetik*, Vol. IV, pp. 1–247, Ed. by P. E. Becker. Stuttgart; Thieme.

Macklin, M. (1927). "Hereditary Abnormalities of the Eye." *Can. med. Ass. J.*, **17,** 327, 421, 1136, 1191.

Vogt, A., Wagner, H., and Schläpfer, H. (1940). "Erbbiologie und Erbpathologie des menschlichen Auges." In *Handbuch des Erbbiologie des Menschen*, Ed. by G. Just, Vol. III, pp. 575–689. Berlin; Springer.

Waardenburg, P. J. (1932). *Das menschliche Auge und seine Erbanlagen.* The Hague; Nijhoff.

— (1950). "Twin Research in Ophthalmology." *Documenta Ophth.*, **4,** 153.

— Franceschetti, A., and Klein D. (1961–63). *Genetics and Ophthalmology*, Vol. I 1961, Vol. II 1963, Vol. III in preparation. Oxford; Blackwell.


### REFERENCES IN THE TEXT


Alajmo, B., and Rubino, A. (1935). *Rass. ital. Ottol.*, **4,** 445.

Algan, B. (1957). *Bull. Soc. Ophtal. Fr.*, **70,** 436.

Alström, C. H., Hallgren, B., Nilsson, L. B., and Åsander, H. (1959). *Acta psychiat. scand.*, **34,** Suppl. 129.

Almaric, M. P. (1960). *Bull. Soc. Ophtal. Fr.*, **73,** 195.

Andersen, S. R. (1946). *Acta ophthal.*, **24,** 99.

Anderson, B. (1948). *Trans. Am. Ophthal. Soc.*, **46,** 326.

Andersson, R., and Kassman, T. (1968). *Acta ophthal.*, **46,** 441.
Appel, B., and Messina, S. J. (1942). *New Engl. J. Med.*, **226,** 915.
Ashton, N., and Sorsby, A. (1951). *Br. J. Ophthal.*, **35,** 751.
Atwool, W. F. (1895). *Roy. Ophthal. Hosp. Res.*, **14,** 260.
Auzicchio, G. de Vincentis M. (1950). *G. ital. oftal.*, **3,** 118.
Bakwin, H., and Eiger, M. S. (1956). *J. Paediat.*, **49,** 558.
Bamatter, F., and Lamy, M. (1957). *Probl. act. Ophthal.*, **1,** 597.
Barabas, A. P. (1966). *Br. med. J.*, **2,** 682.
Barbeau, A. (1968). *J. Genét. hum.*, Suppl. 15, 49.
Beattie, P. H. (1947). *Br. J. Ophthal.*, **31,** 649.
Beaumont, W. M. (1900). *Trans. Ophthal. Soc. U.K.*, **20,** 258.
Becker, B., and Hahn, K. A. (1964). *Am. J. Ophthal.*, **57,** 543.
Becker, F. (1935). *Klin. Mbl. Augenheilk.*, **95,** 547.
Beighton, P. (1968). *Proc. R. Soc. Med.*, **61,** 987.
Bell, Julia (1933). *Ann. Eugen.*, **5,** 311.
— (1933 *et seq.*). *Treasury of Human Inheritance*, Vol. II, Ed. by K. Pearson and later by L. S. Penrose. Cambridge University Press.
Bergstedt, M. S., Johansson, S., and Muller, R. (1962). *Neurology, Minneapolis*, **12,** 124.
Berliner, M. L. (1939). *Archs. Ophthal.*, **22,** 97.
Bernard, J., Bessis, M., and Seligman, M. (1960). *Presse méd.*, **68,** 563.
Berryman, M. L. (1953). Thesis, Geneva.
Bietti, G. (1937). *Boll. Oculist.*, **16,** 1159. *Klin. Mbl. Augenheilk.*, **99,** 737.
Biro, I. (1939). *Ophthalmologica*, **98,** 43.
Blatt, N. (1924). *Arch. Ophthal.*, **114,** 604. *Z. Augenheilk.*, **53,** 325.
Boehringer, H. R., Dietezle, P., and Landolt, E. (1960). *Ophthalmologica*, **139,** 330.
van Bogaert, L. (1934). *Bull. Acad. r. Méd. Belg.*, **14,** 323.
— (1948). In *Modern Trends in Ophthalmology—2*, Ed. by A. Sorsby. London; Butterworths.
— and Borremans, P. (1936). *Annls. Méd.*, **39,** 54.
— and de Savitsch, F. (1937). *Encéphale*, **32,** 113.
Bonting, S. L., Carravaggio, L. L., and Couras, P. (1961). *Expl. Eye Res.*, **1,** 14.
Bradburne, A. A. (1912). *Trans. Ophthal. Soc. U.K.*, **32,** 142.
— (1916). *Ophthal. Rev.*, **35,** 65.
Braendstrup, P. (1941). *Acta ophthal.*, **19,** 272.
van den Breggen, F. (1915). *Nederl. Tydschr. geneesk.*, **59,** 1874.
Bremer, F. W. (1926). *Dt. Z. Nervenheilk.*, **95,** 7.
Brown, N. J., Corner, B. D., and Dodgson, M. C. H. (1954). *Archs. Dis. Childh.*, **29,** 48.
Brownell, R. D. and Wolter, J. R. (1964). *Archs. Ophthal.*, **71,** 481.
Bruce, G. M., Denning, C. R., and Spaller, H. F. (1960). *Archs Ophthal.*, **63,** 391.
Brückner, A. (1906). *Arch. Augenheilk.*, **55,** 23.
Brunner, W. (1930). *Arch. Ophthal.*, **124,** 1.
Bücklers, M. (1938). In *Handbuch der Erbkrankheiten*, Vol. 5, Ed. by A. Gutt. Leipzig; Thieme. See also *Die Erblichen Hornhautdystrophien.* Stuttgart; Ferdinand Enke.
— (1949). *Klin. Mbl. Augenheilk.*, **114,** 386.
— and Gilch, T. (1938). Quoted by Bücklers (1938) p. 82.
Bürki, E. (1942). *Ophthalmologica*, **101,** 257.
Burn, R. A. (1950). *Br. J. Ophthal.*, **34,** 65.
Butler, T. H. (1938). *Trans. Ophthal. Soc. U.K.*, **57,** 42.
Calhoun, F. P. (1919). *Am. J. Ophthal.*, **2,** 255.
Cameron, E. P. (1926). *Br. J. Ophthal.*, **10,** 384.
Cameron, P. B. (1950). *Archs Ophthal.*, **43,** 818.
Casa, D. (1955). *Acta Genet. med. Gemell.*, **4,** 230.
Chase, H. B., and Chase, E. B. (1941). *J. Morph.*, **68,** 279.
Chassigneux, J., and Chome, J. (1960). *Presse méd.*, **68,** 563.
Clark, F. C. (1919). *Archs Ophthal.*, **48,** 475.

Clarke, E. (1898). *Trans. Ophthal. Soc. U.K.*, **18,** 136.
Clarke, J. M. (1910). *Br. med. J.*, **1,** 150.
Clausen, W. (1921). *Klin. Mbl. Augenheilk.*, **67,** 116.
— (1928). *Klin. Mbl. Augenheilk.*, **81,** 135.
Cockayne, E. A. (1936). *Br. J. Ophthal.*, **20,** 569.
Collier, M. (1962). *Annls Oculist.*, **195,** 512. *Archs Ophtal. Paris*, **22,** 376. *Clin. Ophthal.*, No. 1.
Condon, R. A., and Somerville-Large, L. B. (1955). *Trans. Ophthal. Soc. U.K.*, **75,** 709.
Coover, D. H. (1910). *Ophthalmoscope*, **8,** 259.
Coverdale, H. (1948). *Br. J. Ophthal.*, **32,** 669.
Cowan, A. (1936). *Am. J. Ophthal.*, **19,** 287.
Crone, R. A. (1952). Thesis, Amsterdam.
Crouzon, O., and Béhague, P. (1920). *Bull. Mem. Soc. med. Hôp., Paris*, **44,** 372.
Curtius, F. (1933). *Multiple Sklerose und Erbanlage*. Leipzig; Thieme.
— and Schlotter, H. (1934). *Dt. Z. Nervenheilk.*, **134,** 44.
Danis, P. (1948). *Annls. Oculist.*, **181,** 148.
Darnforth, E. (1929). *Archs. Derm. Syph.*, **12,** 86.
Davenport, R. C. (1927). *Br. J. Ophthal.*, **11,** 443.
Davidson, S. I. (1960). *Br. J. Ophthal.*, **44,** 590.
Debusmann, W. Quoted by A. Franceschetti and D. Klein (1949). *Acta ophthal.*, **27,** 143.
Desvignes, P., and Vigo, N. I. (1955). *Bull. Soc. Ophtal. Paris*, **4,** 220.
Diethelm, W. (1947). *Ophthalmologica*, **114,** 16.
DiGeorge, A. M., and Harley, R. D. (1966). *Archs Ophthal.*, **75,** 796.
Doggart, J. H. (1948). *Ocular Signs in Slit-lamp Microscopy*. London; Henry Kimpton.
Dohlman, C. H. (1951). *Acta ophthal.*, **29,** 445.
Dorrell, E. A. (1932). *Roy. Berks. Hosp. Rep.*, p. 122.
Dresner, E., and Montgomery, D. A. D. (1949). *Q. Jl Med.* (N.S.), **18,** 93.
Everett, W. G. (1968). *Am. J. Ophthal.*, **65,** 229.
Falkenheim and Rochliny. Quoted by Goldfeder (1927).
Falls, H. F. (1949). *Am. J. hum. Genet.*, **1,** 94. *Am. J. Ophthal.*, **32,** 41.
— (1951). *Am. J. Ophthal.*, **34,** 41.
— and Cotterman, C. W. (1948). *Archs Ophthal.*, **40,** 685.
— Jackson, J., Carey, J. H., Rukavina, J. G., and Block, W. O. (1955). *Archs Ophthal.*, **54,** 660.
— Kruse, W. T., and Cotterman, C. W. (1949). *Am. J. Ophthal.*, **32,** 6, 53.
Fattovich, G. (1936). *G. Psichiat. Neuropatol.*, **64,** 393.
Felix, C. (1925). *Klin. Mbl. Augenheilk.*, **74,** 710.
Fleischer, B. (1938). In *Handbuch der Erbkrankheiten*, Vol. 5, Ed. by A. Gütt. Leipzig; Thieme.
Forni, S. (1951). *Archs Ophtal. Paris*, **11,** 541.
Forsius, H., and Ericsson, A. (1962). *Acta Genet. med. Gemell.*, **11,** 397.
Franceschetti, A. (1930). In *Kurzes Handbuch der Ophthalmologie*, Vol. 1, Ed. by F. Schieck and A. Brückner. Berlin; Springer.
— (1953). *J. Génét. hum.*, **2,** 283.
— and Bock, R. H. (1950). *Am. J. Ophthal.*, **33,** 227.
— and Klein, D. (1941). *Arch. Julius Klaus-Stift. Vererb-Forsch.*, **16,** 469.
— — (1947). *Arch. Julius Klaus-Stift. Vererb-Forsch.*, **22,** 93.
— (1948). *Revta. oto-neuro-oftal. Cirug. neurol. sud-am.*, **30,** 109.
— — (1961). In *Genetics and Ophthalmology*, p. 957. Ed. by P. J. Waardenburg, A. Franceschetti and D. Klein. Oxford; Blackwell.
— — and Guttman, A. (1950). *Arch. Julius Klaus-Stift. Vererb-Forsch.*, **25,** 550.
— and Zwahlen, P. (1944). *Bull. schweitz. Akad. med. Wiss.*, **1,** 60.
— de Morsier, G., and Klein, D. (1945). *Arch. Julius Klaus-Stift. Vererb-Forsch.*, **20,** 60.

Franceschetti, A., François, J., and Babel, J. (1963). *Les hérédo-dégénérescences rétiniennes* Paris; Masson.
François, J. (1949). *Annls Oculist*, **182,** 409.
— (1961). *Heredity in Ophthalmology*. St. Louis; Mosby.
— (1966). *Annls Oculist.*, **199,** 545.
— (1968). *J. Génet. hum.*, Suppl. **15,** 133.
— and Neetens, A. (1956). *Bull. Soc. belge Ophtal.*, **114,** 641.
— and Rabey, M. (1952). *Annls Oculist.*, **185,** 784.
— and De Rouck, A. (1960). *Ophthalmologica*, **140,** 1.
— — (1961). Quoted by Franceschetti, François and Babel (1963).
Frank-Kamenetzki, S. G. (1925). *Klin. Mbl. Augenheilk.*, **74,** 133.
Fraser, G. R., and Friedmann, A. I. (1967). *The Causes of Blindness in Childhood.* Baltimore; Johns Hopkins Press.
— — (1968). *Br. med. J.*, **2,** 732.
Fried, K., Feinmesser, M., and Tsitsianov, J. (1969). *J. med. Gen.*, **6,** 132.
Friedburg, D. (1968). *Klin. Mbl. Augenheilk.*, **152,** 379.
Friedman, B. (1939). *Archs Ophthal.*, **22,** 271.
Friedman, M., and Wright, E. (1952). *Am. J. Ophthal.*, **35,** 1017.
Fröhlich, R. J. (1924). *Arch. Rass.-u. GesBiol.*, **15,** 249.
Frykholm, R. (1935). *Klin. Mbl. Augenheilk.*, **94,** 76.
Fukami (1924). Quoted by Waardenburg, Franceschetti and Klein (1961).
Gassler, K. J. (1925). *Arch. Julius Klaus-Stift. Vererb-Forsch.*, **1,** 259.
Gatterbauer, J. (1943). *Klin. Mbl. Augenheilk.*, **109,** 113.
Gedda, L., and Cavalteri, R. (1961). *Proceedings of the Second International Congress on Human Genetics*, Rome, Vol. 2, p. 1070.
Gibbs (1915 and 1916). Quoted by Cockayne (1933). *Inherited Abnormalities of the Skin and its Appendages.* London; Oxford University Press.
Gilch, T. (1937). *Z. KonstitLehre*, **21,** 1.
Godtfredsen, E. (1949). *Acta ophthal.*, **27,** 429.
Goldfeder, A. E. (1927). *Klin. Mbl. Augenheilk.*, **79,** 176.
Gredig, C. (1926). *Arch. Julius Klaus-Stift. Vererb-Forsch.*, **2,** 79.
Gregg, J. B., and Becker, S. F. (1963). *Archs Ophthal.*, **69,** 295.
Griffith, A. D., and Sorsby, A. (1944). *Br. J. Ophthal.*, **28,** 279.
Grimm, R. J., and Tedford, J. (1963). *Am. J. Ophthal.*, **55,** 463.
Grönholm, V. (1921). *Klin. Mbl. Augenheilk.*, **67,** 1.
Gruber, M. (1946). *Ophthalmologica*, **112,** 88.
Gunn, M. (1907). *Trans. Ophthal. Soc. U.K.*, **27,** 221.
Günther, H. (1933). *Endokrinologie*, **13,** 255.
Gütt, A. (Ed.) (1938). *Handbuch der Erbkrankheiten*, Vol. 5. Leipzig; Thieme.
Guttman, A. (1948–50). *Acta genet.*, **1,** 295.
Halbertsma, K. T. A. (1928). *Klin. Mbl. Augenheilk.*, **80,** 794.
Haldane, J. B. S. (1941). *New Paths in Genetics*. London; Allen & Unwin.
Hallgren, B. (1958). *Acta Genet.*, **8,** 97.
— (1959). *Acta psychiat. scand.*, Suppl. **34,** 1.
Haney, W. P., and Falls, H. F. (1961). *Am. J. Ophthal.*, **52,** 53.
Handmann, M. (1929). *Klin. Mbl. Augenheilk.*, **83,** 149.
— (1943). *Klin. Mbl. Augenheilk.*, **109,** 186.
Harman, N. B. (1910). *Trans. Ophthal. Soc. U.K.*, **30,** 264.
Haro, F. S. (1946). *Archs. Ophthal.*, **36,** 89.
Hartung, H. (1926). *Klin. Mbl. Augenheilk.*, **76,** 229.
— (1932). *Klin. Mbl. Augenheilk.*, **88,** 43.
Heath, W. E. (1960). *Br. J. Ophthal.*, **44,** 696.
Heidenreich, J. (1913). Quoted by K. Pearson, E. Nettleship and C. H. Usher (1913).
Heinonen, O. (1927). *Acta ophthal.*, **4,** 278.
Helweg-Larsen, H. F., and Ludvigsen, K. (1946). *Acta derm.-vener.*, **26,** 489.

Hemmes, G. D. (1924). Thesis, Utrecht.
— (1931). *Neederl. Tijdschr. Geneesk.*, **75,** 4738.
Hermann, P. (1958). *Archs Ophtal.*, **18,** 17.
Hines, E. A. (1937). *Ann. intern. Med.*, **11,** 593.
von Hippel, E. (1934). *Ber. dt. ophthal. Ges.*, 309.
Hoare, G. W. (1965). *Br. J. Ophthal.*, **49,** 449.
Hobbs, H. E., Sorsby, A., and Friedman, A. (1959). *Lancet*, **2,** 478.
van der Hoeve, J. (1929). *Bull. Soc. Ophtal. Fr.*, **42,** 310.
— (1932). *Trans. Ophthal. Soc. U.K.*, **52,** 380.
— (1940). In *Modern Trends in Ophthalmology—1*, p. 124. Ed. by F. Ridley and A. Sorsby. London; Butterworths.
Holst, J. C. (1950). *Blind Letsarker i. Norge.* Oslo.
Holth, S., and Berner, O. (1923). *Br. J. Ophthal.*, **7,** 401.
Hooft, C., Delaey, P., Herpol, J., de Loore, F., and Verbeeck, J. (1962). *Helv. paediat. Acta*, **17,** 1.
Horner, W. D. (1876). Quoted in Julia Bell (1933).
Ioannides, Th. (1966). *J. Gén. hum.*, Suppl. **15,** 228.
Iwanov (1928). Reference in *Klin. Mbl. Augenheilk.*, **32,** 541 (1929).
Jablonski, W. (1920). *Dt. med. Wschr.*, **46,** 708.
— (1922). *Klin. Mbl. Augenheilk.*, **68,** 560.
— (1924). *Klin. Mbl. Augenheilk.*, **73,** 320.
Jacobs, H. B. (1957). *Br. J. Ophthal.*, **41,** 31. *Am. J. Ophthal.*, **41,** 40.
Jay, B., Blach, R. K., and Wells, R. S. (1968). *Br. J. Ophthal.*, **52,** 217.
Jensen, V. J. (1958). *Acta ophthal.*, **36,** 71.
Jerndal, T. (1968). *Acta ophthal.*, **46,** 459.
John, I. (1934). *Arch. Ophthal.*, **133,** 60.
Johnson, S. A. M., and Falls, H. F. (1949). *Archs Derm. Syph.*, **60,** 82.
Johnstone, I. L. (1947). *Br. J. Ophthal.*, **31,** 385.
Jonkers, G. H. (1950). *Nederl. Tijdschr. Geneesk.*, **95,** 1471.
Jordan, M. (1955). *Klin. Mbl. Augenheilk.*, **126,** 469.
Joseph, R. (1951). *Br. J. Ophthal.*, **35,** 98.
Kayser, B. (1914). *Klin. Mbl. Augenheilk.*, **52,** 226.
— (1919). *Klin. Mbl. Augenheilk.*, **60,** 349.
Keith, C. G. (1966). *Trans. Ophthal. Soc. U.K.*, **86,** 435.
— (1968). *Proc. R. Soc. Med.*, **61,** 251.
Kerkenezow, N. (1956). *Trans. Ophthal. Soc. Austral.*, **16,** 110.
Kiehle, F. A., and Pugmire, C. (1934). *Archs Ophthal.*, **12,** 75.
Kiloh, L. G., and Nevin, S. (1951). *Brain*, **74,** 115.
Klein, D. (1964). In *Humangenetik*, Ed. by P. E. Becker, Vol. IV, p. 68. Stuttgart; Thieme.
Kleiner, W. (1923). *Arch. Rass.-u. Ges-Biol.*, **15,** 1.
Koby, E. (1923). *Archs Ophtal.*, **40,** 492.
Koch, G. (1940). *Z. ges. Neurol.*, **168,** 614.
Krebs, E., Hartmann, E., and Thiebaut, F. (1930). *Rev. Neurol.*, **37,** 121 and 606.
Kubota, N. (1968). *Acta Soc. ophthal. Jap.*, **72,** 368.
Kurstjens, J. H. (1965). *Documenta Ophth.*, **19,** 1.
Laborne, T. C. (1944). *Ophthalmos*, **3,** 250.
Lambert, R. K., and McDannald, C. F. (1931). *Am. J. Ophthal.*, **14,** 46.
Larsen, V., and Eriksen, A. (1949). *Acta ophthal.*, **27,** 276.
Laughlin, R. C. (1937). *Am. J. Ophthal.*, **20,** 396.
— (1956). *Am. J. Ophthal.*, **41,** 432.
de Lawter, O. (1949). *Med. Ann. Distr. Columbia*, **18,** 398.
van Leeuwen, A. (1949). *Annls. Oculist.*, **182,** 469.
Lindenov, H. (1945). *The Etiology of Deaf-mutism.* (Opera ex Domo Biol, No. 8). Copenhagen; Munksgaard.

Lisch, K. (1937). *Klin Mbl. Augenheilk.*, **110,** 357.
— (1957). *Klin. Mbl. Augenheilk.*, **130,** 49.
Løken, A. C., Hannssen, O., Halvorsen, S., and Jølster, N. J. (1961). *Acta paediat.*, **50,** 177.
Lutman, E. C., and Neel, J. V. (1945). *Archs Ophthal.*, **33,** 341.
Lynch, H. T., Anderson, D. E., and Krush, J. (1968). *Cancer, Philad.*, **21,** 119.
McAlpine, D. (1938). *Brain*, **61,** 430.
McCulloch, C., and McCulloch, R. J. P. (1948). *Trans. Am. Acad. Ophtal. Otolar.*, **52,** 160.
McIlroy, J. H. (1930). *Proc. R. Soc. Med.*, **23,** 285.
Maeda, T. (1934). In *Pedigrees of Hereditary Diseases in the Japanese Race*, Ed. by T. Komai. Kyoto.
Magrader, A. C. (1921). *Am. J. Ophthal.*, **12,** 751.
Makley, T. A. (1956). *Am. J. Ophthal.*, **41,** 768.
Margolis, E. (1962). *Acta genet.*, **12,** 12.
Marlow, F. H., and Faxon, W. L. (1913). Quoted by K. Pearson, E. Nettleship and C. H. Usher (1913).
Maroteaux, P., and Lamy, M. (1963). *Presse mèd.*, **71,** 2091.
Martin, F. (1888). Thesis, Erlangen.
Massimeo, A. (1956). *Bull. Oculist.*, **35,** 824.
Meesmann, A., and Wilke, F. (1939). *Klin. Mbl. Augenheilk.*, **103,** 361.
Meissner, M. (1933). *Z. Augenheilk.*, **80,** 48.
de Mello, A. R. Quoted by Franceschetti and Klein (1948). *Revta oto-neuro-oftal. Cirug. neurol. sud-am.*, **20,** 134.
Miller, S. J. H. (1954). *Trans. Ophthal. Soc. U.K.*, **74,** 349.
— and Paterson, G. D. (1962). *Br. J. Ophthal.*, **46,** 513.
Møllenbach, C. J. (1947). *Medføte defector i øjects indre Linder* (Opera ex Domo Biol. No. 15). Copenhagen; Munksgaard.
Möller, H. M. (1929). *Acta ophthal.*, **7,** 244.
Moon, H. (1876–77). Quoted by Cockayne (1933). *Inherited Abnormalities of the Skin and its Appendages.* London; Oxford University Press.
Moynahan, E. J. (1966). *Proc. R. Soc. Med.*, **59,** 1125.
Münch, O. (1922). *Ber. dt. ophthal. Ges.*, **43,** 241.
Neame, H. (1935). *Proc. R. Soc. Med.*, **28,** 526 (and personal communication).
Nettleship, E. (1907). *Trans. Ophthal. Soc. U.K.*, **27,** 269.
— (1908). *Roy. Ophthal. Hosp. Rep.*, **17,** 1.
— (1909). *Trans. Ophthal. Soc. U.K.*, **29,** 188 (*also* cxvi and cxlix).
— (1912). *Trans. Ophthal. Soc. U.K.*, **32,** 21.
— and Ogilvie, G. M. (1906). *Trans. Ophthal. Soc. U.K.*, **26,** 191.
Niccol, W. (1915). *Ophthalmoscope*, **13,** 224.
Norman, R. M., and Wood, N. (1941). *J. Neurol. Psychiat.*, **4,** 175.
— Urich, H., Tingey, A. H., and Goodbody, R. A. (1959). *J. Path. Bact.*, **78,** 409.
Øther, A. (1968). *Acta ophthal.*, **46,** 79.
Pagenstecher, A. (1925). *Klin. Mbl. Augenheilk.*, **74,** 128.
Parry, H. B., Tansley, K., and Thomson, L. O. (1955). *Br. J. Ophthal.*, **39,** 349.
Parsons, J. H. (1904). *Trans. Ophthal. Soc. U.K.*, **24,** 47.
Pearce, W. G. (1968). *Lancet*, **1,** 1280.
Pearson, K., Nettleship, E., and Usher, C. H. (1913) (Eds.). *A Monograph on Albinism in Man.* Cambridge University Press.
Peter, L. (1926). *Arch. Julius Klaus-Stift. Vererb-Forsch.*, **2,** 143.
Peter, Rosa (1925). *Arch. Ophthal.*, **115,** 29.
Peters, R. (1915). *Klin. Mbl. Augenheilk.*, **55,** 380.
Pfanmüller, F. (1894). Thesis, Giessen. Quoted by Julia Bell (1933).
Phillips, C. I., and Griffiths, D. L. (1969). *Br. J. Ophthal.*, **53,** 346.

Pipkin, A. C., and Pipkin, S. E. (1942). *J. Hered.*, **33,** 419.
Potts, C. R. (1950). *Trans. Am. Ophthal. Soc.*, **48,** 526.
Ptasinska-Urbanska, M. S., and Mitkiewicz-Bochenek, W. (1968). *Annls. Oculist.*, **201,** 431.
Puccionio (1907). Reference in *Klin. Mbl. Augenheilk.* (1908), **46,** 200.
Raiti, S., Plotkin, S., and Newns, G. H. (1963). *Br. med. J.*, **2,** 1625.
Rayner, S. (1962). Report of Institute of Medical Genetics, Uppsala, p. 107.
Redl, Th. (1949). *Klin. Mbl. Augenheilk.*, **114,** 24.
Reese, A. B., and Ellsworth, R. M. (1966). *Archs. Ophthal.*, **75,** 307.
Remky, H., Rix, J., and Klier, K. F. (1965). *Klin. Mbl. Augenheilk.*, **146,** 473.
Renwick, J. H., and Lawler, S. D. (1963). *Ann. hum. Genet.*, **27,** 67.
Ricci, M. A. (1961). *Bull. Soc. Ophtal. Fr.*, 618.
Richter, S. (1967). *Untersuchungen ueber die Hereditāt des Strabismus Concomitans* (Abhandlungen aus dem Gebiete der Augenheilkunde, Band 35). Leipzig; Thieme.
Riedl, F. (1939). *Klin. Mbl. Augenheilk.*, **103,** 169.
Robert, J. M., Schnepp, J., Rougier, I., and Maroteaux, P. (1966). *J. Génét. hum.*, Suppl., **15,** 274.
Roberts, J. A. F., and Sorsby, A. (1951). In *Genetics in Ophthalmology.* London; Butterworths. [Fig. 153 (*d*)]
Robertson, Argyll (1891). *Trans. Ophthal. Soc. U.K.*, **11,** 239.
Romer, A. (1926). *Arch. Julius Klaus-Stift. Vererb-Forsch.*, **2,** 207.
Rose, F. C., and Friedmann, A. J. (1964). *J. med. Gen.*, **1,** 110.
Rosenstein, M. (1925). *Klin. Mbl. Augenheilk.*, **75,** 679.
Rothmund, A. (1868). *Arch. Ophthal.*, **14,** 159.
Rucker, C. W. (1946). *Am. J. Ophthal.*, **29,** 1534.
— (1949). *Am. J. hum. Genet.*, **1,** 52.
Rukavina, J. G., Falls, H. F., Holt, J. F., and Block, W. D. (1959). *J. Bone Jt Surg.*, **41A,** 397.
Rumpf, J. (1937). Thesis, Lausanne.
Rutherford, M. E. (1931). *Br. med. J.*, **2,** 9.
Saebø, J. (1948). *Acta ophthal.*, **26,** 447.
— (1949). *Br. J. Ophthal.*, **33,** 601.
Salleras, A., and Ortiz de Zerate, J. C. (1950). *Br. J. Ophthal.*, **34,** 662.
von Sallmann, L., and Paton, D. (1960). *Archs Ophthal.*, **63,** 421.
Salt, H. B., Wolff, O. H., Lloyd, J. K., Forsbrooke, A. S., Cameron, A. H., and Hubble, D. V. (1960). *Lancet*, **2,** 325.
Sandvig, K. (1961). *Acta ophthal.*, **39,** 33.
Savin, L. H. (1956). *Br. J. Ophthal.*, **40,** 82.
— and Sorsby, A. (1934). *Proc. R. Soc. Med.*, **28,** 525.
Schmid, C. (1924). *Arch. Rass.-u. GesBiol.*, **15,** 263.
Schnyder, W. F. (1926). *Klin. Mbl. Augenheilk.*, **77,** 721.
— (1927). *Klin. Mbl. Augenheilk.*, **79,** 585.
— (1939). *Klin. Mbl. Augenheilk.*, **103,** 494.
Sédan, J., and Roux, A. (1933). *Bull. Soc. Ophtal., Fr.* **46,** 163.
— and Sédan-Bauby, S. (1949). *Bull. Soc. Ophtal. Fr.*, **1,** 29.
Seedorff, K. S. (1949). *Osteogenesis Imperfecta.* Arhus Universitetsforlaget.
Selz, E. (1900). Thesis, Jena. Quoted by Fleischer, 1938.
Senior, B., Friedmann, A. Z., and Braudo, J. L. (1961). *Am. J. Ophthal.*, **52,** 625.
van Senus, A. H. C. (1963). *Documenta ophth.*, **17,** 1.
Siemens, H. W. (1926). *Klin. Mbl. Augenheilk.*, **76,** 769.
Sjögren, H. T. (1931). *Hereditas*, **14,** 197.
Sjögren, T. (1935). *Z. ges. Neurol. Psychiat.*, **152,** 263.
Sjögren, T. (1950). *Confinia neurol.*, **10,** 293.
Smith, M. E., and Zimmerman, L. E. (1968). *Archs Ophthal.*, **79,** 407.
Snell, S. (1903). *Trans. Ophthal. Soc. U.K.*, **23,** 68.

Snell, S. (1908). *Trans. Ophthal. Soc. U.K.*, **28,** 149.
Sorsby, A. (1931). *Proc. R. Soc. Med.*, **25,** 692.
— (1934). *Br. J. Ophthal.*, **18,** 469.
— (1935). *Br. J. Ophthal.*, **19,** 65.
— (1940). *Br. J. Ophthal.*, **24,** 469.
— (1941). *Br. J. Ophthal.*, **25,** 58, 62.
— and Crick, R. P. (1953). *Br. J. Ophthal.*, **37,** 129.
— and Davey, J. B. (1954). *J. Genet.*, **52,** 425.
— — (1955). *Br. J. Ophthal.*, **39,** 257, 385.
— and Fraser, G. R. (1964). *J. med. Genet.*, **1,** 47.
— Leary, G. A., and Fraser, G. R. (1966). *J. med. Genet.*, **3,** 269.
— and Harding, R. (1962). *Vision Res.*, **2,** 139, 149, 157.
— — (1966). *Nature, Lond.*, **210,** 997.
— and Mason, J. E. J. (1949). *Br. J. Ophthal.*, **33,** 67.
— and Nakajima, A. (1958). *Br. J. Ophthal.*, **42,** 563.
— and Williams, C. (1960). *Br. med. J.*, **1,** 293.
— and Wren, N. (1960). *Archs Ophthal.*, **63,** 918.
— Avery, H., and Cockayne, E. A. (1939). *Q. Jl Med.*, N.S., **8,** 51.
— Fraser Roberts, J. A,, and Brain, R. T. (1951). *Documenta ophth.*, **5–6,** 118.
— Newhouse, J. P., and Lucas, D. (1957). *Br. J. Ophthal.*, **41,** 309.
— Sheridan, M., and Leary, G. A. (1962). *Spec. Rep. Ser. med. Res. Coun.*, No. 303. London; H.M.S.O.
— Reading, H. W., and Bunyan, J. (1966). *Nature, Lond.*, **210,** 1011.
— Benjamin, B., Davey, J. B., Sheridan, M., and Tanner, J. M. (1957). "Emmetropia and its Aberrations." *Spec. Rep. Ser. med. Res. Coun.*, No. 293. London; H.M.S.O.
— Franceschetti, A., Joseph, R., and Davey, J. B. (1952). *Br. J. Ophthal.*, **36,** 547.
— Klein, M., Gann, J. H., and Siggins, G. (1951). *Br. J. Ophthal.*, **35,** 1.
— Koller, P. C., Attfield, M., Davey, J. B., and Lucas, D. R. (1954). *J. expl. Zool.*, **125,** 171.
— Savory, M., Davey, J. B., and Fraser, R. J. L. (1956). *Br. J. Ophthal.*, **40,** 144.
Sourdille, M. E. (1925). *Bull. Mém. Soc. fr. Ophtal.*, **38,** 229.
Stadlin, W., and Klein, D. (1948). *Annls Oculist.*, **181,** 692.
Stähli, J. (1925). *Klin. Mbl. Augenheilk.*, **75,** 465.
Stainer, E. (1913). Quoted by K. Pearson, E. Nettleship and C. H. Usher (1913).
Stankovič, J. (1961). *Klin. Mbl. Augenheilk.*, **139,** 165.
Staz, I. (1941). *Br. J. Ophthal.*, **25,** 167.
Stein, R., Lazar, M., and Adam, A. (1968). *Am. J. Ophthal.*, **66,** 67.
Stewart, D. D. S. (1929). *Br. med. J.*, **1,** 101.
Streiff, E. B. (1947). *Arch. Julius Klaus-Stift. Vererb.-Forsch.*, **22,** 356.
— (1949). *Ophthalmologica*, **118,** 815.
— and Zwahlen, P. (1946). *Ophthalmologica*, **111,** 129.
Tertsch, H. (1913). Quoted by K. Pearson, E. Nettleship and C. H. Usher (1913).
Thannhauser, S. J. (1950). *Lipoidoses.* Oxford University Press.
Theodore, F. H. (1939). *Archs Ophthal.*, **21,** 626.
Thompson, A. H., and Cashell, W. G. T. (1935). *Proc. R. Soc. Med.*, **28,** 1415.
Thorson, J. C., and Bell, W. E. (1959). *Archs Ophthal.*, **62,** 833.
Tizzard, T. (1933). *Proc. R. Soc. Med.*, **27,** 253.
Town, A. E. (1943). *Archs. Ophthal.*, **29,** 767.
Traquair, H. M. (1941). *Archs Ophthal.*, **26,** 165.
Trevor-Roper, F. D. (1952). *Br. J. Ophthal.*, **36,** 107.
Unger. Quoted by Julia Bell (1933). *Ann. Eugen.*, **5,** 311.
Usher, C. H. (1914). *Roy. Ophthal. Hosp. Rep.*, **19,** 130.
— (1921). *Br. J. Ophthal.*, **5,** 289.
— (1927). *Br. J. Ophthal.*, **11,** 417.
— (1932). *Biometrica*, **24,** 1.

Usher, C. H. (1935). *Biometrica*, **27**, 5. *Trans. Ophthal. Soc. U.K.*, **55**, 164.
Verrey, A., and Jéquier, M. (1949). *Bull. Soc. Ophtal. Fr.*, **62**, 171.
Vogt, A. (1922). *Klin. Mbl. Augenheilk.*, **69**, 121.
— (1924). *Ber. dt. Ophthal. Ges.*, **44**, 67.
— (1925). In *Handbuch der ges. Augenheilkunde* (Graefe-Saemisch), 3rd. ed., Vol. III. Berlin; Springer.
— (1931). *Lehrbuch und Atlas der Spaltlampenmikroskopie*, 2nd ed., Vol. II. Berlin; Springer.
— (1933). *Klin. Mbl. Augenheilk.*, **90**, 441.
— (1938). *Klin. Mbl. Augenheilk.*, **100**, 597.
— Wagner, H., Ricner, H., and Meyer, G. (1939). *Arch. Julius Klaus-Stift. Vererb-Forsch.*, **14**, 475.
Waaler, G. H. M. (1927). *Acta ophthal.*, **5**, 309.
Waardenburg, P. J. (1913). Thesis, Utrecht.
— (1924). *Genetica*, **6**, 487.
— (1932). *Das menschliche Auge und seine Erbanlagen*. The Hague; Nijhoff.
— (1938). *Klin. Mbl. Augenheilk.*, **101**, 925.
— (1948). In *Modern Trends in Ophthalmology—2*, Ed. by A. Sorsby. London; Butterworths.
— (1949). Quoted in Waardenburg, Franceschetti and Klein (1961).
— Franceschetti, A., and Klein, D. (1961). *Genetics and Ophthalmology*. Oxford; Blackwell.
Wagner, H. (1938). *Klin. Mbl. Augenheilk.*, **100**, 840.
Wagner, P. (1956). *Klin. Mbl. Augenheilk.*, **129**, 772.
Walsh, E. B. (1947). *Clinical Neuro-ophthalmology*. Baltimore; Williams & Wilkins.
Warburg, M., and Andersen, S. R. (1968). *Acta ophthal.*, **46**, 372.
Weech, A. A. (1927). *Bull. Johns Hopk. Hosp.*, **40**, 73.
Weekers, R., Gouguard-Rion, C., and Gouguard, L. (1955). *Bull. Soc. belge Ophtal.*, **110**, 255.
Westerlund, E. (1947). *Clinical and Genetic Studies on the Primary Glaucoma Diseases* (Opera ex Domo Biol, No. 12). Copenhagen; Munksgaard.
Weyert, F. (1890). *Klin. Mbl. Augenheilk.*, **28**, 325.
White, B. V., and Fulton, M. N. (1937). *J. Hered.*, **28**, 177.
Wilson, W. M. G. (1949). *Can. med. Ass. J.*, **60**, 580.
Witkop, C. J., Shankle, C. H., Graham, J. B., Murray, M. R., Ruckangel, D., and Byerle, B. H. (1960). *Archs Path.*, **70**, 696.
Wold, K. C. (1949). *Archs Ophthal.*, **43**, 225.
Wolff, E. (1929–30). *Proc. R. Soc. Med.*, **23**, 623.
Wolfflin, E. (1923). *Arch. ges. Physiol.*, **201**, 214.
— (1949). *Z. menschl. Vererb-Konstit.*, **129**, 243.
Worth, C. (1906). *Trans. Ophthal. Soc. U.K.*, **26**, 141.
Yanoff, M. (1968). *Archs Ophthal.*, **79**, 291.
Ziegler, L., and Griscom, J. M. (1915). *Trans. Am. Ophthal. Soc.*, **14**, 356.
Ziprkowski, L., Krakavski, A., Adams, A., Costeff, H., and Sade, J. (1962). *Arch. Derm. Syph.*, **86**, 530.
Zonca, G. Quoted by Franceschetti and Klein (1948).

## INDEX

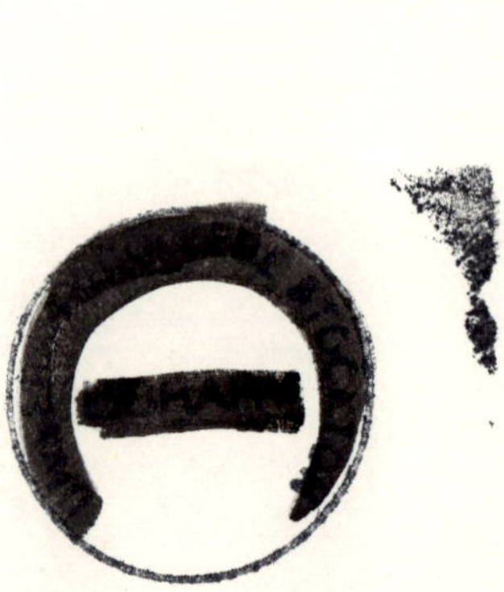